P9-ELS-182

NURSING SERIES

Cardiovascular Nursing:
A Comprehensive Overview

2nd Edition

WESTERN® SCHOOLS

By
Karen M. Marzlin, DNP, RN, CCNS, CCRN-CMC
Cynthia L. Webner, DNP, RN, CCNS, CCRN-CMC

30 contact hours will be awarded upon successful completion of this course.

Western Schools is accredited as a provider of continuing nursing education by the
American Nurses Credentialing Center's Commission On Accreditation.

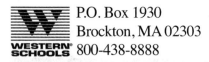
P.O. Box 1930
Brockton, MA 02303
800-438-8888

ABOUT THE AUTHORS

Karen Marzlin, DNP, RN, CCNS, CCRN-CMC, is an acute care Clinical Nurse Specialist practicing with medical cardiology patients in a 56-bed variable staffing CCU. Karen has been a nurse for over 23 years and has spent her entire career working with the cardiac patient. Karen also dedicated 10 years of her career to management and cardiovascular program administration. She has a passion for creating excellence at the bedside that is evident in her daily practice.

Karen M. Marzlin has disclosed that she has no significant financial or other conflicts of interest pertaining to this course book.

Cynthia L. Webner, DNP, RN, CCNS, CCRN-CMC, is an acute care Clinical Nurse Specialist with over 31 years of experience in a wide variety of clinical practice venues surrounding the cardiac patient. Twelve years of her career were dedicated to nursing management and Heart Center administration. She currently practices as a hospital based advanced practice nurse with medical cardiology patients. Cindy has a passion for nursing and the cardiac patient and is committed to learning something new every day.

Cynthia L. Webner has disclosed that she has no significant financial or other conflicts of interest pertaining to this course book.

Karen and Cindy both began their careers as graduates from diploma nursing schools. They both subsequently returned to school and obtained a BSN from Walsh University in Canton, OH, and an MSN as acute care Clinical Nurse Specialists from Duquesne University in Pittsburgh, PA. Karen and Cindy again graduated from Duquesne University in May of 2011 with a Doctor of Nursing Practice degree. They are both supportive of specialty certification and maintain the following certifications through the American Association of Critical Care Nurses Certification Corporation: Certified Clinical Nurse Specialist (CCNS), Certified Critical Care Nurse (CCRN) and Cardiac Medicine Certification (CMC).

ABOUT THE CONTENT EDITOR

Kimberly S. Hodge, MSN, RN, CCRN-CMC, CNS, has been an adult critical care nurse for over 20 years and has practiced in medical, surgical, trauma, oncology, cardiac medical, and cardiac surgical ICUs, as well as acute hemodialysis, the emergency department, and critical care transport. She has been a CCRN since 1993 and was one of the first to achieve sub-specialty certification in cardiac medicine (CMC) from the American Association of Critical Care Nurses (AACN). Kimberly currently practices as a critical care clinical nurse specialist at St. Francis Hospital in Indiana and is responsible for four units specializing in adult medical-surgical, neurology/neurosurgical, and cardiac medicine services.

Kimberly S. Hodge has disclosed that she has no significant financial or other conflicts of interest pertaining to this course book.

Nurse Planners: Amy Bernard, MS, BSN, RN-BC, Anne Manton, PhD, RN, PMHNP-BC, FAAN, FAEN
The planners have disclosed that they have no significant financial or other conflicts of interest pertaining to this course book.
Copy Editor: Dorothy Terry
Indexer: Sylvia Coates

Western Schools' courses are designed to provide nursing professionals with the educational information they need to enhance their career development. The information provided within these course materials is the result of research and consultation with prominent nursing and medical authorities and is, to the best of our knowledge, current and accurate. However, the courses and course materials are provided with the understanding that Western Schools is not engaged in offering legal, nursing, medical, or other professional advice.

Western Schools' courses and course materials are not meant to act as a substitute for seeking out professional advice or conducting individual research. When the information provided in the courses and course materials is applied to individual circumstances, all recommendations must be considered in light of the uniqueness pertaining to each situation.

Western Schools' course materials are intended solely for *your* use and *not* for the benefit of providing advice or recommendations to third parties. Western Schools devoids itself of any responsibility for adverse consequences resulting from the failure to seek nursing, medical, or other professional advice. Western Schools further devoids itself of any responsibility for updating or revising any programs or publications presented, published, distributed, or sponsored by Western Schools unless otherwise agreed to as part of an individual purchase contract.

Products (including brand names) mentioned or pictured in Western School's courses are not endorsed by Western Schools, the American Nurses Credentialing Center (ANCC) or any state board.

ISBN: 978-1-57801-431-6

A dedication from the authors, Karen Marzlin and Cynthia Webner

Firstly, to our God and creator,
by whom we are fearfully and wonderfully designed.

To our loving families who are always supportive.

To our Heart Center clinical colleagues
who continually engage with us and raise the bar for clinical excellence.

Finally, to Nathan, the most wonderful gift from God,
who is also on the journey of life long learning.

COURSE INSTRUCTIONS
IMPORTANT: Read these instructions *BEFORE* proceeding!

COMPLETING THE FINAL EXAMINATION

Enclosed with your course book you will find a FasTrax® answer sheet. Use this answer sheet to respond to all the final exam questions that appear in this course. If the course has less than 100 questions, leave any remaining answer circles on the FasTrax answer sheet blank.

Be sure to fill in circles completely using **blue or black ink.** The FasTrax grading system will not read pencil. If you make an error, you may use correction fluid (such as Wite-Out®) to correct it.

FasTrax answer sheets are preprinted with your name and address and the course title. If you are completing more than one course, be sure to record your answers on the correct corresponding answer sheet.

A PASSING SCORE

The final exam is a multiple choice exam. You must score 70% or better in order to pass this course and receive a certificate of completion. Should you fail to achieve the required score, an additional FasTrax answer sheet will be sent to you so that you may make a second attempt to pass the course. You will be allowed three chances to pass the same course without incurring additional charges. After three failed attempts, your file will be closed.

COURSE EVALUATIONS

The Course Evaluation provided in this course book is a critical component of the course and must be completed and submitted with your final exam. Responses to evaluation statements should be recorded in the right hand column of the FasTrax answer sheet, in the section marked "Evaluation." Evaluations provide Western Schools with vital feedback regarding courses. Your feedback is important to us; please take a few minutes to complete the evaluation.

To provide additional feedback regarding this course, Western Schools services, or to suggest new course topics, use the space provided on the Important Information form found on the back of the FasTrax instruction sheet included with your course. Return the completed form to Western Schools with your final exam.

SUBMITTING THE COMPLETED FINAL EXAM

For your convenience, Western Schools provides a number of exam grading options. Full instructions and complete grading details are listed on the FasTrax instruction sheet provided with this course. If you are mailing your answer sheet(s) to Western Schools, we recommend you make a copy as a back-up.

COURSE COMPLETION TIME FRAMES AND EXTENSIONS

You have two (2) years from the date of purchase to complete this course. If you are not able to complete the course within 2 years, a six (6) month extension may be purchased. If you have not completed the course within 30 months from the original enrollment date, your file will be closed and no certificate will be issued.

CHANGE OF ADDRESS?

In the event that your address changes prior to completing this course, please call our customer service department at 1-800-618-1670, so that we may update your file.

WESTERN SCHOOLS GUARANTEES YOUR SATISFACTION

If any continuing education course fails to meet your expectations, or if you are not satisfied for any reason, you may return the course materials for an exchange or a refund (less shipping and handling) within 30 days. Software, video, and audio courses must be returned unopened. Textbooks must not be written in or marked up in any other way.

Thank you for using Western Schools to fulfill your continuing education needs!

WESTERN SCHOOLS
P.O. Box 1930
Brockton, MA 02303
800-438-8888
www.westernschools.com

WESTERN SCHOOLS
COURSE EVALUATION

CARDIOVASCULAR NURSING:
A COMPREHENSIVE OVERVIEW

INSTRUCTIONS: Using the scale below, please respond to the following evaluation statements. All responses should be recorded in the right-hand column of the FasTrax answer sheet, in the section marked "Evaluation." Be sure to fill in each corresponding answer circle completely using blue or black ink. Leave any remaining answer circles blank.

A	B	C	D
Agree Strongly	Agree Somewhat	Disagree Somewhat	Disagree Strongly

OBJECTIVES: Upon completing this course, the reader will be able to

1. Recall the basic structures of the heart and their physiologic functions.
2. Discuss ways pharmacology is used to improve myocardial performance.
3. Describe the key pharmacological agents used to preserve and increase myocardial oxygen supply.
4. Discuss the impact of risk factors on the development of coronary heart disease.
5. Discuss the scope of coronary heart disease management throughout the continuum of presentation, from stable angina through acute myocardial infarction.
6. Discuss the indications for, and the benefits and potential complications of, cardiac revascularization.
7. Describe current strategies for the management of heart failure.
8. Recognize the three main types of cardiomyopathy and their physiological differences.
9. Recognize aortic valve disease and identify its impact on the body.
10. Recognize mitral valve disease and identify its impact on the body.
11. Discuss the implications and current management strategies of atrial fibrillation.
12. Recognize the indications for cardiac pacemakers and defibrillators and the impact of these devices on a patient.

COURSE CONTENT

13. The course materials were presented in a well organized and clearly written manner.
14. The course content was presented in a fair, unbiased and balanced manner.
15. The course expanded my knowledge and enhanced my skills related to the subject matter.
16. I intend to apply the knowledge and skills I've learned to my nursing practice. (Select the appropriate response below.)

        A. Yes   B. Unsure   C. No   D. Not Applicable

ATTESTATION

17. By submitting this answer sheet, I certify that I have read the course materials and personally completed the final examination based on the material presented. Mark "A" for Agree and "B" for Disagree.

Note: To provide additional feedback regarding this course, Western Schools services, or to suggest new course topics, use the space provided on the Important Information form found on the back of the FasTrax instruction sheet included with your course.

CONTENTS

FIGURES AND TABLES

Chapter 6

Chapter 7

Chapter 8

ABBREVIATIONS

BY CHAPTER

Chapter 1

ACE	angiotensin-converting enzyme
ATP	adenosine triphosphate
AV	atrioventricular
CHD	coronary heart disease
Hb	hemoglobin
LAD	left anterior descending artery
LCX	left circumflex artery
MI	myocardial infarction
O_2	oxygen
PDA	posterior descending artery
RAAS	renin-angiotensin-aldosterone system
RCA	right coronary artery
S_1	first heart sound
S_2	second heart sound
SA	sinoatrial
SaO_2	arterial oxygen content

Chapter 2

ACE	angiotensin-converting enzyme
ADH	antidiuretic hormone (arginine vasopressin)
AMP	adenosine monophosphate
ARBs	angiotensin II receptor blockers
AV	atrioventricular
ß1	beta 1
$ß_2$	beta 2

BNP	brain natriuretic peptide or B-type natriuretic peptide
FDA	U.S. Food and Drug Administration
HCM	hypertrophic cardiomyopathy
HCTZ	hydrochlorothiazide
IV	intravenous
MI	myocardial infarction
PDE	phosphodiesterase
RAAS	renin-angiotensin-aldosterone system

Chapter 3

ACS	acute coronary syndrome
ADP	adenosine diphosphate
apo A-I	apolipoprotein A-I
Apo-B	apolipoprotein B
APSAC	anisoylated plasminogen streptokinase activator complex (anistreplase)
aPTT	activated partial thromboplastin time
DNA	deoxyribonucleic acid
DVT	deep vein thrombosis
FDA	U.S. Food and Drug Administration
GI	gastrointestinal
GP	glycoprotein
HDL-C	high-density lipoprotein cholesterol
HIT	heparin-induced thrombocytopenia
INR	International Normalized Ratio
IV	intravenous
LDL-C	low-density lipoprotein cholesterol
LMWH	low-molecular-weight heparin

MI	myocardial infarction
n-PA	lanoteplase
non-STEMI	non-ST-segment elevation myocardial infarction
PCI	percutaneous coronary intervention
PE	pulmonary embolism
PT	prothrombin time
r-PA	reteplase
STEMI	ST-segment elevation myocardial infarction
TNK-t-PA	tenecteplase
t-PA	tissue plasminogen activator
UFH	unfractionated heparin
VLDL-C	very-low-density lipoprotein cholesterol

Chapter 4

ACC/AHA	American College of Cardiology/American Heart Association
ACE	angiotensin-converting enzyme
AHA	American Heart Association
ATP-III	Adult Treatment Panel
BMI	body mass index
CAD	coronary artery disease
CHD	coronary heart disease
DASH	dietary approaches to stop hypertension
DBP	diastolic blood pressure
FDA	U.S. Food and Drug Administration
Hb	hemoglobin
HDL-C	high-density lipoprotein cholesterol
hs-CRP	high-sensitivity C-reactive protein
LDL-C	low-density lipoprotein cholesterol
Lp(a)	lipoprotein (a)
MI	myocardial infarction
NSAIDS	nonsteroidal anti-inflammatory drugs
RAAS	renin-angiotensin-aldosterone system
SBP	systolic blood pressure

Chapter 5

ACE	angiotensin-converting enzyme
ACS	acute coronary syndrome
ADLs	activities of daily living
AV	atrioventricular
BNP	B-type natriuretic peptide or brain natriuretic peptide
CABG	coronary artery bypass grafting
CAD	coronary artery disease
CHD	coronary heart disease
CK	creatine kinase
CTA	computed tomography angiogram
ECG	electrocardiogram
ED	emergency department
EMS	emergency medical services
FDA	U.S. Food and Drug Administration
HCM	hypertrophic cardiomyopathy
IV	intravenous
LAD	left anterior descending artery
LMWH	low-molecular-weight heparin
MET	metabolic equivalent
MI	myocardial infarction
non-STEMI	non-ST-segment elevation myocardial infarction
NSAIDS	nonsteroidal anti-inflammatory drugs
PCI	percutaneous coronary intervention
PDA	posterior descending artery
PHQ	patient health questionnaire
PTCA	percutaneous transluminal coronary angioplasty
RCA	right coronary artery
ROM	range-of-motion
SA	sinoatrial
SSRIs	selective serotonin reuptake inhibitors

STEMI	ST-segment elevation myocardial infarction
UA	unstable angina
UFH	unfractionated heparin

Chapter 6

ACS	acute coronary syndrome
ARDS	acute respiratory distress syndrome
BARI	Bypass Angioplasty Revascularization Investigation
CABG	coronary artery bypass grafting
CHD	coronary heart disease
CK	creatine kinase
COPD	chronic obstructive pulmonary disease
CT	computed tomography
ECG	electrocardiogram
EPO	erythropoietin
FDA	U.S. Food and Drug Administration
GP	glycoprotein
IABP	intra-aortic balloon pump
IV	intravenous
LAD	left anterior descending artery
LIMA	left internal mammary artery
LMWH	low-molecular-weight heparin
MI	myocardial infarction
MIDCAB	minimally invasive coronary artery bypass grafting
MRSA	methicillin-resistant Staphylococcus aureus
NPO	nothing by mouth
NSAIDS	nonsteroidal anti-inflammatory drugs
OPCAB	off-pump coronary artery bypass grafting
PCI	percutaneous coronary intervention
POBA	plain old balloon angioplasty
PTCA	percutaneous transluminal coronary angioplasty

RBC	red blood cell
RCA	right coronary artery
RIMA	right internal mammary artery
SANDBAG	Standards of Angioplasty Nursing Techniques to Diminish Bleeding Around the Groin
STEMI	ST-segment elevation myocardial infarction
TMLR	transmyocardial laser revascularization
UA	unstable angina
UFH	unfractionated heparin

Chapter 7

ACC	American College of Cardiology
ACE	angiotensin-converting enzyme
ACE-I	angiotensin-converting enzyme inhibitors
ADLs	activities of daily living
AHA	American Heart Association
ARBs	angiotensin II receptor blockers
BNP	brain natriuretic peptide or B-type natriuretic peptide
CAD	coronary artery disease
CHD	coronary heart disease
CM	cardiomyopathy
CMS	Centers for Medicare & Medicaid Services
CNS	central nervous system
CRT	cardiac resynchronization therapy
DC	discontinue
DM	diabetes mellitus
ECF	extracellular fluid
ECG	electrocardiogram
EF	ejection fraction
FDA	U.S. Food and Drug Administration
HF	heart failure
HTN	hypertension

ICDs	implantable cardioverter-defibrillators		PVCs	premature ventricular contractions
IV	intravenous		RAAS	renin-angiotensin-aldosterone system
LV	left ventricular		RCM	restrictive cardiomyopathy
LVH	left ventricular hypertrophy		S_1	first heart sound
MI	myocardial infarction		S_2	second heart sound
NSAIDs	nonsteroidal anti-inflammatory drugs		S_3	third heart sound
NYHA	New York Heart Association		S_4	fourth heart sound
RAAS	renin-angiotensin-aldosterone system		SAM	systolic anterior motion
S_1	first heart sound		WHO	World Health Organization
S_2	second heart sound			

Chapter 9

ACC	American College of Cardiology
ACE	angiotensin-converting enzyme
AHA	American Heart Association
CHD	coronary heart disease
ECF	extracellular fluid
ECG	electrocardiogram
S_1	first heart sound
S_2	second heart sound
S_3	third heart sound
S_4	fourth heart sound

The following from the left column:

S_3	third heart sound
S_4	fourth heart sound
SOB	shortness of breath
SNS	sympathetic nervous system

Chapter 8

ACC	American College of Cardiology
ACE	angiotensin-converting enzyme
AHA	American Heart Association
ARVC	arrhythmogenic right ventricular cardiomyopathy
CAD	coronary artery disease
CHD	coronary heart disease
CRT	cardiac resynchronization therapy
DCM	dilated cardiomyopathy
ECF	extracellular fluid
ECG	electrocardiogram
ESC	European Society of Cardiology
HCM	hypertrophic cardiomyopathy
HOCM	hypertrophic obstructive cardiomyopathy
ICDs	implantable cardioverter-defibrillators
MI	myocardial infarction
MRI	magnetic resonance imaging
NYHA	New York Heart Association
PASA	percutaneous alcohol septal ablation

Chapter 10

ACC	American College of Cardiology
ACE	angiotensin-converting enzyme
AHA	American Heart Association
AV	atrioventricular
ECF	extracellular fluid
ECG	electrocardiogram
INR	International Normalized Ratio
MI	myocardial infarction
S_1	first heart sound
S_2	second heart sound
S_3	third heart sound

Chapter 11

ACE	angiotensin-converting enzyme
AV	atrioventricular
CHD	coronary heart disease
DC	direct current
ECG	electrocardiogram
FDA	U.S. Food and Drug Administration
HCM	hypertrophic cardiomyopathy
HOCM	hypertrophic obstructive cardiomyopathy
ICDs	implantable cardioverter-defibrillators
INR	international normalized ratio
IV	intravenous
K+	potassium
MI	myocardial infarction
NA+	sodium
PAC	premature atrial contraction
PLAATO	percutaneous left atrial appendage transcatheter occlusion
RCM	restrictive cardiomyopathy
SA	sinoatrial
TEE	transesophageal echocardiogram
TIA	transient ischemic attack
TP	threshold potential
TRP	transient receptor potential
WPW	Wolff-Parkinson-White

Chapter 12

ACC	American College of Cardiology
AHA	American Heart Association
AV	atrioventricular
BPEG	British Pacing and Electrophysiology Group
CRT	cardiac resynchronization therapy
CPR	cardiopulmonary resuscitation
DCM	dilated cardiomyopathy

ECG	electrocardiogram
EOL	end of life
EMS	emergency medical system
ERI	elective replacement interval
FDA	U.S. Food and Drug Administration
HRS	Heart Rhythm Society
ICDs	implantable cardioverter-defibrillators
LVEF	left ventricular ejection fraction
MI	myocardial infarction
MRI	magnetic resonance imaging
NASPE	North American Society of Pacing and Electrophysiology
NYHA	New York Heart Association
SA	sinoatrial
SSS	sick sinus syndrome
VF	ventricular fibrillation
VT	ventricular tachycardia

PRETEST

1. Begin this course by taking the pretest. Circle the answers to the questions on this page, or write the answers on a separate sheet of paper. Do not log answers to the pretest questions on the FasTrax test sheet included with the course.

2. Compare your answers to the PRETEST KEY located at the end of the Pretest. The pretest key indicates the chapter where the content of that question is discussed. Make note of the questions you missed, so that you can focus on those areas as you complete the course.

3. Complete the course by reading the chapters and completing the exam questions at the end of each chapter. Answers to these exam questions should be logged on the FasTrax test sheet included with the course.

Note: Choose the one option that BEST answers each question.

1. The heart has several layers, including the endocardium, myocardium, and epicardium. The myocardium is the

   a. inner surface of the heart chambers and valves.

   b. smooth outer layer of the heart that contains a network of coronary arteries and veins.

   c. thick middle layer of the heart that contains cardiac muscle fibers.

   d. thin fibrous sac that surrounds the heart.

2. The mitral valve is located between the

   a. aorta and the left ventricle.

   b. right atrium and the right ventricle.

   c. right ventricle and the pulmonary artery.

   d. left atrium and the left ventricle.

3. One of the primary types of medications used to decrease preload is

   a. diuretics.

   b. beta-blockers.

   c. calcium channel blockers.

   d. digoxin.

4. Preventing the conversion of angiotensin I to angiotensin II best describes the action of

   a. ACE inhibitors.

   b. angiotensin receptor blockers.

   c. calcium channel blockers.

   d. nitrates.

5. Nicotinic acid and fibric acid derivatives are most effective in lowering

   a. high-density lipoprotein cholesterol.

   b. low-density lipoprotein cholesterol.

   c. triglycerides.

   d. C-reactive protein.

6. Aspirin, glycoprotein IIb/IIIa inhibitors, and clopidogrel are all medications that can be utilized for

   a. thrombolytic therapy.

   b. antiplatelet therapy.

   c. fibrinolytic therapy.

   d. anticoagulation therapy.

7. People with known coronary heart disease are considered to be in the highest risk group for having a future coronary event. What other group of patients have the same risk as those with coronary heart disease?

    a. Patients with low HDL cholesterol
    b. Patients with type 2 diabetes
    c. Patients with a first degree relative who has heart disease
    d. Patients with high blood pressure

8. The single most important modifiable cardiovascular risk factor is

    a. hypertension.
    b. high cholesterol.
    c. diabetes mellitus.
    d. smoking.

9. Angina that is described as increasing in severity and frequency is referred to as

    a. unstable angina.
    b. stable angina.
    c. Prinzmetal's angina.
    d. new-onset angina.

10. The most reliable diagnostic test used to determine the presence of coronary artery disease is

    a. electrocardiography.
    b. cardiac angiography.
    c. stress testing.
    d. nuclear imaging.

11. In a patient with an acute ST segment elevation, how many minutes from the time the patient comes in contact with emergency medical services is the goal for PCI reperfusion?

    a. 30 minutes
    b. 60 minutes
    c. 90 minutes
    d. 120 minutes

12. The second most common cause of mortality related to cardiac bypass surgery is

    a. cardiac dysrhythmias.
    b. sternal wound infection.
    c. postoperative stroke.
    d. intraoperative myocardial infarction.

13. The most common cause of left ventricular dysfunction resulting in heart failure is

    a. hypertensive heart disease.
    b. valvular heart disease.
    c. rheumatic heart disease.
    d. ischemic coronary heart disease.

14. According to the New York Heart Association Classification, a patient with class III heart failure is described as

    a. comfortable at rest but less-than-ordinary activity results in fatigue, palpitations, dyspnea, or anginal pain.
    b. free from fatigue, palpitations, dyspnea, and anginal pain during ordinary activity.
    c. comfortable at rest but ordinary activity results in fatigue, palpitations, dyspnea, or anginal pain.
    d. having symptoms of cardiac insufficiency at rest.

15. Dilated cardiomyopathy is defined as

    a. rigidity of the cardiac walls, resulting in a decreased ability of the chamber walls to expand during cardiac filling.

    b. enlarged cardiac chambers with an impaired ability to contract, resulting in systolic dysfunction.

    c. an increase in muscle mass, resulting in a decrease in ventricular filling and a decrease in cardiac output.

    d. enlarged cardiac chambers with an impaired ability to contract, resulting in diastolic dysfunction.

16. The most common cause of aortic stenosis in patients 70 years of age and older is

    a. rheumatic heart disease.

    b. infective endocarditis.

    c. senile degenerative calcification.

    d. congenital valve disease.

17. Mitral facies is a pinkish purple discoloration of the cheeks that is common in patients with

    a. severe mitral stenosis.

    b. severe mitral regurgitation.

    c. severe aortic stenosis.

    d. severe aortic regurgitation.

18. Atrial fibrillation that comes on spontaneously and terminates itself is called

    a. persistent atrial fibrillation.

    b. permanent atrial fibrillation.

    c. temporary atrial fibrillation.

    d. paroxysmal atrial fibrillation.

19. Class II antiarrhythmic medications used to control heart rate in patients with atrial fibrillation include

    a. calcium channel blockers.

    b. beta-blockers.

    c. potassium channel blockers.

    d. sodium channel blockers.

20. A patient with permanent pacemakers should be aware that

    a. the use of a microwave oven may damage the pacemaker.

    b. the use of a microwave oven by someone else in his or her presence is acceptable as long as the person with the pacemaker does not touch the microwave.

    c. the use of a microwave oven will not harm the pacemaker.

    d. he or she should leave the room when a microwave oven is running.

PRETEST KEY

1.	C	chapter 1	6.	B	chapter 3	11.	C	chapter 5	16.	C	chapter 9
2.	D	chapter 1	7.	B	chapter 4	12.	C	chapter 6	17.	A	chapter 10
3.	A	chapter 2	8.	D	chapter 4	13.	D	chapter 7	18.	D	chapter 11
4.	A	chapter 2	9.	A	chapter 5	14.	A	chapter 7	19.	B	chapter 11
5.	C	chapter 3	10.	B	chapter 5	15.	B	chapter 8	20.	C	chapter 12

INTRODUCTION

The prevention of cardiovascular disease should begin at birth. From birth, the delicate inner layer of our vessels (the endothelium) begins the fight to combat a wide variety of insults that can damage cells and vessel walls. This damage begins a progression of cardiovascular disease that may disable and ultimately end life. Prevention is the first step to cardiovascular health. Unfortunately, too many people wait until disease progression is well under way before taking notice.

Coronary heart disease is responsible for 1 in every 5 deaths in the United States and is the number one killer in both men and women. Every 25 seconds, someone suffers from a coronary event. Although the incidence of coronary heart disease is decreasing, it still causes approximately one death per minute in the U.S. (American Heart Association, 2010). Although many advances have recently been made in cardiovascular medicine, they have not been enough to move cardiovascular death from the top of the list. Many people believe that intracoronary stenting and open-heart surgery can solve the problem of heart disease; unfortunately, these procedures only resolve the end result of the problem. Without risk factor modification, the process continues. In many cases, before intracoronary stenting and open-heart surgery are options, irreversible damage to the heart occurs, resulting in a decline in cardiac activity. Damage to the myocardium can also result from processes that do not involve blockage of the coronary arteries, including hypertension and valvular disease.

Because of its prevalence, nurses commonly care for patients who have, or are at risk for, cardiovascular disease. This book provides information to support nurses working in a variety of settings who care for patients with cardiovascular disease. The purpose of this course is to serve as a reference for nurses working in noncardiovascular specialties, and to provide nurses who desire to work in the cardiovascular arena with a good introductory text. The curriculum begins with a foundation of cardiovascular anatomy and physiology. When normal cardiovascular functioning is understood, the learner can then move forward to understanding pathophysiology. The content of the chapters on cardiovascular medications and risk factors is referenced throughout the rest of the text, as cardiovascular disease processes are discussed. Nursing application points are highlighted throughout the text to assist in identifying key issues in the care of patients with cardiovascular disease.

Heightened awareness is the first step toward impacting this devastating disease. Nurses with knowledge open the door to early recognition and treatment of cardiovascular disease. The astute nurse can make the difference between a life that is cut short by cardiovascular disease and one that is long and healthy.

A note about the terminology used in *Cardiovascular Nursing: A Comprehensive Overview*, 2nd Edition: Throughout nursing and healthcare literature, the terms *dysrhythmia* and *arrhythmia* are used interchangeably. This text will adopt the term *dysrhythmia* instead of *arrhythmia*, as the use of the letter *a* at the beginning of a word (in most accepted medical terminology) signifies the absence of something. Since patients with cardiac rhythm disturbances do in fact have a rhythm, we believe that the word *dysrhythmia* is the more accurate terminology. The term *arrhythmia* was retained when referring to pharmacology and specific classes of medications to represent the continued current verbiage.

CHAPTER 1

CARDIAC ANATOMY AND PRINCIPLES OF PHYSIOLOGY

CHAPTER OBJECTIVE

After completing this chapter, the learner will be able to recall the basic structures of the heart and their physiologic functions.

LEARNING OBJECTIVES

After completing this chapter, the learner will be able to

1. identify the layers of the heart wall.

2. explain the structural difference between atrioventricular valves and semilunar valves.

3. describe systole and diastole and their purpose in the cardiac cycle.

4. describe the anatomy of the coronary arteries.

5. recognize the components of the cardiac conduction system.

6. define the components of cardiac output.

7. describe how the heart and lungs form a cardiopulmonary circuit that delivers oxygen to body tissues.

8. explain the role of the autonomic nervous system in regulating the heart and blood pressure.

9. explain the role of the renin-angiotensin-aldosterone system in regulating blood pressure.

INTRODUCTION

Cardiac anatomy and physiology form an important foundation for understanding all aspects of cardiovascular nursing. A solid physiological basis for the understanding of cardiovascular disease and treatments allows the nurse to link knowledge to practice in a more meaningful way.

BASIC CARDIAC ANATOMY

The heart is a hollow, muscular, four-chambered organ. It is positioned in the mediastinum (middle of the thoracic cavity) between the lungs, just above the diaphragm. The heart is attached to the thorax by the great vessels. The great vessels include the aorta, pulmonary artery, inferior vena cava, and superior vena cava. The adult heart is approximately 5 inches by 3.5 inches by 2.5 inches (Dennison, 2007), or approximately the size of a person's fist. The tip of the left ventricle forms the apex (bottom) of the heart. The apex is located at approximately the fifth intercostal space, at the midclavicular line. The base, or top, of the heart is located at approximately the second intercostal space (see Figure 1-1).

Cardiac Chambers

The right and left atria (upper chambers) are separated by a mass of connective tissue called the *interatrial septum*. The right and left atria are low-pressure, thin-walled chambers that receive blood

1

FIGURE 1-1: LOCATION OF HEART IN CHEST

Pericardial sac

Xiphoid process

Note. From *Atlas of Anesthesia: Critical Care* by N. Yeston and R. Kirby. Edited by R. Miller (series editor) and R. Kirby. Copyright 1997, by Current Medicine. Used with permission from Images. MD.

and act as reservoirs. The right atrium receives deoxygenated blood from the venous system via the inferior and superior venae cavae, as well as from the coronary sinus (the primary coronary vein). The left atrium receives oxygenated blood from the pulmonary veins after the blood has traveled through the lungs (see Figure 1-2).

The right and left ventricles (lower chambers) are the pumping chambers of the heart and receive blood from the atria. The ventricles are separated by the interventricular septum. The right ventricle is a thin-walled, low-pressure pump that receives deoxygenated blood from the right atrium. This ventricle pumps blood into the pulmonary artery, which carries the blood to the lungs to exchange carbon dioxide for oxygen. The left ventricle is a thick-walled, high-pressure pump that receives oxygenated blood from the left atrium and pumps blood into the aorta for distribution throughout the circulatory system.

FIGURE 1-2: LEFT FRONTAL VIEW OF THE HEART

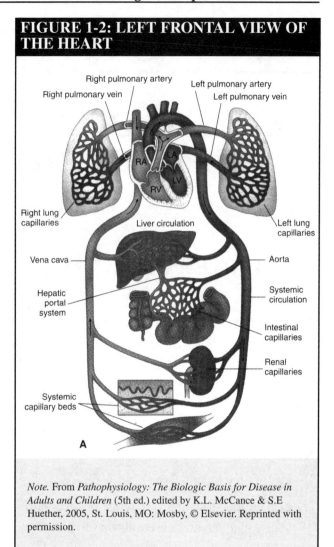

Note. From *Pathophysiology: The Biologic Basis for Disease in Adults and Children* (5th ed.) edited by K.L. McCance & S.E Huether, 2005, St. Louis, MO: Mosby, © Elsevier. Reprinted with permission.

Clinical Application

Because the right ventricular wall is thinner than the left ventricular wall, the right ventricle fails more easily in response to elevated pulmonary pressures than the left ventricle does to elevated systemic pressures. Therefore, patients can have acute right-sided heart failure as a result of pulmonary hypertension.

Layers of the Heart

The three layers of the heart are the endocardium, myocardium, and epicardium. The pericardium is an additional layer that surrounds the heart (see Figure 1-3).

FIGURE 1-3: LAYERS OF THE HEART WALL

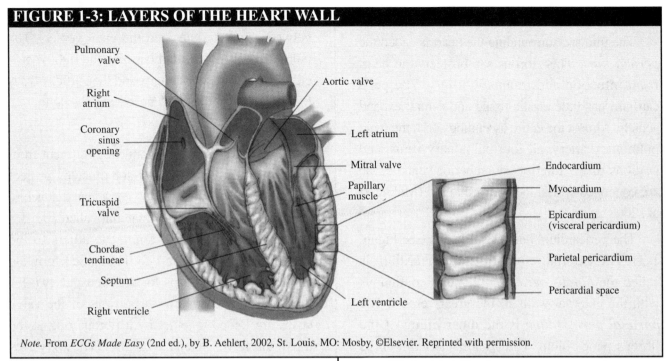

Note. From *ECGs Made Easy* (2nd ed.), by B. Aehlert, 2002, St. Louis, MO: Mosby, ©Elsevier. Reprinted with permission.

Endocardium

The endocardium is a serous membrane consisting of connective tissue, elastic fibers, and a thin layer of epithelial cells that form a smooth surface for the movement of blood and prevention of clot formation. The endocardium is the inner surface of the heart chambers and valves, and also covers the walls of the vessels of the entire vascular system, creating a closed circulatory system.

Clinical Application

Inflammation of the endocardium or heart valves is called endocarditis. Endocarditis can affect both native valves and prosthetic valves.

Myocardium

The myocardium is the thick middle layer of the heart. The largest layer of the heart, the myocardium contains cardiac muscle fibers that have the ability to contract as well as conduct electrical stimuli. The myocardium of the ventricles is thicker than the myocardium of the atria. The left ventricle has the thickest myocardium because of the high pressure in the aorta that the ventricle must pump against to eject its contents. As patients develop myocardial hypertrophy (increased cell size), this layer of the heart becomes larger.

Clinical Application

Damage to the myocardial layer of the heart results in a decreased ability for the heart to contract, resulting in an impaired ability to eject blood from the ventricles. The myocardial layer of the heart can be damaged as a result of a myocardial infarction (MI) or from an inflammatory process (myocarditis).

Epicardium

The epicardium is the smooth outer layer of the heart that contains the network of coronary arteries and veins, the autonomic nerves, the lymphatic system, and fat tissue. Coronary blood vessels that supply the myocardium and endocardium with oxygen-rich blood must cross the epicardium before passing through the myocardium and, finally, entering the endocardium. Increased age and obesity increase the amount of fat tissue in the epicardial layer, resulting in an increase in the amount of tissue that must be supplied with oxygen-rich blood before supplying the myocardium and endocardium (Malouf, Edwards, Tajik, & Seward, 2008).

Pericardium

The thin sac surrounding the heart is called the *pericardium*. This fibrous sac protects the heart from infection and traumatic injury. The pericardium has little elastic tissue and cannot expand acutely. Almost the entire ascending aorta, the main pulmonary artery, all four pulmonary veins, and portions of the inferior and superior venae cavae are contained within the pericardial sac (Malouf et al., 2008).

The pericardium has several layers (see Figure 1-3). The external cover of the pericardium is called the *fibrous pericardium* and is continuous with the external walls of the great vessels. The *parietal pericardium* is the inner lining of the fibrous pericardium. The *visceral pericardium* is another name for the epicardium. This inner lining of the pericardium forms the outer lining of the heart and great vessels. The space between the parietal and visceral layers of the pericardium contains a small amount (approximately 10 to 30 ml) of lubricating fluid (Bond, 2010). This fluid prevents friction between the epicardium and the fibrous pericardium during each cardiac contraction. Pericardial disease can interfere with the ability of the ventricles to fill during diastole. Pericarditis is inflammation of the pericardium.

Clinical Application

If the aorta ruptures or dissects, the pericardium can rapidly fill with blood. Rapid filling of the pericardial sac results in the inability of the heart to relax and fill. This can produce fatal results, including cardiac tamponade and death.

Cardiac Valves

The four cardiac valves located within the heart are designated as either *atrioventricular* (AV) *valves* or *semilunar valves* (see Figure 1-4). The valves located between the atria and ventricles are AV valves. The tricuspid valve is located between the right atrium and right ventricle, and the mitral valve is located between the left atrium and left ventricle. The two semilunar valves are located between the ventricles and the great vessels. The pulmonic valve is located between the right ventricle and the pulmonary artery, and the aortic valve is located between the left ventricle and the aorta.

Atrioventricular Valves

The AV valves are anatomically different from the semilunar valves. Papillary muscles project from the inner surface of the ventricle and attach to delicate strands of fibrous material called *chordae tendineae*. The chordae tendineae attach to the valve leaflets (see Figure 1-5). The leaflets form the valve cusps (three cusps for the tricuspid, two for the mitral). The uppermost portions of the valve cusps are joined together by a fibrous ring at the top of the valve, called the *annulus*. The AV valves open passively during diastole, forming a funnel-like shape that allows blood to flow from the atria to the ventricles. At the end of diastole, ventricular pressure increases and forces the valve leaflets to come together and close the valve opening between the atrium and the ventricle. As the ventricle contracts to eject blood, the papillary muscles contract to prevent the valve leaflets from prolapsing into the atrium. The closure of the leaflets prevents the backward flow of blood from the ventricle to the atrium. At the end of systole, when the ventricle relaxes, the AV valves open again and the cycle is repeated.

Clinical Application

During an acute MI of the left ventricle, the papillary muscle of the mitral valve can become weakened and potentially rupture. If the papillary muscle ruptures, the mitral valve can no longer maintain unidirectional blood flow. As a result, blood backs up into the left atrium and pulmonary vasculature during ventricular contraction, causing acute left-sided heart failure and potential pulmonary edema.

FIGURE 1-4: VALVES AND CHAMBERS OF THE HEART

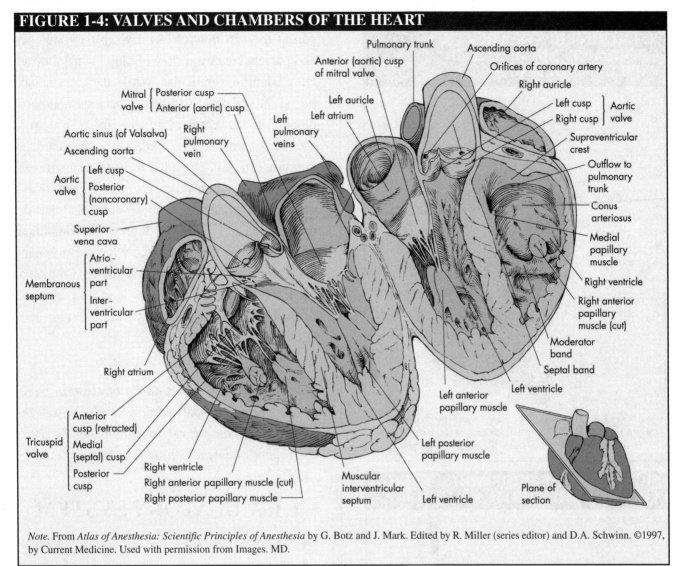

Note. From *Atlas of Anesthesia: Scientific Principles of Anesthesia* by G. Botz and J. Mark. Edited by R. Miller (series editor) and D.A. Schwinn. ©1997, by Current Medicine. Used with permission from Images. MD.

Semilunar Valves

Each semilunar valve consists of an annulus and three cusps (see Figure 1-6). The pulmonic and aortic valves have the same structure; however, the aortic valve leaflets are heavier and thicker because of the increased pressure system in the left side of the heart. The pulmonic valve is located between the right ventricle and the pulmonary artery, and the aortic valve is located between the left ventricle and the aorta. These valves function by pressure changes in the heart and the great vessels. During diastole, the semilunar valves are closed as the ventricles fill with blood from the atria. As the AV valves close and systole begins, the ventricles begin to contract. When the pressure in the ventricles is greater than the pressure on the other side of the semilunar valves, the valves are forced open and blood is ejected out of the ventricles into the great vessels. When ventricular ejection is complete, the pressure in the ventricles is less than the pressure in the great vessels, and the semilunar valves close tightly. Tight closure prevents the backward flow of blood from the great vessels to the ventricles. The cycle then begins again.

Clinical Application

When auscultating the heart, the first heart sound (S_1), referred to as "lub," is associated with closure of the AV valves. The second heart sound (S_2), referred to as "dub," is associated with closure of the semilunar valves. These two sounds together form the "lub-dub" heard during cardiac auscultation.

FIGURE 1-5: MITRAL VALVE AND THE RELATIONSHIPS OF THE CUSPS, CHORDAE TENDINEAE, AND PAPILLARY MUSCLES

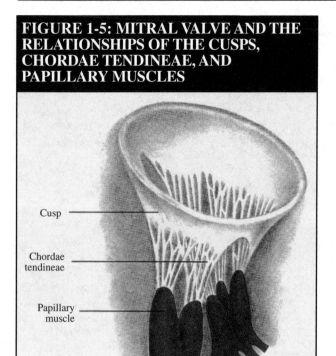

Cusp

Chordae
tendineae

Papillary
muscle

Note. From *Critical Care Nursing: Diagnosis and Management* (2nd ed.), by L.A. Thelan, J.K. Davie, L.D. Urden, and M.E. Lough, 1994, St. Louis, MO: MO: Mosby, ©Elsevier. Reprinted with permission.

FIGURE 1-6: INFERIOR AND SUPERIOR VIEWS OF THE AORTIC VALVE

Inferior View   Superior View

Note. From *Critical Care Nursing: Diagnosis and Management* (2nd ed.), by L.A. Thelan, J.K. Davie, L.D. Urden, and M.E. Lough, 1994, St. Louis, MO: MO: Mosby, ©Elsevier. Reprinted with permission.

Clinical Application

S_1 ("lub") represents the beginning of ventricular systole, or contraction, and S_2 ("dub") represents the beginning of ventricular diastole, or relaxation.

When cardiac valves function correctly, they permit forward flow of blood when they are open and prevent backward flow of blood when they are closed. During ventricular systole, the tricuspid and mitral valves close to prevent backward flow of blood from the ventricles into the atria. During ventricular systole, all blood forced from the ventricles during ejection is propelled forward through open pulmonic and aortic valves into the pulmonary and systemic vascular beds. During ventricular diastole, the tricuspid and mitral valves open, allowing filling of the ventricles from the atria. When the pulmonic and aortic valves close properly during ventricular diastole, they prevent the backward flow of blood from the pulmonary and systemic vascular beds into the ventricles.

Clinical Application

An aortic valve that does not close properly results in a backward flow of blood from the aorta into the left ventricle, reducing the stroke volume of the previous contraction.

CIRCULATORY SYSTEM

The heart and blood vessels work together for one primary purpose: the delivery of oxygen and other nutrients to the cellular level. The capillaries are the location where oxygen and nutrients are exchanged.

Arterial System

Oxygenated blood leaves the left ventricle and travels to the tissue level via the systemic arterial system. Arteries are made up of elastic tissue that allows them to respond to the high pressures associated with the force of left ventricular contraction. Large arteries also contain smooth muscle.

All arteries have three layers of tissue that surround the open lumen (see Figure 1-7). The inner layer, called the *intima*, has a thin lining of endothelium that contains epithelial cells. The intima decreases resistance to flow and minimizes

FIGURE 1-7: CROSS-SECTION OF AN ARTERY AND A VEIN

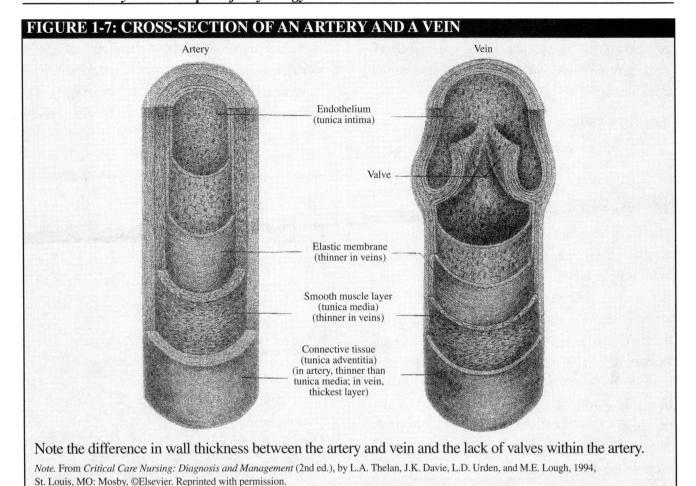

Artery   Vein

Endothelium
(tunica intima)

Valve

Elastic membrane
(thinner in veins)

Smooth muscle layer
(tunica media)
(thinner in veins)

Connective tissue
(tunica adventitia)
(in artery, thinner than
tunica media; in vein,
thickest layer)

Note the difference in wall thickness between the artery and vein and the lack of valves within the artery.

Note. From *Critical Care Nursing: Diagnosis and Management* (2nd ed.), by L.A. Thelan, J.K. Davie, L.D. Urden, and M.E. Lough, 1994, St. Louis, MO: Mosby, ©Elsevier. Reprinted with permission.

the chance of platelet aggregation (a component of clotting). The *media* (the middle layer) is composed of smooth muscle and elastic connective tissue. The media is responsible for changes in the diameter of the vessel, as needed, to assist with blood pressure control. The fibrous outer layer, called the *adventitia,* is designed to protect the vessel and provide connection to other internal structures. Arteries have the ability to expand or contract in response to the body's cardiac output needs.

Arterioles

The large arteries carry blood from the aorta to the rest of the body. The arteries divide and become smaller as they move away from the aorta. The smallest arteries branch into arterioles. Arterioles connect to the capillary bed. At the arteriole level of the capillary is smooth muscle that is referred to as the *precapillary sphincter.* The arterioles and the precapillary sphincters regulate blood flow to the

capillaries. This regulation of blood flow is primarily determined by the oxygen needs of the tissue through a process called *autoregulation.* When oxygen needs increase, the arterioles dilate. This dilation decreases resistance to flow and results in increased flow to the capillaries (Darovic, 2002).

Capillary System

When oxygenated blood reaches the capillary level, oxygen and other nutrients are exchanged. Because capillary walls are only one cell thick, gases and nutrients pass through the walls easily. Miles of capillaries are located near almost all body cells. The capillaries contain no smooth muscle (Bridges & Schmelz, 2010); therefore, capillary tone depends on the tone of the vessel just before and after the capillary. Four pressures influence the movement of fluids across capillary membranes: capillary hydrostatic pressure, interstitial hydrostatic pressure, capillary oncotic pressure, and interstitial colloidal oncotic pressure (Opie, 2004). After oxygen and nutrients are exchanged for waste products, deoxygenated blood is returned to the right atrium from the capillaries via the venous system.

Venous System

The venous system is a lower-pressure system than the arterial system. Because veins are not subject to the high pressures of the arterial system, their walls are much thinner than those of arteries. Thinner walls allow for much more distensibility. At any given time, the venous system generally holds 60% to 80% of the body's total blood volume (Bridges & Schmelz, 2010). The venous system also regulates the amount of blood returning to the heart. Vasoconstriction of veins increases blood flow to the heart by decreasing the amount of blood held in the vascular bed. Vasodilation decreases blood flow to the heart by increasing the vascular bed to hold more volume. The venous system is strongly influenced by gravity and relies on one-way valves that help prevent backward flow of blood through the low-pressure venous system (see Figure 1-7). These venous valves are absent in a small percentage of people and can be damaged by age or by catheter insertion (Malouf et al., 2008). Venous return is also augmented by contraction of skeletal muscles, which compress veins and help to propel blood forward.

Clinical Application

Weakened vein valves cause varicose (dilated) veins. Age, prolonged standing, and pregnancy contribute to varicose veins.

Clinical Application

In right-sided heart failure, venous valves are important in maintaining the unidirectional flow of blood back to the right side of the heart.

Normal Circulatory Patterns

The thoracic aorta arises from the aortic valve and is divided into three segments: ascending aorta, aortic arch, and descending thoracic aorta. The origin of the coronary arteries is located in the ascending aorta, immediately above the aortic valve. The location of the origin of the coronary arteries allows them to receive blood that is rich in oxygen. The aortic arch has three branches: the brachiocephalic artery, the left common carotid artery, and the left subclavian artery (see Figure 1-8). These branches are responsible for blood flow from the heart to the upper torso, neck, head, brain, and the arms.

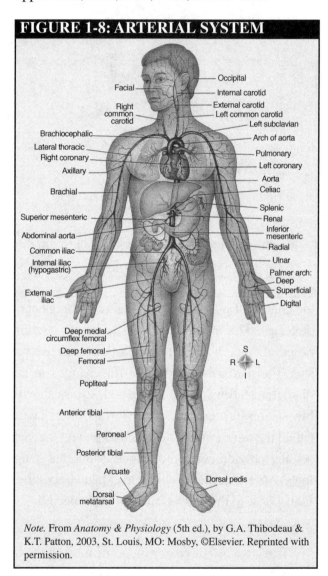

FIGURE 1-8: ARTERIAL SYSTEM

Note. From *Anatomy & Physiology* (5th ed.), by G.A. Thibodeau & K.T. Patton, 2003, St. Louis, MO: Mosby, ©Elsevier. Reprinted with permission.

The thoracic aorta, which is located below the aortic arch, branches off to supply blood to the torso, including the thoracic cavity and the lungs. The abdominal aorta supplies blood to the abdominal organs and the kidneys. At approximately the fourth lumbar vertebra, the aorta divides into the internal iliac arteries. The structures of the lower trunk, including the reproductive organs and the legs, receive their blood supply from the internal iliac arteries.

The venous system mimics the arterial system in returning blood to the heart. Prior to entering the heart, the entire venous system enters into either the superior or inferior vena cava. The superior vena cava receives venous blood returning from the head, neck, upper extremities, and thorax. The inferior vena cava receives blood from below the level of the diaphragm, including the abdomen, pelvis, and lower extremities. The superior and inferior venae cavae empty the returning deoxygenated blood into the right atrium. The coronary veins also drain into the coronary sinus, which then empties directly into the right atrium.

Circulation Through the Heart

When deoxygenated blood is received by the right atrium, it moves to the right ventricle through the tricuspid valve during ventricular diastole. After the right ventricle fills, the tricuspid valve closes and the ventricle contracts and ejects the blood through the open pulmonic valve into the pulmonary artery. The pulmonary artery divides into the right and left pulmonary arteries and carries blood to the pulmonary capillaries, where gas exchange occurs. Blood leaving the right ventricle is low in oxygen and high in carbon dioxide. When gas exchange occurs, oxygen enters the blood and carbon dioxide leaves the blood and is exhaled.

The pulmonary veins return oxygenated blood to the left side of the heart via the left atrium. The blood in the left atrium moves through the open mitral valve into the left ventricle during ventricular diastole. At the end of diastole, the mitral valve closes and the left ventricle contracts, forcing the aortic valve open and ejecting the oxygenated blood into the aorta for participation in systemic circulation. (See Figure 1-9.)

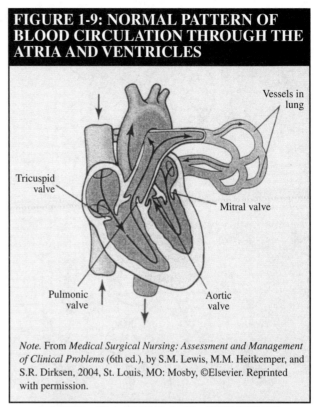

FIGURE 1-9: NORMAL PATTERN OF BLOOD CIRCULATION THROUGH THE ATRIA AND VENTRICLES

Vessels in lung

Tricuspid valve

Mitral valve

Pulmonic valve

Aortic valve

Note. From *Medical Surgical Nursing: Assessment and Management of Clinical Problems* (6th ed.), by S.M. Lewis, M.M. Heitkemper, and S.R. Dirksen, 2004, St. Louis, MO: Mosby, ©Elsevier. Reprinted with permission.

THE CARDIAC CYCLE

*S*ystole, contraction of the heart muscle, results in ejection of blood from the chamber. *Diastole,* relaxation of the heart muscle, allows the chamber to fill. Each of the atria and ventricles undergoes systole and diastole. In a resting adult, each cardiac cycle lasts approximately 0.8 second (Opie, 2004). The efficiency of the cardiac cycle depends on the health of the cardiac muscle, valves, and conduction system. The heart's conduction system provides the timing of events for atrial and ventricular systole (see Figure 1-10).

Ventricular Diastole

Ventricular diastole begins when ventricular contraction is complete. When the pressure in the pulmonary vascular bed and the aorta exceeds the pressure in the right and left ventricles, the semilunar valves close. Simultaneously, the pressure in the filled atria exceeds the pressure in the nearly empty ventricles and the AV valves (tricuspid and mitral valves) open. When the tricuspid and mitral valves open, a rapid, passive filling of the ventricles

FIGURE 1-10: THE CARDIAC CYCLE

Drawings A and B: Ventricular diastole. A. Passive filling of ventricle. B. Active filling of ventricle (atrial kick). Drawings C and D: Ventricular systole. C. Isovolumic contraction. D. Ventricular ejection.

Note. From *Hemodynamic Monitoring: Invasive and Noninvasive Clinical Application* (3rd ed.), by G.O. Darovic, 2002, Philadelphia, PA: Saunders, ©Elsevier. Reprinted with permission.

occurs as blood moves from the atria through the open valves into the ventricles. Approximately 75% of ventricular filling occurs during this passive filling phase. The remainder of ventricular filling occurs with atrial contraction. This contraction of the atria is also known as *atrial systole*. Atrial systole is commonly referred to as *atrial kick* and contributes as much as 25% of the ventricular volume (Bond, 2010).

Clinical Application

When a person is in atrial fibrillation, he or she loses the atrial kick contribution to left ventricular volume. This loss of atrial kick can result in a decrease in stroke volume that is significant enough to cause a decrease in cardiac output and, ultimately, symptoms of decreased perfusion.

Ventricular Systole

After atrial contraction, the pressures in the atria and ventricles equalize, the AV valves partially close, and ventricular systole begins. Ventricular systole has two phases. The first phase is *isovolumic* or *isovolumetric contraction* (Darovic, 2002), so named because the volume of blood in the ventricles does not change during this phase. During isovolumic contraction, the ventricular walls tense and press toward the center of the ventricular cavity. This tensing of the walls increases the pressure in the ventricles. When the pressure in the ventricles exceeds that in the atria, the AV valves close quickly, preventing backward flow of blood into the atria. In order for ejection of the ventricular contents to occur, the myocardial walls of the ventricles must develop enough pressure to force the semilunar (aortic and pulmonic) valves open. When the pressure in the ventricles exceeds the pressure in the aorta and pulmonary artery, the aortic and pulmonic valves open.

The second phase of systole is *ejection,* during which blood is ejected into the systemic and pulmonary circulation. The semilunar valves close at the end of systole, when the pressure in the arteries exceeds the pressure in the ventricles. Normally, ventricular diastole (ventricular filling) is two times longer than ventricular systole (ventricular emptying).

Clinical Application

As heart rate increases, ventricular diastolic time shortens, while ventricular systolic time essentially stays the same. Therefore, an increased heart rate decreases the time available to fill the ventricles. This decrease in ventricular filling can lead to reduced cardiac output and signs of poor perfusion. Tachycardia, therefore, has the potential to lead to decreased perfusion of end organs.

Contractility

The atria and ventricles have contractile muscle cells called *myocytes.* Without functioning myocytes, the myocardium cannot contract. The remainder of the cardiac cells are either pacemaker cells or cells capable of excitability and conductivity. The adult heart has approximately 19 billion cardiac cells (Bond, 2010). Millions of cardiac cells are lost with each year of life. If a person lives to 100 years of age, he or she will have lost approximately two thirds of his or her original heart cells (Opie, 2004). Cardiac muscle cells differ from skeletal muscle cells in that they are shorter, broader, and more interconnected. Intercalated disks form junctions between cardiac muscle cells, allowing them to function as integrated units. The junctions serve as electrical connections, joining muscle fibers in a single unit capable of rapidly conducting an impulse. These connections allow the atria and ventricles to contract almost simultaneously.

Cardiac muscle cells are also more metabolically active, require more energy, and experience more prolonged contractions than do skeletal muscle cells. This prolonged contraction prevents impulses from coming rapidly enough to produce a sustained contraction, thereby preventing cardiac muscle from running low on adenosine triphosphate (ATP) and becoming fatigued (Opie, 2004). The process of myocardial contraction utilizes the ATP molecules for energy.

The contractile property of the cardiac muscle cell comes from the *myofibril.* Myofibrils consist of repeating units called *sarcomeres* and contain protein units responsible for contraction (Bond, 2010). Cardiac muscle fibers contain transverse tubules, also called *T tubules,* that are extensions of the cell membranes. A significant amount of calcium enters the cell through the T tubules from the interstitial fluid surrounding the cells. Without this additional calcium coming through the T tubules, the force of myocardial contraction would be greatly reduced (Opie, 2004).

Clinical Application

The amount of extracellular calcium ions affects the amount of calcium available to enter the cardiac cells via the T tubules. Therefore, low extracellular calcium ions can negatively affect the force of myocardial contraction.

CORONARY ARTERIES

The coronary arteries begin in the epicardial layer of the heart. These arteries then travel through the myocardium and, ultimately, to the endocardium to provide oxygen-rich blood to the entire cardiac musculature (see Figure 1-3). During systole, as the heart contracts, blood flow through the coronary arteries is markedly reduced due to compression of the vessels.

Therefore, coronary artery perfusion occurs primarily during diastole, when the ventricles are relaxed. Also during diastole, oxygenated blood ejected from the left ventricle to the aorta enters the coronary arteries through two small openings, above the closed aortic valve. These small openings are located in the right and left aortic sinuses. From the openings flow the left and right coronary artery systems (see Figure 1-11).

Clinical Application

Coronary circulation begins with the epicardium and reaches the endocardium last; therefore, myocardial ischemia and infarction begin in the endocardium.

Clinical Application

A thickened myocardial wall (hypertrophy) results in decreased flow of oxygen-rich blood to the deep myocardium and endocardial layer.

Clinical Application

Coronary artery perfusion can be compromised if diastole is shortened due to a rapid heart rate.

Left Coronary Artery System

The left main coronary artery, which supplies oxygenated blood to the largest portion of the myocardium, travels a short distance before dividing into the *left anterior descending artery* (LAD) and *left circumflex artery* (LCX) (see Figure 1-12).

Left Anterior Descending Artery

The LAD supplies oxygenated blood to the anterior wall of the left ventricle, with some perfusion of the right ventricle as well. The septal perforating branches of the LAD supply oxygenated blood to the septum and the bundle branches, whereas the diagonal branches supply oxygenated blood to the anterior left ventricular free wall (see Figure 1-12 and Table 1-1).

Left Circumflex Artery

The LCX supplies oxygenated blood to the lateral wall of the left ventricle and the left atrium. The LCX may also supply oxygenated blood to the inferior wall of the left ventricle in some people. The sinoatrial (SA) node receives oxygenated blood from the nodal branch of the LCX in 45% of the population (Bond, 2010; Malouf et al., 2008),

---

FIGURE 1-11: AORTIC VALVE

(A) Anterior view of aortic valve   (B) Valve open   (C) Valve closed

Note that the right coronary artery arises from the right aortic sinus (cusp) and the left coronary artery arises from the left aortic sinus (cusp).

Note. From *Clinically Oriented Anatomy* (4th ed.), by K.L. Moore and A.F. Dalley, II, 1999, Philadelphia, PA: Lippincott Williams & Wilkins. Reprinted with permission from Lippincott Williams & Wilkins (http//lww.com).

and the AV node receives its oxygenated blood from the LCX in 10% of the population (Bond, 2010) (see Figure 1-12 and Table 1-1).

Right Coronary Artery System

The right coronary artery (RCA) comes from the right side of the aorta. The RCA supplies oxygenated blood to the right atrium and right ventricle as well as the inferior and posterior walls of the left ventricle in most people. The nodal branch of the RCA supplies oxygenated blood to the SA node in 55% of the population (Bond, 2010; Malouf et al., 2008) and the AV nodal branch of the RCA supplies oxygenated blood to the AV node in about 90% of the population (Bond, 2010). The posterior branch of the left bundle branch system receives oxygenated blood from the RCA and the LAD (see Figure 1-12 and Table 1-1).

Dominance

The term *right* or *left dominance* refers to the vessel (LCX or RCA) from which the posterior descending artery (PDA) arises. In 70% of the population, the PDA arises from the RCA (Malouf et al., 2008). In the remainder of the population, the PDA arises from the LCX. The PDA supplies oxygenated blood to the posterior portions of the right and left ventricles as well as the posterior one third of the septum.

Collateral Circulation

Collateral circulation provides communication between the major coronary arteries and their branches. When stenosis of one artery produces a pressure gradient, the collateral vessels can dilate over time and provide a natural bypass for blood flow beyond the stenosis.

The coronary arterioles lie within the myocardium and supply blood to the capillaries. The capillary system is also referred to as the *microcirculation.* Abnormalities in microcirculation can cause cardiac symptoms in the presence of normal epicardial coronary arteries.

FIGURE 1-12: ANTERIOR VIEW OF THE HEART SHOWING THE LOCATIONS OF THE CORONARY ARTERIES

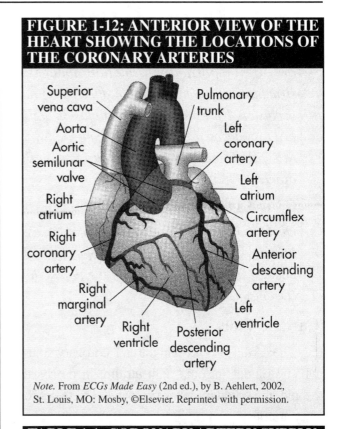

Note. From *ECGs Made Easy* (2nd ed.), by B. Aehlert, 2002, St. Louis, MO: Mosby, ©Elsevier. Reprinted with permission.

TABLE 1-1: CORONARY ARTERY SUPPLY

Coronary Artery	Circulation Supplied To
Left anterior descending artery	Anterior left ventricle Anterior two thirds of septum Bundle of His and bundle branches
Left circumflex artery	Left atrium SA node (45% of population) AV node (10% of population) Lateral left ventricle Posterior left ventricle Posterior septum (20% of population)
Right coronary artery	Right atrium SA node (55% of population) AV node (90% of population) Inferior left ventricle Posterior septum (80% of population) Right ventricle Posterior left ventricle Left posterior bundle branch

Clinical Application

The location of occlusion of a coronary artery provides important information about the structures of the myocardium affected by the occlusion. For example, a total occlusion of the LAD produces a left ventricular anterior wall MI with potential for right and left bundle branch blocks.

Clinical Application

Occlusion of the RCA commonly produces AV heart blocks because the RCA supplies the AV node in approximately 90% of the population (Dennison, 2007).

Cardiac Veins

The cardiac veins drain into the coronary sinus, which empties into the right atrium. In nearly all people, the coronary veins run parallel to the coronary arteries.

ACTION POTENTIAL AND THE CARDIAC CONDUCTION SYSTEM

Action Potential

The action potential is a series of events that results in a change of the electrical charge inside a cell from negative (resting) to positive (stimulated), and back to negative. This change in electrical charge is the result of a difference in the concentration of ions across the cell membrane. The ions primarily responsible for cardiac function are sodium, potassium, and calcium. The cardiac action potential consists of *polarization* (resting state), *depolarization* (stimulation of the cardiac muscle cell), and *repolarization* (return of the cell to a resting state). As depolarization occurs, normal healthy cardiac muscle cells respond with contraction of the muscle. However, depolarization does not guarantee contraction. If a cardiac muscle cell has been damaged, normal contraction might not occur, even when the

cell is stimulated. Additionally, an abnormal level of sodium, potassium, or calcium can adversely affect the action potential.

Conduction System

Contraction of the chambers of the heart in a coordinated fashion is necessary for normal function of the heart. The cardiac conduction system allows for this systematic approach (see Figure 1-13).

SA Node

Stimulation of cardiac muscle cells is normally initiated in a small group of pacemaker cells located in the center of the SA node. The SA node is the natural pacemaker of the heart and sets a heart rate of 60 to 100 beats per minute. External nervous system stimulation is not necessary for SA node activity but can impact it. The SA node is located near the coronary sinus and close to the junction of the superior vena cava and the right atrium (Opie, 2004). The SA node is supplied by the RCA in 55% of the population. The LCX supplies the SA node in the remaining 45% of the population. From the SA node, depolarization travels through the right atrial tissue via internodal pathways and through the left atrial tissue via *Bachmann's bundle.* From the internodal pathways, the impulse travels to the AV node.

AV Node

The AV node slows conduction from the atria to the ventricles. Conduction is slowed to assure that the ventricles are relaxed at the time of atrial contraction, allowing them to fill completely before contracting. The AV node is located in the right atrium, just above the insertion of the tricuspid valve (Opie, 2004).

AV Junction

From the AV node, the electrical impulse travels along the *bundle of His.* The AV node and the bundle of His are surrounded by tissue known as the *AV junction.* The AV junction contains pacemaker cells

FIGURE 1-13: NORMAL CARDIAC CONDUCTION SYSTEM

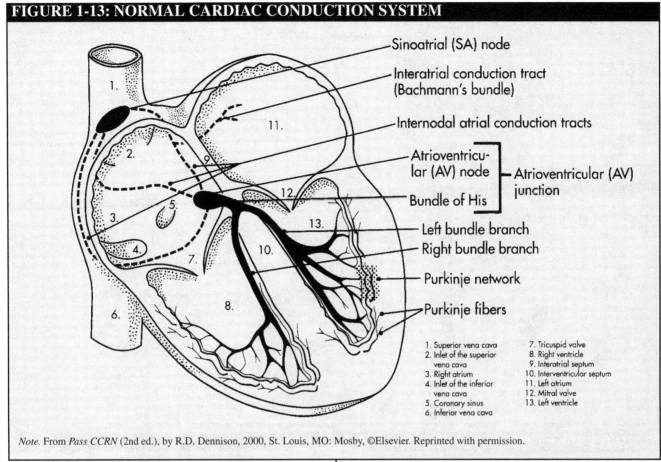

- Sinoatrial (SA) node
- Interatrial conduction tract (Bachmann's bundle)
- Internodal atrial conduction tracts
- Atrioventricu-lar (AV) node
- Bundle of His
- Atrioventricular (AV) junction
- Left bundle branch
- Right bundle branch
- Purkinje network
- Purkinje fibers

1. Superior vena cava
2. Inlet of the superior vena cava
3. Right atrium
4. Inlet of the inferior vena cava
5. Coronary sinus
6. Inferior vena cava
7. Tricuspid valve
8. Right ventricle
9. Interatrial septum
10. Interventricular septum
11. Left atrium
12. Mitral valve
13. Left ventricle

Note. From *Pass CCRN* (2nd ed.), by R.D. Dennison, 2000, St. Louis, MO: Mosby, ©Elsevier. Reprinted with permission.

and will initiate a heart rate of 40 to 60 beats per minute if no impulse is received from the SA node.

Bundle Branches

The bundle of His divides into the right and left bundle branches. The *right bundle branch* carries the impulse to the right ventricle. The *left bundle branch* divides into the left posterior bundle branch and the left anterior bundle branch. The left posterior bundle branch carries the impulse to the posterior and inferior left ventricle; the left anterior bundle branch carries the impulse to the anterior and superior left ventricle.

Purkinje Fibers

From the bundle branches, the impulse travels to the *Purkinje fibers,* where depolarization is carried through the subendocardial layers of the heart. The *Purkinje network* is also the location of the heart's third group of pacemaker cells. If no impulse is received through the normal conduction

patterns, the Purkinje system will initiate a heart rate of 20 to 40 beats per minute.

HEMODYNAMIC PRINCIPLES AND VENTRICULAR FUNCTION

Cardiac Output

Perfusion of the body with oxygenated blood is dependent on cardiac output. *Cardiac output* is the amount of blood ejected by the left ventricle every minute. Heart rate and stroke volume are the primary determinants of cardiac output (see Figure 1-14). Stroke volume has three components: *preload, afterload,* and *contractility.* Changes in heart rate, preload, afterload, or contractility change cardiac output (see Table 1-2). Additionally, increasing any one of these factors increases myocardial oxygen demand. *Stroke volume* is the volume of blood ejected by the left ventricle with each beat. Each

FIGURE 1-14: DETERMINANTS OF CARDIAC OUTPUT

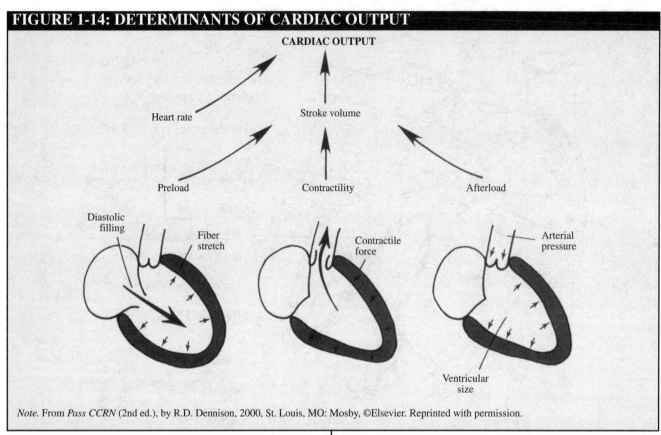

Note. From *Pass CCRN* (2nd ed.), by R.D. Dennison, 2000, St. Louis, MO: Mosby, ©Elsevier. Reprinted with permission.

TABLE 1-2: KEY DEFINITIONS RELATING TO CARDIAC OUTPUT

Cardiac output	Volume of blood ejected by ventricle every minute Cardiac output = Heart rate x Stroke volume
Stroke volume	Volume of blood ejected by ventricle each beat Stroke volume = Preload + Afterload + Contractility
Ejection fraction	Percent of volume in ventricle ejected with each beat
Preload	Stretch on the ventricular myocardial fibers at the end of ventricular diastole; determined by the volume in the ventricle at the end of diastole
Afterload	Pressure the ventricle must overcome to eject its contents
Contractility	Ability of the ventricle to pump independent of preload or afterload

ventricle holds about 150 ml when full and ejects about 50% to 60% of its volume with each beat (Dennison, 2007). The percentage of volume ejected with each beat is termed the *ejection fraction.*

Clinical Application

Patients with decreased contractility from a previous MI have lower ejection fractions and reduced stroke volumes. Patients with low ejection fractions and reduced stroke volume have the potential to exhibit signs of decreased perfusion to the end organs.

Determinants of Cardiac Output

Heart Rate

Heart rate is defined as the number of times the heart beats every minute. Normal heart rate in an adult ranges from 60 to 100 beats per minute. During exercise, heart rate naturally increases to meet the increased metabolic needs of the body. Heart rate also decreases as the body's needs decrease, such as during sleep. However, extremely slow heart rates (less than 40 beats per minute) and extremely high heart rates (greater than 150 beats per minute) experienced over a prolonged period can negatively affect cardiac output. Rapid heart rates do not allow adequate time for ventricular filling, and slow heart rates do not provide an adequate volume of ejected blood per minute.

Preload

Preload, one of the determinants of stroke volume, is defined as the stretch on the ventricular myocardial fibers at the end of ventricular diastole. The volume of blood filling the ventricles causes the myocardium to stretch. According to Starling's law, the larger the volume of blood in the ventricle at the end of diastole (within physiologic limits), the greater the energy of the subsequent contraction (Opie, 2004). Therefore, as the filling of the ventricle increases, the strength of the subsequent contraction also increases, resulting in a greater stroke volume.

Venous return to the heart determines the amount of blood that enters the ventricles and stretches myocardial fibers. The amount of venous blood returned to the right atrium ultimately enters the right and left ventricles. It is this volume of blood that produces the stretch in the ventricles during diastole. If venous return decreases, as with hypovolemia, preload decreases. When preload decreases, stroke volume decreases.

Clinical Application

Evaluation of a patient's fluid status gives a clinician a good indication of preload. A patient experiencing extracellular fluid deficit will have a decreased preload, whereas a patient with extracellular fluid overload will have an increased preload.

Afterload

Afterload, another component of stroke volume, is the workload of the ventricle, or the pressure the ventricle must overcome to eject its contents. Afterload is affected by anatomical structures as well as physiological changes that may impede the ejection of ventricular contents. These structures and changes include aortic or pulmonic valve func-

tion, arterial or pulmonary arterial pressures (vascular resistance), compliance of vascular walls, and diastolic pressure in the great arteries. If the ventricular contents are to be ejected, the pressure in the ventricles must become great enough to force the aortic and pulmonic valves open. A stenotic valve is much more difficult to open due to the abnormalities in the valve. Therefore, aortic or pulmonic stenosis increases afterload.

The overall resistance the left ventricle must pump against, known as *systemic vascular resistance,* is determined primarily by the systemic arterioles (Opie, 2004). When the arterioles dilate, systemic vascular resistance decreases; when they constrict, systemic vascular resistance increases. Arterioles respond to systemic changes and vasoconstrict or vasodilate depending on the hemodynamic needs of the body. Noncompliant vascular walls (as exist in hypertension) do not relax easily and increase afterload. The vascular resistance the right ventricle must pump against is the *pulmonary vascular resistance.* It is determined by the pulmonary artery pressures.

Blood pressure is not equal to systemic vascular resistance. It is a product of cardiac output and systemic vascular resistance. However, blood pressure is a noninvasive method of evaluating systemic vascular resistance. Generally, as diastolic pressure rises, so does systemic vascular resistance.

Clinical Application

Patients with untreated hypertension have a continuous increase in afterload, resulting in increased left ventricular workload. Sustained increased workload eventually causes the left ventricle to fail.

Contractility

The third and final component of the stroke volume equation is *contractility.* Contractility is the ability of the ventricle to contract independent of preload or afterload. Contractility is referred to as the *inotropic state of the myocardium* and is a major component of systole. During ventricular contraction, the sarcomere (repeating unit of the myofibril), or cardiac muscle, shortens (Bond, 2010). The extent of myofibril shortening determines the velocity of the ejection of the myocardial contents. Damage to the myocardial muscle cells, as occurs in MI, decreases the ability of the myofibrils to shorten and impairs the ability of the ventricle to contract. Overstretch of the myofibrils also results in myofibrils that can no longer shorten effectively.

Additional Factors Contributing to Cardiac Output

The shape of the left ventricle is designed to provide a contraction that is generally an inward movement. This inward movement occurs simultaneously among all walls of the ventricle. This normal inward contraction of the ventricle is referred to as *normal muscular synergy* (Darovic, 2002). The normally coordinated contraction may become uncoordinated due to a variety of conditions. For example, the ventricle may become damaged due to ischemic heart disease or aneurysms. Abnormalities in conduction, such as bundle branch blocks and ventricular ectopy, can also alter normal contraction patterns. Finally, changes in ventricular size caused by dilation or fibrosis can also alter normal muscular synergy. This *dyssynergy* can result in an increase in the energy needed for contraction and a decrease in cardiac output.

Additionally, both ventricles are designed to contract simultaneously. *Ventricular dysynchrony* occurs when the right and left ventricles do not contract at the same time. This dysynchrony is commonly demonstrated by a bundle branch block pattern on an electrocardiogram. If the right and left ventricles do not contract in unison, cardiac output and performance are compromised.

Clinical Application

Dilated cardiomyopathy results from myocardial fibrils that have been overstretched and can no longer shorten normally. Therefore, patients with dilated cardiomyopathy have decreased contractility.

THE CARDIOPULMONARY CIRCUIT AND DELIVERY OF OXYGEN

The heart and lungs work together to form the cardiopulmonary circuit (see Figure 1-15). The purpose of the cardiopulmonary circuit is to deliver oxygen to all the tissues of the body. The amount of oxygen delivered to the tissues is determined by three factors:

- cardiac output
- hemoglobin level
- oxygen saturation.

Under normal conditions, approximately 1,000 ml of oxygen are delivered to the tissues each minute via the arterial system and the tissues of the body extract approximately 25% of the oxygen delivered to them (Dennison, 2007), leaving approximately a 75% reserve. If the cardiopulmonary circuit fails to deliver enough oxygen to meet the needs of the tissues, the amount left in the reserve diminishes. The oxygen reserve is measured by assessing the percent of oxygen saturation of venous blood.

Myocardial Oxygenation

The balance of myocardial oxygen supply and demand is key in providing cardiac muscle with the proper amount of oxygen to maintain optimum function (Figure 1-16). The ability of the myocardium to contract effectively is directly related to the amount of oxygen that is supplied to the heart. The myocardium is unique because the left ventricle extracts approximately 75% of the oxygen that is delivered, as opposed to the 25% that is normally extracted by other tissues (Darovic, 2002). Two thirds of oxygen extraction occurs during isovolumic contraction (Darovic, 2002). Because

FIGURE 1-15: SCHEMATIC OF THE CARDIOPULMONARY CIRCUIT

Note. From *Pass CCRN* (2nd ed.), by R.D. Dennison, 2000, St. Louis, MO: Mosby, ©Elsevier. Reprinted with permission.

FIGURE 1-16: FACTORS INFLUENCING MYOCARDIAL SUPPLY AND DEMAND

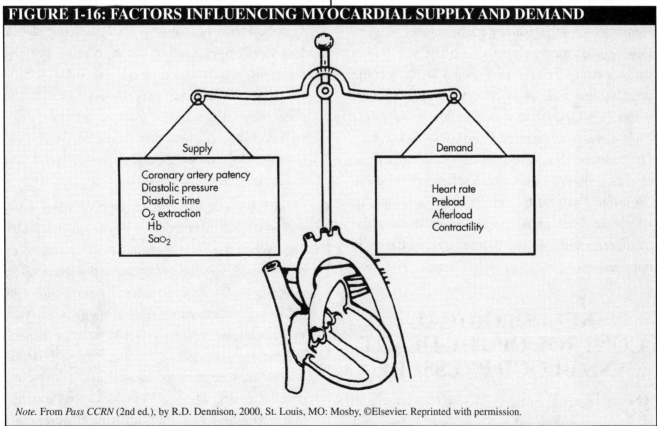

Note. From *Pass CCRN* (2nd ed.), by R.D. Dennison, 2000, St. Louis, MO: Mosby, ©Elsevier. Reprinted with permission.

there is little oxygen reserve to be utilized during periods of increased need, the myocardium becomes very dependent on flow from the coronary arteries. The body inherently changes the diameter of the coronary arteries to change the delivery of oxygen. As myocardial oxygen demand increases, the coronary arteries dilate, if able, to deliver more oxygen-rich blood to the myocardium. As myocardial oxygen demand increases, so must the myocardial oxygen supply. Myocardial oxygen demand increases with an increase in any of the four components of cardiac output (heart rate, preload, afterload, or contractility). If myocardial oxygen supply cannot be increased during periods of increased demand, then ischemia occurs.

Clinical Application

In patients with coronary heart disease (CHD), narrowed blood vessels are often unable to dilate enough to provide the necessary oxygen supply and, therefore, angina occurs during periods of increased metabolic demand. The inability to adequately dilate is why stable angina generally occurs with activity and subsides when activity is stopped.

Myocardial oxygen supply depends on cardiac output, hemoglobin level, and oxygen saturation. Hemoglobin is the primary transporter of oxygen. Low hemoglobin levels can exacerbate ischemia in patients with CHD. If hemoglobin levels become critically low, ischemia can occur, even in patients without CHD. Oxygen saturation levels also affect the delivery of oxygen to myocardial tissue. Oxygen saturation levels can drop during periods of critical illness. Low oxygen saturation levels are commonly caused by pulmonary conditions, in which the diffusion of oxygen across the alveolar membrane and into the pulmonary capillaries is impaired.

NEUROLOGICAL CONTROL OF THE HEART AND BLOOD PRESSURE

Both branches of the *autonomic nervous system* (the sympathetic nervous system and the parasympathetic nervous system) innervate the heart. The *sympathetic nervous system* allows the body to function under stress, and the *parasympathetic nervous system* helps the body conserve and restore resources. Both branches of the autonomic nervous system contribute to regulation of the major components of cardiac output. Because blood pressure is the product of cardiac output and systemic vascular resistance, it is also impacted by the autonomic nervous system.

Sympathetic Nervous System (Adrenergic Response)

The sympathetic nervous system has two key neurotransmitters, or messengers: epinephrine and norepinephrine. These neurotransmitters, also called *catecholamines,* are released in response to excitation or stress. The excitation or stress can be caused by something as simple as waking up, to something as severe as extreme fright. Epinephrine is also called *adrenaline.* The major effects of epinephrine release are increased heart rate, increased stroke volume, increased contractility, increased systolic blood pressure with decreased diastolic blood pressure (resulting in an increase in pulse pressure), and increased blood flow to the extremities (Opie, 2004). Norepinephrine is also called *nonadrenaline.* The major effects of norepinephrine include increased heart rate, increased systolic and diastolic blood pressures, and decreased blood flow to the extremities (Opie, 2004).

Sympathetic nerve fibers supply the SA node, AV node, and myocardium of the atria and ventricles. When the neurotransmitters are activated by the sympathetic nervous system, the exact effect depends on the specific receptors stimulated (see Table 1-3). Beta1-adrenergic receptors are located in the heart and, when stimulated, cause an increase in heart rate, conductivity, and contractility. Beta2-adrenergic receptors are located in the lungs and periphery and, when stimulated, cause bronchial and peripheral vasodilation. Alpha1-adrenergic receptors are located in the vessels of vascular smooth muscle and affect the tone of the small arterioles responsible for determining systemic vascular resistance. Stimulation of alpha receptors

TABLE 1-3: ADRENERGIC RECEPTOR LOCATION AND RESPONSE		
Receptor	**Location of Receptor**	**Response to Stimulation**
Alpha1	Vascular smooth muscles	Vasoconstriction
Beta1	SA node, AV node, and myocardium	Increased heart rate Increased conduction Increased contractility
Beta2	Vascular and bronchial smooth muscles	Bronchodilation Vasodilation
Dopaminergic	Vascular smooth muscle (renal, coronary, and mesenteric)	Vasodilation

results in arterial vasoconstriction and, ultimately, an increase in blood pressure. Alpha1 and beta2 stimulation oppose each other in the periphery and oppositely affect systemic vascular resistance. The net result of sympathetic nervous system stimulation on alpha- and beta-receptors depends on the degree to which each receptor is stimulated. In general, alpha-receptors are more sensitive to norepinephrine and beta-receptors are more sensitive to epinephrine (Gold Standard/Elsevier, 2010). The renal, mesenteric, and coronary blood vessels also contain dopaminergic receptors. Stimulation of dopaminergic receptors results in vasodilation.

Clinical Application

The high sensitivity of beta-receptors to epinephrine is the reason epinephrine is used during cardiac resuscitation in patients with pulseless rhythms.

Parasympathetic Nervous System (Vagal Response)

The parasympathetic nervous system innervates the SA node, AV node, AV junction, and myocardium of the atria (Dennison, 2007). There is minimal parasympathetic innervation of the ventricles. When the parasympathetic nervous system is stimulated, the response is called a *cholinergic,* or *vagal,* response. Acetylcholine is the neurotransmitter that is released when parasympathetic nerve fibers are stimulated. It binds to parasympathetic receptors. Cholinergic receptors are classified into two types: *nicotinic* and *muscarinic* (Bridges,

2010). Parasympathetic receptors located in the heart and smooth muscles are called *muscarinic receptors.*

Clinical Application

Atropine interferes with the effects of the parasympathetic nervous system. Therefore, atropine will only have an effect on slow heart rates that are the result of parasympathetic stimulation, such as a vagal response. Atropine will not work on heart blocks that occur at a level below the AV node. This is because there are not adequate numbers of parasympathetic fibers below the level of the AV node. Atropine will have no effect in the post heart transplant patient because vagus nerve innervation is lost.

Clinical Application

Atropine is likely to be ineffective in treating slow heart rates after a cardiac transplantation. This is because the transplanted heart lacks innervation by parasympathetic nervous system (Gold Standard/Elsevier, 2010).

Stimulation of the parasympathetic nervous system decreases heart rate and slows conduction. It has very little effect on the force of ventricular contraction because of the minimal innervation of the parasympathetic nervous system in the ventricles. When the parasympathetic nervous system is stimulated, acetylcholine is released, resulting in a cholinergic, or vagal, response. Acetylcholine directly inhibits the SA node, thus decreasing heart rate. Stimulation of the parasympathetic nervous system also causes vasodilation due to nitric oxide release from the endothelium (Opie, 2004). Venous vasodilation decreases preload, and arterial vasodilation decreases afterload. Vagal tone is more pronounced during sleeping hours. When blood pressure is elevated, the feedback from the baroreceptors (discussed below) causes parasympathetic stimulation, which results in a slower heart rate, decreased force of contraction, and vasodilation. These effects result in lower cardiac output and blood pressure.

Clinical Application

The activation of the parasympathetic nervous system during an acute hypertensive crisis explains the reflex bradycardia commonly seen in this clinical situation. Conversely, low blood pressure causes reflex tachycardia.

Baroreceptors

Baroreceptors (also called *pressure receptors* or *mechanoreceptors*) are specialized nerve tissues located in the aortic arch and carotid sinus (the origin of the internal carotid artery) (McCance, 2006). They function as sensors in the nervous system and are sensitive to wall tension within the arterial vessels. An increase or decrease in wall tension and pressure sends signals to the medulla, the vasomotor center in the brain stem, via the *afferent pathways* (Opie, 2004). The medulla interprets the information it receives from the baroreceptors and transmits information back to the heart and blood vessels via motor nerves called *efferent pathways* (Opie, 2004). Impulses from this center control the diameter of blood vessels. When blood pressure is increased, baroreceptors recognize the increased wall tension and send a message to inhibit the sympathetic nervous system and stimulate the parasympathetic nervous system. Heart rate slows and veins and arteries dilate throughout the system. These changes result in decreased blood pressure. When blood pressure decreases, wall tension decreases. The opposite

effects (increased heart rate and vasoconstriction) occur with stimulation of the sympathetic nervous system.

Clinical Application

When the vagal maneuver of carotid massage is performed, baroreceptors in the carotid arteries are stimulated to slow conduction from the SA node through the AV node and, therefore, heart rate is decreased.

Chemoreceptors

The carotid arteries also contain chemoreceptors. These receptors respond to changes in blood chemistry, including arterial oxygen content, arterial carbon dioxide levels, and arterial pH (Opie, 2004). As blood pressure lowers to a critical point, the delivery of oxygen also decreases to a critical point. As oxygen delivery decreases, carbon dioxide levels increase. When stimulated by an elevated arterial carbon dioxide level, chemoreceptors send a message to the vasomotor center to stimulate cardiac activity via the sympathetic nervous system. Heart rate increases and vasoconstriction occurs, causing an increase in blood pressure with a resultant increase in oxygenation.

Role of the Renin-Angiotensin-Aldosterone System

Renin is released from the kidneys in response to low circulating volume, low cardiac output, or poor kidney perfusion. Activation of the sympathetic nervous system and increased catecholamines stimulate renin release. In response to renin, angiotensin I is converted to angiotensin II in the presence of angiotensin-converting enzyme (ACE). ACE is found in the capillary bed of the lungs and other tissues. The important end results of the renin-angiotensin-aldosterone system (RAAS) are caused by the effects of circulating angiotensin II. Angiotensin II has three primary effects:

1. arterial vasoconstriction

2. stimulation of thirst

3. stimulation of the adrenal cortex to secrete aldosterone (aldosterone increases sodium and water reabsorption).

As the blood vessels constrict and water is reabsorbed and retained, blood pressure increases and perfusion to the body, including the kidneys, improves. This increased perfusion then decreases the production of renin by the kidneys.

Clinical Application

The end results of stimulation of the RAAS include arterial vasoconstriction and aldosterone secretion. Arterial vasoconstriction increases afterload, and aldosterone secretion increases preload. These effects are clinically important in patients with heart failure who have chronic stimulation of the RAAS.

CONCLUSION

An understanding of basic anatomy and physiology of the heart is essential for all healthcare professionals. The heart is a complex, intricate pump with one purpose: the forward propulsion of blood to perfuse the body and remove waste products. Many anatomical and physiological factors can impact how well the heart fulfills its purpose. Even in people without heart disease, the cardiovascular system may not always work optimally. It is the responsibility of all healthcare professionals to recognize the impact of treatments, medications, and other interventions on this carefully designed system.

EXAM QUESTIONS

CHAPTER 1
Questions 1-9

Note: Choose the one option that BEST answers each question.

1. The inner surface of the heart chambers and valves that also covers the walls of the vessels of the vascular system is the

    a. pericardium.

    b. epicardium.

    c. myocardium.

    d. endocardium.

2. Atrioventricular valves are anatomically different from semilunar valves in that they have

    a. two cusps instead of three cusps.

    b. three cusps instead of two cusps.

    c. papillary muscles and chordae tendineae.

    d. a valve annulus.

3. During ventricular diastole, the

    a. atrioventricular valves are open as the ventricles fill from the atria.

    b. atrioventricular valves are closed as the ventricles fill from the atria.

    c. semilunar valves are open as the ventricular contents are ejected.

    d. semilunar valves are closed as the ventricular contents are ejected.

4. In most people, the coronary artery that supplies the inferior wall of the left ventricle and the AV node is the

    a. left main coronary artery.

    b. left circumflex artery (LCX).

    c. left anterior descending artery (LAD).

    d. right coronary artery (RCA).

5. In normal cardiac conduction, depolarization begins at the SA node. One fact about the SA node is that

    a. it is located in the left ventricle and is damaged to some extent during every MI.

    b. sudden cardiac death occurs if the SA node is blocked.

    c. it is the natural pacemaker and sets a heart rate of 60 to 100 beats per minute.

    d. the SA node receives its blood supply from the LAD in approximately 90% of the population.

6. The major determinants of cardiac output include

    a. heart rate, preload, afterload, and contractility.

    b. heart rate, blood pressure, arterial oxygen saturation, and contractility.

    c. blood pressure, contractility, arterial oxygen saturation, and preload.

    d. afterload, preload, contractility, and blood pressure.

7. The actual delivery of oxygen to tissues is
    determined by cardiac output as well as by the
    amount of

    a. glucose in the blood.

    b. hemoglobin and the oxygen saturation of
        the hemoglobin.

    c. white blood cells interfering with delivery
        of oxygen.

    d. cholesterol in the blood.

8. Stimulation of alpha1 receptors results in

    a. vasodilation and increased blood pressure.

    b. vasodilation and decreased blood pressure.

    c. vasoconstriction and decreased blood
        pressure.

    d. vasoconstriction and increased blood
        pressure.

9. The RAAS helps the regulation of blood
    pressure by producing

    a. angiotensin II and causing dilation when
        blood pressure is high.

    b. angiotensin II and causing vasoconstriction
        when blood pressure is low.

    c. vasopressin and causing dilation when
        blood pressure is high.

    d. vasopressin and causing vasoconstriction
        when blood pressure is low.

CHAPTER 2

CARDIOVASCULAR PHARMACOLOGY AND HEMODYNAMIC FUNCTION

CHAPTER OBJECTIVE

After completing this chapter, the learner will be able to discuss ways pharmacology is used to improve myocardial performance.

LEARNING OBJECTIVES

After completing this chapter, the learner will be able to

1. list pharmacological options available to increase or decrease the major components of cardiac output and myocardial oxygen demand.

2. define the mechanism of action, key indications, and key nursing considerations for medications that affect the cardiovascular system.

INTRODUCTION

Cardiovascular pharmacology is a complex subject, and one that grows and changes daily with the addition of each new body of research. This chapter looks at how cardiovascular pharmacology affects hemodynamic function. Pharmacology specific to the treatment of certain cardiac conditions will be discussed in later chapters.

This chapter is divided into two subsections. Section one provides an overview of pharmacological options to manipulate the major determinants of cardiac output and myocardial oxygen demand.

The section surveys the options available to manipulate preload, afterload, contractility, and heart rate. The purpose of this section is to provide a "big picture" look at the effects of pharmacological agents on these determinants of myocardial performance.

Section two takes a closer look at the major groups of cardiovascular medications and, in some cases, individual medications. This section presents more information about the mechanism of action, results, and key nursing considerations of these medications. In addition to impacting the major hemodynamic parameters, many medications have complex actions that provide additional cardiovascular benefits. These additional actions will be discussed in this section.

The primary goal of cardiovascular pharmacology is to improve cardiac performance. This goal is achieved in a variety of ways, including manipulating the major components of cardiac output and myocardial oxygen demand. In clinical practice, these four components (heart rate, preload, afterload, and contractility) are sometimes manipulated with intravenous (IV) agents in emergency situations, such as cardiogenic shock; however, they are also commonly manipulated in chronic disease management with oral medications.

OVERVIEW OF CARDIOVASCULAR PHARMACOLOGY

Pharmacology to Alter Preload

Definition

Preload is the stretch on the ventricle at the end of diastole. The volume of blood in the ventricle causes this stretch. Optimal preload is necessary for optimal cardiac performance.

Increasing Preload

When preload is too low, cardiac output decreases. Hemorrhagic shock is an example of a clinical situation in which preload drops acutely. Preload is also low when an extracellular fluid deficit exists due to dehydration or when excessive venous vasodilation occurs. When venous vasodilation occurs, blood is pulled away from the heart and preload decreases. The pharmacological options for increasing preload are outlined in Table 2-1.

Decreasing Preload

When preload is too high, a stretch beyond normal physiologic limits can cause a decrease in the force of contraction. In addition, increased preload causes an increase in myocardial oxygen demand. Patients with heart failure are at risk for having extracellular fluid overload and may need therapy acutely and on a continual basis to decrease preload. Table 2-2 outlines the pharmacological options for decreasing preload.

Pharmacology to Alter Afterload

Definition

Afterload is the resistance that the ventricle must overcome to eject its contents. Systemic vascular resistance measures left ventricular afterload.

TABLE 2-1: PHARMACOLOGICAL CONSIDERATIONS FOR INCREASING PRELOAD	
Options	**Specific Agents/Key Information**
1. Administer extracellular fluid expander	• Isotonic crystalloids, such as 0.9% sodium chloride and lactated Ringer's solution • Colloids, such as albumin, dextran, and hetastarch • Blood or blood products
2. Decrease dose or stop drugs that cause venous vasodilation	• Nitroglycerin, nesiritide, and morphine sulfate (venous vasodilation pools blood away from the heart and decreases preload)

TABLE 2-2: PHARMACOLOGICAL CONSIDERATIONS FOR DECREASING PRELOAD	
Options	**Specific Agents/Key Information**
1. Stop or decrease fluid	
2. Diuretics	• Loop diuretics such as furosemide reduce extracellular circulating volume
3. Angiotensin-converting enzyme (ACE) inhibitors	• Interfere with the physiologic response of the renin-angiotensin-aldosterone system (RAAS) (aldosterone secretion decreases, as do sodium and water retention) • ACE inhibitors end in "pril," such as captopril
4. Aldosterone antagonists	• Spironolactone and eplerenone • Directly block aldosterone and decrease sodium and water retention
5. Venous vasodilators	• Intravenous (IV) nitroglycerin, nesiritide, and morphine sulfate (venous vasodilation pools blood away from the heart and decreases preload)

Systemic vascular resistance also plays a major role in maintaining blood pressure.

Increasing Afterload

An increase in afterload is not a desired effect in patients with heart disease; therefore, medications to increase afterload are only given in emergency situations. For example, medications to increase afterload are indicated when hypotension is unresponsive to fluids or other treatment and blood pressure is dangerously low. Pharmacological options for increasing afterload are listed in Table 2-3. *Vasopressors* is the term given to medications used to increase afterload.

Decreasing Afterload

High afterload impedes cardiac output and also increases myocardial oxygen demand. Decreasing afterload is a goal of therapy for all patients with heart failure, left ventricular dysfunction, and hypertension. Table 2-4 lists a variety of pharmacological options used in the reduction of afterload.

Pharmacology to Alter Contractility

Definition

Contractility is the actual ability of the ventricle to contract independently of preload or afterload. However, in clinical practice, alterations in preload and afterload have an impact on contractility. In addition, other systemic factors, such as acid base balance and electrolyte levels, can also impact contractility. Contractility is known to be impaired in cardiac patients who have left ventricular dysfunction and low ejection fractions.

Increasing Contractility

Inotropes are medications that increase contractility. Patients who have significant left ven-

TABLE 2-3: PHARMACOLOGICAL CONSIDERATIONS FOR INCREASING AFTERLOAD	
Options	**Specific Agents/Key Information**
1. Sympathomimetics to stimulate the alpha receptors of the sympathetic nervous system	• Dopamine • Norepinephrine • Phenylephrine • Epinephrine
2. Arginine vasopressin (antidiuretic hormone [ADH])	• Vasoconstrictive and antidiuretic effect • Promotes reabsorption of water • Restores catecholamine sensitivity

TABLE 2-4: PHARMACOLOGICAL CONSIDERATIONS FOR DECREASING AFTERLOAD	
Options	**Specific Agents/Key Information**
1. Smooth muscle relaxants	• Nitroprusside • Hydralazine
2. Calcium channel blockers	• Dihydropyridine calcium channel blockers (ending in "ine"), such as amlodipine, have strong arterial vasodilator properties
3. Alpha receptor blockers	• Labetalol (combination alpha- and beta-blocker) • Prazosin and terazosin
4. ACE inhibitors	• Interrupt the RAAS and limit production of angiotensin II, a potent arterial vasoconstrictor • Medications ending in "pril"
5. Angiotensin II receptor blockers (ARBs)	• Directly block the effects angiotensin II • Medications ending in "sartan," such as valsartan
6. Phosphodiesterase (PDE) inhibitors	• Milrinone (used as an IV inotrope but also has arterial vasodilator properties)

tricular dysfunction may need the support of an IV inotrope to increase contractility if they are unable to maintain a cardiac output sufficient to meet the demands of the body. Patients in acute cardiogenic shock or patients in end-stage heart failure have known left ventricular dysfunction. Because inotropic agents substantially increase myocardial oxygen demand, it is important to correct problems with preload or afterload before administering an inotropic agent to improve cardiac output.

Table 2-5 outlines agents used to increase myocardial contractility.

Decreasing Contractility

Oral medications are commonly prescribed to decrease contractility and, therefore, decrease myocardial oxygen demand. A common indication for these medications is angina. Options for decreasing contractility are listed in Table 2-6.

Pharmacology to Alter Heart Rate

Overview

Cardiac output is heart rate multiplied by stroke volume. Increasing heart rate can be an effective strategy for increasing cardiac output. However, if heart rate becomes too rapid, the ventricles do not have time to adequately fill, and cardiac output decreases.

Increasing Heart Rate

In clinical practice, heart rate is only intentionally increased to improve cardiac output when it is below the normal rate and the patient is symptomatic. If heart rate is normal, it is not increased to a faster rate to increase cardiac output because an increase in heart rate also produces an increase in myocardial oxygen demand. Pharmacological options for increasing heart rate are listed in Table 2-7.

Decreasing Heart Rate

During a dysrhythmia in which the heart rate is high and the patient is symptomatic, medications can be used to decrease heart rate. Medications that decrease heart rate are also given to patients with

TABLE 2-5: PHARMACOLOGICAL CONSIDERATIONS FOR INCREASING CONTRACTILITY	
Options	**Specific Agents/Key Information**
1. Sympathomimetics that stimulate the beta1 (ß1) receptors of the sympathetic nervous system	• Dobutamine (most commonly used because it is a predominant ß1 stimulator) • Other sympathomimetics may have inotropic properties, even if not used primarily for an inotropic purpose
2. PDE inhibitors	• Milrinone (used as an IV inotrope but also has arterial and venous vasodilator properties)
3. Cardiac glycosides	• Digoxin (weak inotrope and is never used IV to support left ventricular dysfunction; exerts weak inotropic properties when given orally)

TABLE 2-6: PHARMACOLOGICAL CONSIDERATIONS FOR DECREASING CONTRACTILITY	
Options	**Specific Agents/Key Information**
1. Beta-blockers that block the ß1 receptors of the sympathetic nervous system	• Metoprolol • Carvedilol • "olol" medications ** Note: Medications that block ß1 receptors may also have properties that cause ß2 and alpha-receptor blockade*
2. Calcium channel blockers	• Diltiazem • Verapamil

normal heart rates when there is a desire to further decrease myocardial oxygen demand. Patients with angina often take medications that reduce their heart rates in order to decrease myocardial oxygen demand and prevent symptoms. Table 2-8 describes the pharmacological options for decreasing heart rate.

Clinical Application

There are many oral agents that manipulate the components of cardiac output and myocardial oxygen demand. Nurses should consider the hemodynamic impact of oral medications used in chronic conditions as well as the hemodynamic impact of IV medications used in acute conditions.

A CLOSER LOOK AT CARDIOVASCULAR MEDICATIONS

Sympathomimetics

Sympathomimetics are medications that stimulate the sympathetic nervous system and can be used to increase heart rate, contractility, and afterload. Different sympathomimetics have different dominant actions, depending on the receptors they stimulate:

- Beta1 (ß1) receptors are located in the heart. ß1 stimulation results in an increase in heart rate and contractility.

- Beta2 (ß2) receptors are located in the lungs and periphery. ß2 stimulation causes bronchial

TABLE 2-7: PHARMACOLOGICAL CONSIDERATIONS FOR INCREASING HEART RATE

Options	Specific Agents/Key Information
1. Parasympatholytics (lysis of the parasympathetic nervous system)	• Atropine (most commonly used pharmacological agent to increase heart rate)
2. Sympathomimetics that stimulate the ß1 receptors of the sympathetic nervous system	• Epinephrine • Dopamine

Note: The nonpharmacological intervention of pacing the heart with either an external, temporary, or permanent pacemaker is commonly the preferred method of increasing heart rate to a set and controlled rate.

TABLE 2-8: PHARMACOLOGICAL CONSIDERATIONS FOR DECREASING HEART RATE

Options	Specific Agents/Key Information
1. Beta-blockers that block the ß1 receptors of the sympathetic nervous system	• Metoprolol and carvedilol • "olol" medications • Class II antiarrhythmics*
2. Calcium channel blockers	• Diltiazem and Verapamil • Class IV antiarrhythmics*
3. Cardiac glycosides	• Digoxin
4. Unclassified antiarrhythmics	• Adenosine (slows or stops conduction through the atrioventricular [AV] node)
5. Other antiarrhythmics	• Class I and class III antiarrhythmics* • Used to establish or maintain a normal rhythm and therefore control heart rate

* Vaughan-Williams classification system

vasodilation and peripheral vasodilation in skeletal muscle.

- Alpha1 receptors are located in the arterioles. Alpha1 stimulation causes arteriole vasoconstriction and increases afterload.

- Dopaminergic receptors are located in the renal and mesenteric beds. When stimulated, these receptors dilate the renal and mesenteric arteries.

Boxes 2-1 to 2-3 list specific sympathomimetics by purpose and receptor stimulation. Tables 2-9 to 2-13 take a closer look at five of the sympathomimetics most commonly used in cardiovascular nursing.

BOX 2-1: ALPHA RECEPTOR STIMULATORS USED TO INCREASE AFTERLOAD

- Dopamine
- Phenylephrine
- Norepinephrine
- Epinephrine

BOX 2-2: BETA1 RECEPTOR STIMULATORS USED TO INCREASE CONTRACTILITY

- Dobutamine (most commonly used sympathomimetic for inotropic purposes)
- Epinephrine
- Norepinephrine (used primarily as a vasopressor but also has inotropic properties)
- Dopamine (used primarily as a vasopressor but also has inotropic properties)

BOX 2-3: BETA1 RECEPTOR STIMULATORS USED TO INCREASE HEART RATE

- Epinephrine
- Dopamine

Non-Sympathomimetic Medications Used as Vasopressors and Inotropes

Arginine vasopressin is a non-sympathomimetic medication that can be used as a vasopressor. Because it is an antidiuretic hormone, there is an obvious antidiuretic effect. Its other actions are complex and not fully understood. Although it is a vasoconstrictor, it does allow for regional vasodilation to vital organs. Arginine vasopressin can be used in refractory hypotension not responsive to sympathomimetics. It can help to restore the patient's sensitivity to catecholamines. Exogenous arginine vasopressin is not titrated like other vasopressors but, rather, is administered at a consistent low dose during the course of treatment.

Milrinone, a phosphodiesterase inhibitor, is a non-sympathomimetic medication that can be used as an inotrope. It creates a positive inotropic effect by increasing availability of calcium by inhibiting the degradation of cyclic adenosine monophospate (AMP) (Gold Standard/Elsevier, 2010). In addition, this inotropic medication has simultaneous venous and arterial vasodilator effects as a result of its action on vascular as well as cardiac muscle. Thus, milrinone has the added benefit of decreasing preload and afterload. Milrinone can be used in patients with acute heart failure who need inotropic support. Additionally, milrinone has a positive effect on diastolic function (Gold Standard/Elsevier, 2010). Patients receiving milrinone must be closely monitored because potential side effects include ventricular dysrhythmias and exacerbation of accelerated ventricular rate in patients with atrial dysrhythmias (Gold Standard/Elsevier, 2010).

Medications That Affect The Renin-Angiotensin-Aldosterone System

Three groups of medications directly affect the remin-angiotensin-aldosterone system (RAAS): angiotensin-converting enzyme (ACE) inhibitors, angiotensin II receptor blockers (ARBs), and aldosterone antagonists.

ACE Inhibitors

ACE inhibitors prevent the conversion of angiotensin I to angiotensin II by inhibiting the angiotensin-converting enzyme. Angiotensin II is a potent arterial vasoconstrictor; therefore, ACE inhibitors promote arterial vasodilation by preventing the formation of angiotensin II. This arterial vasodilation reduces afterload.

TABLE 2-9: EPINEPHRINE

What receptors are stimulated?	• ß1 and ß2 (at low doses) • Alpha receptors (at high doses)
What are the resultant actions?	• Increased contractility (positive inotrope) • Increased automaticity • Bronchodilation • Selective vasoconstriction
When and why is it used?	• Advanced cardiac life support; first-line drug for cardiac standstill • Anaphylactic shock • Hypotension or profound bradycardia
What are special nursing considerations?	• Instant onset • Peak 20 minutes • 1 mg IV every 3 to 5 minutes during cardiac standstill

(Gold Standard/Elsevier, 2010; Opie & Gersh, 2009)

TABLE 2-10: DOBUTAMINE

What receptors are stimulated?	• Primarily ß1 • Some alpha receptor stimulation • Modest ß2 (more ß2 than alpha)
What are the resultant actions?	• Increased contractility (positive inotrope) • Increased AV node conduction • Modest vasoconstriction
When and why is it used?	• Used as an inotrope with modest afterload reduction
What are special nursing considerations?	• Onset 1 to 2 minutes • Peak 10 minutes • Blood pressure is variable: ß2 causes vasodilation • Increased cardiac output increases blood pressure

(Gold Standard/Elsevier, 2010; Opie & Gersh, 2009)

TABLE 2-11: DOPAMINE

What receptors are stimulated?	• Dopaminergic and some ß1 at low doses • ß1 at moderate doses • Pure alpha stimulation at high doses (> 10 mcg/kg/min)
What are the resultant actions?	• Increased contractility at small and moderate doses • Increased conduction • Vasoconstriction at high doses • Does not treat or prevent renal failure at low doses
When and why is it used?	• Refractory hypotension • Shock
What are special nursing considerations?	• IV onset 1 to 2 minutes • Peak 10 minutes • Maximal effects at 20 mcg/kg/min • Large IV line or central line • Phentolamine (alpha blocker) for infiltrate

(Gold Standard/Elsevier, 2010; Opie & Gersh, 2009)

TABLE 2-12: NOREPINEPHRINE

What receptors are stimulated?	• Primarily alpha stimulation • Some ß1
What are the resultant actions?	• Potent vasoconstriction (vasopressor) • Some increased contractility (positive inotrope)
When and why is it used?	• Refractory hypotension • Shock • Used as vasopressor but has inotropic properties
What are special nursing considerations?	• Rapid IV onset • Duration 1 to 2 minutes (blood pressure checks every 2 minutes while titrating) • Large IV line or central line • Phentolamine (alpha blocker) for infiltration of IV site

(Gold Standard/Elsevier, 2010; Opie & Gersh, 2009)

TABLE 2-13: PHENYLEPHRINE (SYNTHETIC COMPOUND)

What receptors are stimulated?	• Direct effect is dominant alpha stimulation • No substantial ß1 effect at therapeutic doses • Indirect effect: causes release of norepinephrine
What are the resultant actions?	• Potent vasoconstriction (vasopressor)
When and why is it used?	• Refractory hypotension
What are special nursing considerations?	• Rapid IV onset • Duration of action 10-15 minutes • Large IV line or central line • Phentolamine (alpha blocker) for infiltration of IV site

(Gold Standard/Elsevier, 2010)

The formation of angiotensin II also stimulates the release of aldosterone from the adrenals. Aldosterone informs the body to retain sodium and, therefore, water while excreting potassium. Angiotensin II also stimulates the release of arginine vasopressin (ADH), which causes additional vasoconstriction and water reabsorption. When angiotensin II formation is inhibited, the release of aldosterone and vasopressin decrease and preload and afterload further decrease.

Because of the positive effects of decreasing afterload and preload, ACE inhibitors decrease the workload of the left ventricle. In addition to interfering with the formation of angiotensin II, ACE inhibitors block the breakdown of bradykinin, which directly supports vasodilation. Therefore, this action has an additional positive effect in patients with heart failure. ACE inhibitors are cen-

tral to the management of heart failure. They are also used after myocardial infarction (MI) to prevent heart failure development. ACE inhibitors can decrease mortality in patients with an ejection fraction of less than 40% after an MI by decreasing left ventricular remodeling (Antman et al., 2004). The process of left ventricular remodeling will be discussed further in Chapter 7. Additionally, ACE inhibitors are used to treat nephropathy as well as hypertension in patients with diabetes and other high-risk features (Opie & Gersh, 2009).

ACE inhibitors also help to prevent many of the other negative effects of angiotensin II. Additional effects of ACE inhibitors include:

1. reduction in left ventricular hypertrophy

2. improvement in endothelial function via increased release of nitric oxide

3. reduction in oxidative stress

4. decrease in inflammatory response

5. promotion of antithrombotic environment via a decrease in fibrinogen

6. decrease in intra glomerular pressure, glomerular fibrosis, and glomerular protein leak.

(Opie & Gersh, 2009)

The positive effects of ACE inhibitors commonly take weeks to months to be seen.

The four potential major side effects of ACE inhibitors can best be understood by relating the effect to the physiological action of ACE inhibitors.

1. *Hypotension:* Hypotension is a potential adverse effect caused by the vasodilatory effects of blocking angiotensin II formation.

2. *Hyperkalemia:* Hyperkalemia is a potential adverse effect caused by the decreased release of aldosterone from the adrenals. Aldosterone tells the body to hold on to sodium and to excrete potassium. Because of the risk of hyperkalemia, electrolyte levels and renal function must be monitored carefully during initiation and maintenance of ACE inhibitors.

3. *Angioedema/Chronic Cough:* The development of acute angioedema can be a life-threatening complication and is related to the increased circulating levels of bradykinin. The previous development of angioedema is an absolute contraindication for the administration of an ACE inhibitor. Eighty-five to 90% of patients can tolerate long-term ACE inhibitor therapy (Hunt et al., 2009). However, a small percentage of patients develop a dry persistent cough related to increased bradykinin, requiring them to stop taking ACE inhibitors.

4. *Renal Dysfunction:* Although ACE inhibitors have an overall renoprotective effect, they can cause adverse renal function in patients with chronic and severe low cardiac output states, those with severe sodium or volume depletion,

and those with preexisiting renal disease. These patients have been relying on efferent arteriole vasoconstriction to help support adequate glomerular filtration. The initiation of ACE inhibitors results in efferent arteriole vasodilation. Bilateral renal artery stenosis places the patient at high risk for acute renal dysfunction because afferent arteriole vasodilation is limited and glomerular filtration is dependent on efferent vasoconstriction. A slight increase in creatinine that stabilizes after initiation of an ACE inhibitor is not a contraindication for continued administration (Opie & Gersh, 2009).

General contraindications for ACE inhibitor administration include:

• systolic blood pressure less than 80 mm Hg

• elevated serum potassium

• creatinine greater than 3 mg/dl

• previous angioedema

• bilateral renal artery stenosis

• pregnancy.

(Hunt et al., 2009)

ACE inhibitors end with "pril." Box-2-4 lists available ACE inhibitors.

BOX 2-4: ACE INHIBITORS

• Benazepril	• Lisinopril
• Captopril	• Quinapril
• Enalapril	• Ramipril
• Fosinopril	

Angiotensin II Receptor Blockers

ARBs directly block angiotensin II after it is formed and therefore have similar hemodynamic effects as ACE inhibitors. This section will discuss the differences with ARBs. Current guidelines indicate the use of ARBs when ACE inhibitors are unable to be tolerated due to intractable cough or angioedema. ARBs do not produce a cough because they do not promote increased bradykinin levels. Although angioedema is less common in patients taking ARBs, there are some patients who will develop angioedema with both ACE inhibitors and ARBs. Therefore, great caution must be used in administering an ARB to a patient with a history of angioedema (Hunt, et al., 2009; Opie & Gersh, 2009). Except for the cough, ARBs have side effects and precautions similar to ACE inhibitors.

The lack of increased bradykinin levels may decrease the effectiveness of ARBs in the management of heart failure because bradykinin is responsible for additional vasodilator effects beneficial in the treatment of heart failure. Research comparing the benefits of ACE inhibitors and ARBs is ongoing. However, current heart failure guidelines still recommend ACE inhibitors as the preferred medication for patients with current or prior symptoms and with reduced left ventricular dysfunction (Hunt, et al., 2009). In select patients, ARBs may be used in place of ACE inhibitors as first-line agents.

There are other pathways to angiotensin II formation in addition to the ACE pathway. For this reason, there is also ongoing research regarding the possible added benefits of concomitant ARB and ACE inhibitor use (Heart Failure Society of America, 2004). Current guidelines do not indicate the addition of an ARB to patients already taking an ACE inhibitor and aldosterone antagonist because of the high risk of hyperkalemia. ARBs end with "sartan." Candesartan was the first ARB approved by the U.S. Food and Drug Administration (FDA) for the use in the treatment of heart failure (Hunt et al., 2009). Box 2-5 lists available ARBs.

BOX 2-5: ANGIOTENSIN II RECEPTOR BLOCKERS

• Candesartan	• Eprosartan
• Irbesartan	• Losartan
• Telmisartan	• Valsartan

Aldosterone Antagonists

Aldosterone is a mineralocorticoid hormone released from the adrenal cortex as part of the end result of the action of the RAAS. Aldosterone informs the body to hold onto sodium, and therefore water, and to excrete potassium. For this reason, aldosterone antagonists are sometimes referred to as potassium-sparing diuretics. ACE inhibitors indirectly affect the release of aldosterone, whereas aldosterone antagonists directly block aldosterone. The end result is a decrease in sodium and water retention and, therefore, a decrease in preload.

Aldosterone is thought to play an even larger role in cardiovascular function. Some additional potential effects of aldosterone blockade include:

• minimized release of catecholamines

• improved endothelial function

• antithrombotic effects

• decreased vascular inflammation and myocardial fibrosis.

(Hunt et al., 2009; Opie & Gersh, 2009)

Two aldosterone antagonists are available: spironolactone and eplerenone. Spironolactone is a nonselective agent that blocks aldosterone and also exhibits an antiandrogenic effect in both men and women. This antiandrogenic effect can cause gynecomastia in men (Gold Standard/Elsevier, 2010). Low-dose spironolactone has been shown to decrease mortality in patients with severe heart failure who are already taking an ACE inhibitor (Soine, 2010).

Eplerenone is a selective aldosterone antagonist that does not have the associated side effect of gynecomastia in men. Eplerenone is indicated in patients with left ventricular dysfunction after MI and those with diabetes to prevent progression of heart failure, recurrent MI, and sudden cardiac death (Antman et al., 2004; Gold Standard/Elsevier, 2010). Both spironolactone and eplerenone can cause hyperkalemia, especially when given with an ACE inhibitor.

Beta-Blockers

Beta-blockers can block the ß1 or ß2 receptors of the sympathetic nervous system. When beta-blockers block ß1 receptors, a decrease in heart rate and contractility results. When they block ß2 receptors, bronchial and peripheral vasoconstriction occur. Therefore, caution should be used when administering beta-blockers to patients with restrictive airway disease or peripheral vascular disease.

Clinical Application

Many patients with cardiac disease have coexisting peripheral vascular disease. If a nonselective blocker is prescribed, the patient may experience an increase in intermittent claudication associated with the peripheral vascular disease. This effect is related to the blockage of ß2.

Beta-blockers are widely prescribed in cardiovascular medicine and are indicated for a number of cardiovascular disorders. Box 2-6 lists cardiovascular indications for the use of beta-blockers. Beta-blockers are included in the practice guidelines for the management of heart failure, stable angina, and acute coronary syndromes. Their use in these disorders will be discussed in more detail in later chapters.

BOX 2-6: CARDIOVASCULAR INDICATIONS FOR BETA-BLOCKERS

Acute MI

Angina

Aortic dissection

Digoxin-induced ventricular dysrhythmias

Heart failure

Hypertension

Hypertrophic cardiomyopathy (HCM)

Mitral valve prolapse

Post-myocardial infarction

Prolonged QT syndrome

Supraventricular dysrhythmias

Ventricular dysrhythmias

Beta-blockers decrease myocardial oxygen demand by decreasing contractility and heart rate. They also help increase coronary perfusion by increasing diastolic filling time. When used to treat hypertension, beta-blockers prevent reflex tachycardia associated with other vasodilators. Although beta-blockers do not cause direct arterial vasodilation, they decrease contractility and heart rate, which decreases cardiac output. A decrease in cardiac output lowers blood pressure. Some beta-blockers are cardioselective, meaning they predominantly block ß1; others are noncardioselective blocking both ß1 and ß2.

Cardioselective beta-blockers

- Acebutolol
- Atenolol
- Betaxolol
- Bisoprolol (highy ß1 selective)
- Metoprolol
- Esmolol (ultra short acting)

Noncardioselective beta-blockers

- Carvedilol (also has alpha 1 blockade)
- Labetalol (also has alpha blockade)
- Nadolol
- Penbutolol
- Propranolol
- Timolol
- Sotalol (also has class III antiarrhythmic properties)

Contraindications to beta-blocker initiation include severe bradycardia, high-degree AV block, sick sinus syndrome, and acute decompensated heart failure (Gibbons et al., 2002). Caution must be exercised when using beta-blockers in patients with coexisting depression, asthma, or peripheral vascular disease. Caution is particularly important when using noncardioselective beta-blockers in patients with asthma or peripheral vascular disease. Diabetic patients should exercise caution when taking beta-blockers because beta-blockers can mask the symptoms of hypoglycemia. Side effects of beta-blockers include lethargy, fatigue, insomnia, nightmares, impotence, worsening asthma, and worsening claudication (Gibbons et al., 2002).

Beta-blockers are sometimes combined with alpha-blockers. Alpha-blockers produce vasodilation and are indicated in the treatment of hypertension.

Calcium Channel Blockers

Calcium channel blockers decrease the flux of calcium across cell membranes. Calcium channel blockers can be used to decrease heart rate, contractility, and afterload. The mechanisms of action of these three potential effects are:

- *Decreased contractility:* blocks inward flow of calcium in phase two of the cardiac action potential and decreases the force of contractions.

- *Decreased heart rate:* depresses automaticity and velocity and decreases heart rate.

- *Decreased afterload:* relaxes vascular smooth muscle.

All calcium channel blockers have some common effects. For example, they all have some degree of negative inotropic effect. They also reduce coronary and systemic vascular resistance. For these reasons, calcium channel blockers are effective in decreasing myocardial oxygen demand. However, not all calcium channel blockers are created equal and they do not all have the same effects or degree of effect. There are three distinct groups of calcium blockers. Table 2-14 defines the differences between these groups.

Short- and intermediate-acting dihydropyridine calcium channel blockers are not used in the treatment of angina or hypertension because of their questionable safety profile. Nifedipine, an older generation dihydropyridine calcium channel blocker, is contraindicated in unstable angina because of its predominant peripheral arterial vasodilatory effects (Mendoza & Loghin, 2001). Sublingual use of nifedipine has not been acceptable since 1995, when it was shown to have adverse effects related to its unpredictable and sometimes dangerous hemodynamic response (Gibbons et al., 2002).

Decompensated heart failure is a contraindication to the administration of calcium channel blockers. Calcium channel blockers are not indicated in the treatment of heart failure because they have a negative inotropic effect and do not have the added benefit of interrupting neurohormonal responses. Newer generation, longer-acting dihydropyridine calcium channel blockers, such as amlodipine, have more coronary vasodilatory properties and are better tolerated in patients with decreased left ventricular dysfunction. Amlodipine, a coronary vasoselective dihydropyridine calcium channel blocker, is the best-tolerated calcium channel blocker in patients with ischemic cardiomyopathy (Gibbons et al., 2002).

In patients with heart blocks or bradydysrhythmias, the calcium channel blockers that affect heart rate (verapamil and diltiazem) should not be used.

TABLE 2-14: CALCIUM CHANNEL BLOCKERS

	Verapamil	Dihydropyridine calcium channel blockers	Diltiazem
Heart rate	↓	↑ (reflex tachycardia)	↓
AV nodal conduction	↓	Neutral	↓
Contractility	↓	↓	↓
Arterial vasodilation	↑	↑	↑

(Gold Standard/Elsevier, 2010)

Adverse effects of calcium channel blockers include peripheral edema, worsening heart failure, hypotension and constipation (Gold Standard/Elsevier, 2010). In addition, verapamil and diltiazem can cause bradycardia and heart block.

Primary indications for calcium channel blockers include:

- atrial fibrillation or flutter, paroxysmal supraventricular tachycardia: diltiazem or verapamil

- angina (including vasospastic angina): diltiazem or verapamil with nitrates dihydropyridine ("ine") calcium channel blockers with beta-blockers (beta-blocker used to prevent reflex tachycardia)

- hypertension: dihydropyridine ("ine") calcium channel blockers.

Additional indications include:

- hypertrophic cardiomyopathy (HCM): diltiazem and verapamil (avoid dihydropyridine calcium channel blockers)

- treatment and prevention of coronary spasm: dihydropyridine calcium channel blockers.

Other Arterial and Venous Vasodilators

Nitroglycerin and Nitrates

When administered intravenously in low doses, nitroglycerin is a primary venous vasodilator. The dose of a sublingual nitroglycerin tablet is high enough to produce both venous and arterial vasodilation. Low-dose IV nitroglycerin is effective in alleviating chest pain, even though it acts primarily as a venous vasodilator. It works by reducing preload and, therefore, myocardial oxygen demand. This reduction in myocardial oxygen demand can be sufficient to relieve chest pain associated with angina. Higher doses of nitroglycerin produce direct dilation of the large coronary arteries and arterioles. Nitroglycerin also exhibits antithrombotic and antiplatelet effects.

Patients taking oral or topical nitrates can develop a tolerance. To prevent this tolerance, allow a nitrate-free period of 8 to 10 hours per day, preferably during the night (Calagan, Schachter, Kruger, Cameron, & Loghin, 2001). Some patients develop headaches as a result of the vasodilation associated with nitroglycerin.

Clinical Application

Headaches should be treated immediately, because pain increases sympathetic nervous system stimulation and myocardial oxygen demand, potentially worsening ischemia.

Because nitrates decrease preload, they are contraindicated in patients with HCM, who are dependent on adequate preload to maintain their cardiac output. Nitrates and other vasodilators should also be used with extreme caution in patients with aortic stenosis because these patients have a limited ability to increase cardiac output in response to hypotension. Nitrates are also contraindicated in the acute period following a right ventricular MI or an inferior MI because these patients are predisposed to significant drops in blood pressure with nitrates. Nitrates can cause some reflex tachycardia; administration with a beta-blocker can prevent this side effect.

Nitrates also should not be prescribed to patients taking sildenafil (Viagra), or other similar medications, because of the risk of profound hypotension. Rarely, the administration of sublingual nitroglycerin can produce bradycardia and hypotension due to activation of the Bezold-Jarisch reflex (Gibbons et al., 2002). When triggered, this reflex causes a vasovagal response (Bridges, 2010).

Clinical Application

Women, in addition to men, should be assessed for taking sildenafil or sildenfil-like drugs. Both women and men may take sildenafil (trade name Revatio) for the treatment of pulmonary hypertension.

Nitroprusside

Nitroprusside has mixed venous and arterial vasodilative properties; however, it is predominantly an arterial vasodilator. Nitroprusside is indicated in hypertensive crisis and other cardiac emergencies, such as acute mitral regurgitation, acute decompensated heart failure, and acute aortic dissection when immediate afterload reduction is needed. Hypotension is the number one side effect and nursing consideration. Continuous blood pressure monitoring via an arterial line is preferred. Although thiocyanate toxicity can occur, it is not an initial nursing consideration because patients are not at risk unless they have been receiving nitroprusside for several days at high doses (Dennison, 2007).

Nesiritide

Nesiritide is a synthetic brain natriuretic peptide (BNP). BNP is naturally released from the ventricles in heart failure to promote vasodilation and counteract the effects of the RAAS. Nesiritide is a newer vasodilator that has both venous and arterial vasodilative effects. It is used in the management of acute decompensated heart failure to decrease preload and afterload. Nesiritide is administered as a short-term infusion (24 to 48 hours) for patients in heart failure who are demonstrating signs of extracellular fluid overload. Because nesiritide also lowers blood pressure, the patient must have a blood pressure greater than 90 mm Hg systolic. (Gold Standard/Elsevier, 2010). The use of scheduled intermittent nesiritide therapy in the treatment of heart failure is not indicated (Hunt et al., 2009).

Clinical Application

Venous vasodilators reduce preload and potentially cause hypotension. When a patient is hypotensive, preload should be corrected first. This includes administering fluids as well as discontinuing or reducing the dose of venous vasodilators. Although not used predominantly as a venous vasodilator, it is important for nurses to know that morphine sulfate has venous vasodilating properties that result in hypotension as a potential side effect.

Digoxin

Digoxin is a cardiac glycoside that has very complex mechanisms of action. It has weak inotropic properties and also some parasympathetic properties. These parasympathetic properties decrease sympathetic outflow and decrease renin production, which are particularly beneficial when used in the treatment of heart failure.

Digoxin has a narrow therapeutic range, and toxicity can occur at therapeutic levels. Signs and symptoms of toxicity include

- nausea and vomiting

- headache

- confusion

- vision disturbances, such as the appearance of halos or a change in color perception.

To avoid toxicity, low doses of digoxin (0.125 mg per day) are now used in most patients (Hunt et al., 2009). Interactions occur between digoxin and a variety of medications, including other cardiovascular agents. Some cardiovascular agents reduce the clearance of digoxin and predispose the patient to toxicity. These agents include: amiodarone, propafenone, quinidine, felodipine, diltiazem, and verapamil. Other cardiovascular agents, such as nondihydropyridine calcium channel blockers, beta-blockers, and class III antiarrhythmic agents, can potentiate the action of digoxin (Gold Standard/Elsevier, 2010).

Prior to initiation of digoxin, the patient's electrolyte status should be assessed. Low potassium, low magnesium, and high calcium increase the effect of digoxin. Hypokalemia as well as hyperkalemia increase the risk of digoxin toxicity (Gold Standard/Elsevier, 2010). Because digoxin interacts with many other medications, careful assessment of the patient's medication profile is an important nursing intervention.

Dialysis is not effective in treating digoxin toxicity because of the high tissue-binding property of digoxin. Untreated digoxin-toxicity-induced dysrhythmias can be fatal (Dennison, 2007). Dysrhythmias seen with toxicity usually involve increased automaticity with impaired conduction; for example, paroxysmal atrial tachycardia with heart block.

Clinical Application

Digoxin should be withheld in a patient with any clinical signs of digoxin toxicity, even in the presence of a therapeutic digoxin level, until the patient's clinical condition can be thoroughly discussed with the physician.

Diuretics

Diuretic therapy is used to reduce preload in both acute and chronic conditions.

Loop Diuretics

Loop diuretics work in the ascending loop of Henle and result in a loss of water, hyodrogen ions, and electrolytes (potassium, sodium, and chloride). Loop diruretics result in a greater loss of water and less of a loss of potassium and sodium compared to thiazide diuretics. In addition to promoting loss of total body fluid, loop diuretics also promote venous vasodilation, which further helps in the reduction of preload.

Loop diuretics have a rapid onset and short duration of action. They are called *high-ceiling diuretics* because additional benefit can be achieved with higher doses. Although they are not effective in treating acute renal failure, loop diuretics may continue to be effective in the presence of renal dysfunction and may be used to remove excess fluid in a fluid overloaded state. A list of loop diuretics is provided in Box 2-7.

BOX 2-7: LOOP DIURETICS

Bumetanide (Bumex)

Furosemide (Lasix)

Torsemide (Demadex)

Thiazide Diuretics

Thiazide diuretics inhibit reabsorption of sodium and chloride in the distal tubule. They have a delayed onset but longer duration of action than loop diuretics. They are also considered less potent than loop diuretics and they have decreased effectiveness in the presence of renal dysfunction. Thiazide diuretics are considered low-ceiling diuretics because increased effectiveness is not seen with higher doses. A list of thiazide diuretics is found in Box 2-8.

BOX 2-8: THIAZIDE DIURETICS

Bendrofluazide

Benthiazide

Chlorothiazide

Chlorthalidone

Cyclothiazide

Hydrochlorothiazide (HCTZ)

Hydroflumethazide

Indapamide

Metolazone

Polythiazide

Trichlormethiazide

General side effects of thiazide diuretic therapy include:

Blood Chemistry changes:

- Hypokalemia potassium

- Hyperglycemia (blood sugar)

- Hyperuricemia (uric acid)
  - cholesterol
  - triglycerides
  - high-density lipoprotein cholesterol

- Hypercalcemia (calcium; specific to thiazide diuretics)

Other side effects:

- Dizziness

- Decreased glomerular filtration in kidneys related to hypovolemia

- Impaired glucose tolerance

- Gout

- Ventricular dysrhythmias (potassium)

- Ototoxicity (deafness, reversible; specific to loop diuretics).

EMERGING MEDICATIONS

Cardiovascular pharmacology is rapidly changing. New pharmacological agents are under investigation in nearly all classes of medications and for all cardiovascular conditions. A few examples of emerging medications include:

1. Direct renin inhibitors such as Aliskiren, which is currently used in the treatment of hypertension. Aliskiren was the first renin inhibitor approved for use by the FDA and represents a new type of medication used to impact the RAAS (Gold Standard/Elsevier, 2010).

2. Vasopressin 2 Antagonists such as Tolvaptan, an oral medication that works in the renal collecting ducts and can be added to standard IV therapy in the treatment of acute decompensated heart failure. This medication is specifically indicated in heart failure when there is a volume overload state with a low serum sodium level. This medication can only be used in the hospital setting where serum sodium levels can be closely monitored (Gold Standard/Elsevier, 2010).

CONCLUSION

A solid understanding of the hemodynamic impact of pharmacology can be the foundation upon which to apply knowledge to newer agents.

Cardiovascular drugs are commonly used to maximize hemodynamic performance in patients with poor left ventricular function. In addition, many of the same pharmacological agents are used in secondary prevention efforts to interrupt physiological responses leading to disease progression. Nurses play a tremendous role in assisting patients with understanding the benefits of their prescribed pharmacological treatment plans. Patients who truly understand the physiologic benefits of therapy can be empowered to participate in decision-making and the management of their own care.

EXAM QUESTIONS

CHAPTER 2
Questions 10-20

Note: Choose the one option that BEST answers each question.

10. The condition that warrants using medications to decrease preload is

    a. volume depletion from excessive diuretic use.

    b. volume excess from heart failure.

    c. low blood pressure.

    d. any heart condition.

11. Pharmacological options that can be used to increase preload include

    a. IV fluids and cessation of venous vasodilators.

    b. diuretics and venous vasodilators.

    c. any medication that lowers blood pressure.

    d. any medication that increases afterload.

12. Systemic afterload reduction is a primary goal in

    a. septic shock and heart failure.

    b. pneumonia and chronic obstructive pulmonary disease.

    c. septic shock and pneumonia.

    d. heart failure and hypertension.

13. An example of a calcium channel blocker used to dilate arteries and thus decrease afterload is

    a. amlodipine.

    b. hydralazine.

    c. prazosin.

    d. captopril.

14. A nursing consideration when administering medications to increase contractility or heart rate is that the medications

    a. can also cause severe bleeding.

    b. also increase myocardial oxygen demand.

    c. have a very high rate of allergic reactions.

    d. cannot be given to anyone over age 60.

15. Medications that mimic the sympathetic nervous system can cause

    a. increased platelet count, increased red blood cell count, and increased fibrinogen level.

    b. decreased heart rate, decreased afterload, and decreased contractility.

    c. decreased platelet count, decreased red blood cell count, and decreased fibrinogen level.

    d. increased heart rate, increased afterload, and increased contractility.

16. The action of ACE inhibitors is best described as

    a. preventing the initial release of renin.

    b. directly blocking the effects of angiotensin II.

    c. preventing the conversion of angiotensin I to angiotensin II.

    d. directly blocking the effects of aldosterone.

17. A key nursing assessment for a patient taking an ACE inhibitor and an aldosterone antagonist is monitoring the lab values for

    a. potassium.

    b. glucose.

    c. white blood cell count.

    d. phosphorus.

18. Beta-blockers should be used cautiously in patients with reactive airway disease and peripheral vascular disease because blocking of

    a. ß1 receptors can cause bronchial and peripheral vasodilation.

    b. ß2 receptors can cause bronchial and peripheral vasodilation.

    c. ß1 receptors can cause bronchial and peripheral vasoconstriction.

    d. ß2 receptors can cause bronchial and peripheral vasoconstriction.

19. The calcium channel blockers that decrease heart rate are

    a. verapamil and carvedilol.

    b. amlodipine and diltiazem.

    c. diltiazem and verapamil.

    d. amlodipine and captopril.

20. When administering a thiazide diuretic, which of the following blood chemistry abnormalities are a possible direct effect?

    a. Hyperglycemia, hypokalemia, and hypercalcemia

    b. Hyperglycemia, hypokalemia, and hypocalcemia

    c. Hypoglycemia, hypokalemia, and hypercalcemia

    d. Hypoglycemia, hypokalemia, and hypocalcemia

CHAPTER 3

PHARMACOLOGY TO PRESERVE AND INCREASE MYOCARDIAL OXYGEN SUPPLY

CHAPTER OBJECTIVE

After completing this chapter, the learner will be able to describe the key pharmacological agents used to preserve and increase myocardial oxygen supply.

LEARNING OBJECTIVES

After completing this chapter, the learner will be able to

1. describe the benefits of low-density lipoprotein cholesterol reduction.

2. define the lipid-lowering agents most effective in reducing low-density lipoprotein cholesterol.

3. list lipid-lowering agents used to reduce triglycerides and increase high-density lipoprotein cholesterol.

4. discuss the key side effects of and patient education criteria for lipid-lowering therapy.

5. describe the purpose, indications, and potential complications of thrombolytic and fibrinolytic therapy.

6. explain the use of unfractionated heparin and low-molecular-weight heparin.

7. define the three main groups of antiplatelet agents used in the treatment of cardiovascular disease.

INTRODUCTION

Medications used to protect myocardial oxygen supply can be grouped into two categories: those aimed at the long-term prevention of atherosclerotic coronary artery disease and those aimed at the prevention or disruption of clot formation. These medications play a major role in the prevention and treatment of cardiovascular disease.

LIPID-LOWERING MEDICATIONS

Low-Density Lipoprotein Cholesterol

A 1% reduction in total cholesterol reduces the incidence of cardiac events by 2% (Fraker & Fihn, 2007). In addition, a 1% increase in high-density lipoprotein cholesterol (HDL-C) reduces the risk by 2% to 4% (Grundy et al., 2002). Therefore, reduction of low-density lipoprotein cholesterol (LDL-C) is a primary goal in the management of coronary heart disease. In the presence of established coronary artery disease, lipid-lowering therapy should be prescribed with even mild elevations of LDL-C. The effects of various groups of medications on LDL-C levels are outlined in Table 3-1.

Of the available lipid-lowering drugs, the HMG-CoA reductase inhibitors (statins) are the most potent for reducing LDL-C. Other agents that substantially lower LDL-C are bile acid resins and

TABLE 3-1: EFFECTS OF LIPID-LOWERING THERAPY ON LDL-C LEVELS

Class of Medications	% Reduction
HMG-CoA reductase inhibitors (statins)	18% to 60%
Bile acid sequestrants	15% to 30%
Nicotinic acid	15% to 30%
Fibrates	5% to 20%
Intestinal absorption inhibitors	18%
(Berra & Fair, 2010; Grundy et al., 2002)	

nicotinic acid. All three of these drug classes have a dose-dependent effect on LDL-C.

The effect of fibrates on LDL-C is different. Fibrates primarily decrease triglycerides and therefore increase HDL-C. Among the fibrates, fenofibrate has a greater effect on LDL-C reduction than clofibrate or gemfibrozil. However, fibrates tend to normalize LDL-C particle composition, changing the small, dense, atherogenic LDL particles to a larger, less dense, less atherogenic type. This increase in LDL particle size may contribute to an increase in LDL-C level, while still reducing the risk of coronary atherosclerosis (Gold Standard/Elsevier, 2010; Opie & Gersh, 2009).

Triglycerides and High-Density Lipoprotein Cholesterol

Table 3-2 details the effects of lipid lowering medications on triglyceride and HDL-C levels.

The most effective agents for improving triglyceride and HDL-C levels are nicotinic acid (niacin) and the fibrates. Nicotinic acid has a dose-dependent effect; however, side effects may prevent patients from taking a sufficient dose. Fibrates have a fixed-dose effect and do not have the irritating side effects associated with nicotinic acid. Statins, especially simvastatin and atorvastatin, also lower triglycerides and increase HDL-C. Bile acid resins increase HDL-C but may also increase triglycerides. Bile acid sequestrants may actually cause a transient compensatory increase in triglyceride levels (Opie & Gersh, 2009).

Clinical Application

Educating patients on the expected quantifiable improvements in lipid levels associated with drug therapy allows patients to actively participate in decision-making about when to add drug therapy to healthy dietary changes.

Bile Acid Sequestrants (Resins)

Bile acid sequestrants, also called *resins*, include:

- cholestyramine (Questran)
- colestipol (Colestid)
- colesevelam (WelChol).

TABLE 3-2: EFFECTS OF LIPID-LOWERING THERAPY ON TRIGLYCERIDE AND HDL-C LEVELS

Class of Medications	HDL-C	Triglycerides
Nicotinic acid	↑ 15% to 35%	↓ 20% to 50%
Fibrates	↑ 10% to 20%	↓ 20% to 50%
HMG-CoA reductase inhibitors (statins)	↑ 5% to 15%	↓ 7% to 37%
Bile acid sequestrants	↑ 3% to 5%	does not decrease, may even increase
Intestinal absorption inhibitors	↑ 1%	↓ 8%
(Berra & Fair, 2010; Grundy et al., 2002)		

These drugs combine with bile acids in the intestine and form an insoluble complex that is excreted in feces. The low level of bile acids provides feedback to the hepatic circulation to stimulate the production of more bile acids. Because cholesterol is used in the production of bile acids, the liver is also stimulated to produce more cholesterol. Cholesterol, specifically the oxidation of cholesterol from LDL-C, is a major precursor for the formation of bile acids. The body breaks down cholesterol to make bile acids and then compensates by increasing LDL-C receptors to remove LDL-C from circulation (Berra & Fair, 2010). Although the liver is stimulated to produce more cholesterol, this new cholesterol is used to produce more bile acids. A net decrease in total cholesterol and LDL-C results. Bile acid sequestrants have minimal effects on HDL-C and can actually increase triglyceride levels.

Clinical Application

Bile acid sequestrants should be taken with the largest meal of the day because intestinal bile acids are greatest at this time.

The cholesterol-lowering effects usually begin in 24 to 48 hours, and peak effects are achieved within a 2- to 4-week time period (Gold Standard/Elsevier, 2010). Cholestyramine is one of the oldest medications used to treat hyperlipidemia; the U.S. Food and Drug Administration (FDA) first approved it in 1966 (Gold Standard/Elsevier, 2010). Colesevelam is approved for use with statins and produces a synergistic effect.

Side effects of bile acid sequestrants include gastrointestinal (GI) distress and constipation. Constipation is the most common and troublesome side effect. Bile acid sequestrants can bind with other substances (including other medications) in addition to binding to bile acids. Because of this binding potential, bile acid sequestrants interfere with the absorption of fat-soluble vitamins (A, D, and K). It may also accelerate their clearance and lower their effective plasma levels.

Clinical Application

Because of their binding property, bile acid sequestrants should not be taken at the same time as other medications. Advise patients to take other medications 1 hour before or 4 hours after taking bile acid sequestrants.

The use of these medications is contraindicated in patients with biliary obstruction or abnormal intestinal function. Because bile acid sequestrants can increase triglyceride levels, they are also contraindicated in patients with elevated triglycerides. The powder forms of bile acid sequestrants should be mixed with fluids. Bile acid resins are insoluble and form a gritty solution. This may not be pleasing to some patients and can affect compliance with the therapeutic regime. Tablets should not be cut, chewed, or crushed because they are designed to break down in the GI track. Colestipol is not absorbed and therefore has less toxic potential, making it safer for use in children and pregnant women (Gold Standard/Elsevier, 2010). Bile acid sequestrants have the potential to decrease the absorption of several medications, including digoxin, warfarin, thiazide diuretics, and thyroxin. They also can impair the absorption of vitamin K (Opie & Gersh, 2009).

Nicotinic Acid (Niacin)

Also called *niacin,* nicotinic acid is a B complex vitamin. Because niacin is used in the enrichment of refined flour, niacin deficiency is rare in our country today. Dietary requirements for niacin can be met by the intake of either nicotinic acid or nicotinamide. As vitamins, both of these substances have identical functions. However, as pharmacological agents, they are very different. In addition to being a vitamin, niacin has additional dose-related pharmacological effects not seen with nicotinamide (Gold Standard/Elsevier, 2010).

In peripheral circulation, niacin dilates the cutaneous blood vessels and increases blood flow to the face, neck, and chest. Niacin may cause a release of histamine or prostacyclin that is responsible for this vasodilatation and the classic "flush" associated with niacin use. This vasodilatation can also produce pruritus, headaches, or other pain. Histamine can also increase gastric acid secretion, increasing the likelihood of GI side effects.

Niacin was the first lipid-lowering agent shown to decrease mortality in myocardial infarction (MI) patients (Gold Standard/Elsevier, 2010).

Nicotinic acid-related agents include:

• Niacor

• Slo-Niacin

• Niaspan

Decreased very-low-density lipoprotein cholesterol (VLDL-C) production is one of the primary actions of niacin (Berra & Fair, 2010). One explanation for this result is that niacin decreases the lipolysis of triglycerides in adipose tissue, thereby reducing the transport of free fatty acids to the liver and decreasing hepatic triglyceride synthesis (Gold Standard/Elsevier, 2010). Decreased triglyceride synthesis results in a reduction of VLDL-C production. Lowered LDL-C cholesterol can be a result of decreased VLDL-C production; alternatively, niacin may promote increased clearance of LDL-C precursors.

Niacin also raises HDL-C levels through a mechanism that is not fully understood but is related to increased levels of apolipoprotein A-I (apo A-I) and lipoprotein A-I and a decrease in levels of apolipoprotein B (Apo-B). Women may have better results than men when taking niacin at the same dose (Gold Standard/Elsevier, 2010).

The effects of niacin on the reduction of cholesterol are unrelated to nicotinamide and its role as a vitamin. Therapeutic dosing to achieve lipid lowering is up to 4 g daily which is started in lower doses (100 mg twice daily) to reduce side effects. Therapeutic benefit may be seen in doses as low as 1.5 to 2 g daily (Opie & Gersh, 2009). Side effects of niacin include flushing, GI distress, hyper-

glycemia, gout, and liver toxicity. Flushing and dyspepsia are likely to limit adherence to therapy. Flushing usually subsides within 2 weeks on a stable dose. When given 30 minutes before niacin, aspirin (325 mg) may also blunt the flushing response (Berra & Fair, 2010). Niacin should be administered with food to minimize GI side effects.

Fibrates

Also called *fibric acid agents,* fibrates include:

• clofibrate (Atromid-S)

• fenofibrate (Tricor)

• gemfibrozil (Lopid)

The mechanism of action for these medications is complex and not fully understood; however, they stimulate lipoprotein lipase activity, which increases catabolism and clearance of triglycerides. They also decrease hepatic triglyceride production. In addition, they may also decrease cholesterol synthesis, increase the mobilization of cholesterol from tissues, enhance the removal of cholesterol from the liver, and increase cholesterol excretion in feces. They decrease VLDL-C synthesis and significantly reduce triglycerides. Fibrates also raise HDL-C levels (Gold Standard/Elsevier, 2010).

Fibrates are the drug of choice for type III hyperlipidemia and hypertriglyceridemia (Grundy et al., 2002). They are also the first line medications to reduce the risk of pancreatitis in patients with very high levels of triglycerides (Opie & Gersh, 2009). Fibrates decrease triglycerides by 25% to 50% and increase HDL-C in the presence of hypertriglyceridemia. However, they have variable effects on LDL-C. Despite this, fibrates, particularly fenofibrate, may increase the production of larger, less-dense LDL particles, which helps to promote LDL metabolism and reduce the number of smaller, more-dense particles associated with atherosclerosis. Fenofibrate also reduces lipoprotein (a) and serum fibrinogen, which is an independent risk factor for thrombosis (Gold Standard/Elsevier, 2010). Serum triglyceride levels begin to fall within 2 to 5 days, with maximal effects achieved within 3 weeks (Gold Standard/Elsevier, 2010).

Side effects of fibrates include dyspepsia, rash, alopecia, fatigue, headache, impotence, anemia, myositis flulike syndrome, cholelithiasis, and abnormal liver function test results (Opie & Gersh, 2009). Because fibrates are renally excreted, they are contraindicated in patients with severe renal disease. They are also contraindicated in patients with hepatic disease or preexisting gallbladder disease.

Combining a fibrate with a statin raises safety concerns because of the potential for myopathy and overt rhabdomyolysis. One fibrate (fenofibrate), however, does not interfere with the catabolism of statins (Grundy et al., 2002). Concomitant use of gemfibrozil with a statin increases the risk of rhabdomyolysis (Opie & Gersh, 2009). However, almost all reports of such adverse effects have occurred in situations in which the drug combination should have been avoided. Fibrates and statins should not be combined in the following situations:

- when high doses of statins, particularly simvastatin 80 mg per day or atorvastatin 80 mg per day, are used

- in patients with renal insufficiency because fibrates are renally excreted and plasma levels are increased in patients with renal insufficiency, thereby increasing the risk for drug-drug interactions

- in patients taking any agent that interferes with clearance of statins (for example, the immunosuppressive agent tacrolimus has this effect)

- in patients older than 70 years of age because of general increased problems with renal and hepatic function

(Grundy et al., 2002).

HMG-CoA Reductase Inhibitors

Also known as *statins,* HMG-CoA reductase inhibitors have been widely studied in various clinical trials. The landmark Scandinavian Simvastatin Survival Study showed that simvastatin for secondary prevention not only reduced lipid levels but also reduced future coronary events and overall mortality. Primary prevention studies have shown that statins reduce the need for coronary revascularization and reduce the risk of coronary mortality and morbidity (Opie & Gersh, 2009). All medications in this group have been shown to reduce the risk of cardiovascular disease in clinical trials. Statins are usually used as first line agents because of their proven predictable results, overall safety profile, and ability to be well tolerated by most patients. Statins may have effects other than lipid lowering that play a role in their cardiovascular protective abilities. Some of these proposed additional benefits include: improving endothelial function, contributing to an antithrombotic environment, and inhibiting inflammatory response (Opie & Gersh, 2009). The Jupiter Trial, for example, showed a reduction in cardiovascular events in patients taking rosuvastatin who had normal LDL cholesterol levels but high levels of high sensitivity C reactive protein (Ridker et al., 2008). Examples of HMG-CoA reductase inhibitors include:

- lovastatin (Mevacor)

- simvastatin (Zocor)

- pravastatin (Pravachol)

- fluvastatin (Lescol)

- atorvastatin (Lipitor).

- rosuvastatin (Crestor)

Lovastatin was the first HMG-CoA reductase inhibitor introduced (Gold Standard/Elsevier, 2010). Lovastatin and simvastatin are administered in an inactive form and require hydrolysis to be activated. The mechanism of action of statins involves the inhibition of HMG-CoA reductase which catalyzes an early step in cholesterol synthesis. These inhibitors reduce the quantity of mevalonic acid, a precursor to cholesterol. Cholesterol levels in liver cells are reduced, and the body responds with increased hepatic uptake of LDL-C from the circulation. The result is a decrease in total cholesterol, LDL-C, triglycerides, and apo B. Some statins also increase HDL-C (Opie & Gersh, 2009).

The effect of HMG-CoA reductase inhibitors is dose dependent. The most active time for cholesterol biosynthesis is during the very early morning hours. For this reason, it is generally recommended to give statins late in the evening, prior to bedtime. However, not all medications in this group are clinically affected by the administration time. For example, the effects of atorvastatin on LDL-C reduction are not impacted by the time of day it is administered (Gold Standard/Elsevier, 2010). Higher doses of the most potent statins are generally needed to decrease triglyceride levels.

Atorvastatin at the maximal dose has the greatest LDL-C lowering effect of all the HMG-CoA reductase inhibitors. Atorvastatin has a longer half-life and greater hepatic selectivity than the other HMG-CoA reductase inhibitors, which might explain its greater LDL-C lowering ability. At maximal doses, LDL-C can be lowered by 60% (Gold Standard/Elsevier, 2010). Clinical benefits of atorvastatin have been seen in patients with acute coronary syndrome (ACS), high-risk hypertensive patients, and patients with type II diabetes. The PROVE-IT Study showed that high dose atorvastatin (80 mg/day) reduced LDL-C to a very low level and also reduced the number of adverse clinical events in those patients with recent ACS (Opie & Gersh, 2009).

Fluvastatin has some properties that differ from other medications in its class. For example, it has a short half-life, is highly bound to proteins, and does not cross the blood-brain barrier. Some researchers claim that fluvastatin is less likely than other HMG-CoA reductase inhibitors to cause systemic side effects (Gold Standard/Elsevier, 2010).

Side effects of HMG-CoA reductase inhibitors range in their severity from minor to serious.

Minor effects include:

- headache
- GI effects
- potential worsening of cataracts.

Serious effects include:

- myopathy (ranges in presentation)
    - myalgia and fatigue
    - objective myopathy
    - rhabdomyolysis
- hepatic failure.

Although there is a small risk of these serious side effects, special precautions are important to assure patient safety. Statins are contraindicated in patients with acute or chronic liver disease. Liver function studies should be assessed at baseline, after 12 weeks of therapy, and every 6 months thereafter. A baseline creatinine kinase should also be assessed to aid, if needed, in the future diagnosis of myopathy (Opie & Gersh, 2009). Patients must be instructed to immediately report signs and symptoms related to the potential serious side effects to their physicians, including:

- muscle aching or weakness
- decreased or brown urine
- fever blistering or loosening of the skin
- skin rash or itching
- yellowing of the skin or eyes.

Statins can be combined with nicotinic acid, bile acid sequestrants, and even fibrates if necessary. Caution must be used, however, if combining with fibrates due to the increased risk of rhabdomyolysis. Predisposing factors to the development of myopathy and potential rhabdomyolysis include the co-administration of statins with certain other medications, including fibrates, niacin, cyclosporine, erythromycin, and azole antifungal agents. Combination of a statin with a fibrate is the most acknowledged combination for increasing the risk of rhabdomyolysis (Opie & Gersh, 2009). Specific factors to consider when combining a statin with a fibrate were discussed in the section about fibrate therapy.

Grapefruit juice contains an agent that slows the activity of the liver enzyme that metabolizes some of the agents in this class, particularly simvastatin and atorvastatin. Therefore, grapefruit juice consumption can increase the expected drug levels of a given dose and increase the risk of rhabdomyolysis. Patients should be instructed not to consume large quantities of grapefruit juice when taking these drugs.

Clinical Application

Coadministration of certain medications with HMG-CoA reductase inhibitors can cause rhabdomyolysis. Instruct patients to report all medications they are taking to each prescribing physician.

Intestinal Absorption Inhibitors

Intestinal absorption inhibitors are the newest class of lipid-lowering medications. These medications can be used alone or in combination with HMG-CoA reductase inhibitors. In 2002, ezetimibe was the first intestinal absorption inhibitor to be approved by the FDA. Ezetimibe blocks the absorption of cholesterol in the small intestine and therefore decreases the delivery of intestinal cholesterol to the liver. This results in a decrease of cholesterol stores in the liver and a subsequent increase in blood clearance of cholesterol (Gold Standard/Elsevier, 2010). In 2007 the ENHANCE Trial raised some concern regarding the efficacy of ezetimibe in combination with statin therapy. A statement from the American College of Cardiology in January 2008 stated that "clinical management should not be made based on the ENHANCE trial alone and that combination therapy with ezetimibe remains a reasonable approach for patients on high dose statins who have not reached goal or who can not tolerate statins at higher doses" (Raible, 2008).

DRUGS THAT AFFECT COAGULATION

Coagulation Overview

The coagulation system has two primary purposes:

- to protect the integrity of the vessels and prevent harmful bleeding
- to maintain the fluid state of the blood.

These two goals must be achieved simultaneously to maintain health.

Clotting can be initiated by activation of either the intrinsic or extrinsic pathways of the clotting cascade. The intrinsic pathway is initiated by vessel injury and direct exposure to collagen. The extrinsic pathway is triggered by the endothelial release of tissue factor. Both pathways initiate the common pathway, through which a fibrin stable clot is produced.

In the common pathway:

- Prothrombin is converted to thrombin.
- Thrombin permits the conversion of fibrinogen to fibrin.
- A fibrin stable clot forms.

This fibrin stable clot, sometimes called a *red clot,* is the cause of most ST-segment elevation myocardial infarctions (STEMIs).

Platelets also respond to vessel injury through the processes of adhesion, activation, and aggregation. Platelet aggregation can be large enough to form a platelet plug, a white clot that seals a damaged vessel. This white clot is a primary culprit in unstable angina. In addition to the independent formation of a platelet plug, platelets also release components necessary for the clotting process in the intrinsic pathway and contain a fibrin-stabilizing factor that is important in the final stage of the common pathway, prior to stable clot formation. Platelets cross-link with fibrinogen via the glycoprotein (GP) IIb/IIIa receptors to form a fibrin mesh, which gives a clot more substance.

Thrombolytics and Fibrinolytics

Two main categories of medications are used to dissolve clots that have already formed: medications that are nonfibrin specific (thrombolytics) and those that are fibrin specific (fibrinolytics). Both types are administered intravenously. Table 3-3 lists agents used to dissolve clots during acute STEMIs. For maximum effectiveness, these medications should be administered within 30 minutes of symptom onset (Antman et al., 2004). Indications and contraindications for these medications are discussed in greater detail in Chapter 5.

Streptokinase was the earliest "clot busting" medication used to dissolve clots during an acute MI. It is a nonenzyme protein made from hemolytic streptococci that works by combining with circulating plasminogen and forming complexes that catalyze plasmin formation. The resultant increase in circulating plasmin creates a systemic lytic state, dissolving recent clots.

Because it is a foreign protein, streptokinase can cause allergic reactions. The most common indications of an allergic reaction include pruritus, urticaria, fever, nausea, flushing, headache, and malaise (Verrier & Deelstra, 2010). In response to receiving streptokinase, patients also produce anti-streptokinase antibodies. Patients with antibodies to streptokinase may not receive the full benefit of the medication; therefore, it is contraindicated in these patients. Patients with antistreptokinase antibodies include those who have received streptokinase within the last 6 months and those who have had recent streptococcal infection (Verrier & Deelstra, 2010).

Anistreplase, also known as *APSAC*, is an altered form of streptokinase that is prepared in vitro (Gold Standard/Elsevier, 2010). It converts circulating plasminogen into plasmin and has systemic lytic effects similar to those of streptokinase. Different from streptokinase, anistreplase is able to be given in an intravenous (IV) bolus over 2 to 5 minutes (Gold Standard/Elsevier, 2010). Because anistreplase contains streptokinase, patients with a severe hypersensitivity to streptokinase should not receive this medication (Gold Standard/Elsevier, 2010). Tissue plasminogen activator (t-PA), a fibrin-specific lytic agent, is a serine protease produced by vascular endothelial cells. It is produced for clinical use using recombinant deoxyribonucleic acid (DNA) techniques. It has a particular affinity for fibrin; specifically, it activates the plasminogen that is bound to fibrin. Alteplase (recombinant t-PA), uses an accelerated dose to achieve more rapid reperfusion. The newer drugs derived from t-PA, reteplase (r-PA), tenecteplase (TNK-t-PA), and lanoteplase (n-PA) are designed for bolus dosing to eliminate medication errors associated with the administration of these types of medications (Verrier & Deelstra, 2010). In the GUSTO I Clinical Trial involving both streptokinase and t-PA, there was an approximate 11.5% to 13.5%

TABLE 3-3: THROMBOLYTIC AND FIBRINOLYTIC AGENTS

Type	Actions/Physiologic Effects	Agents
Fibrin specific	• Plasminogen activation • Rapid clot lysis • Clot specific	• Tissue plasminogen activators (t-PAs) • Alteplase (recombinant t-PA) • Reteplase (bolus dose recombinant t-PA) • Tenecteplase (single bolus dose recombinant t-PA)
Nonfibrin specific	• Systemic lysis • Slow clot lysis • More prolonged, systemic effect	• Streptokinase • Anistreplase (also known as *anisoylated plasminogen streptokinase activator complex,* or APSAC)

rate of error in the administration of these drugs. In the group of patients in which an administration error was made, the mortality at 30 days was higher (Cannon, 2000). For this reason the newer generation fibrinolytic medications have been created to be administered in bolus format and thus help eliminate potential medication errors.

Reteplase and tenecteplase also have very short half-lives. The benefit of a short half-life is decreased risk of bleeding; the disadvantage is an increased likelihood of reocclusion after administration. Tenecteplase is a very fibrin-specific medication that causes minimal systemic bleeding, including intracranial bleeding. Allergic response and hypotension can also occur with t-PA and t-PA-related medications.

All medications in this group have a very narrow window of therapeutic effect. If dosing is too low, clot lysis does not occur and there is no interruption of the MI. If the dose is too high, systemic bleeding can occur. Bleeding commonly occurs at vascular access sites. However, intracranial bleeding can also occur and have devastating effects. The risk of bleeding is weighed against the potential benefit when making decisions about the administration of these medications. Contraindications for these medications are discussed in Chapter 5. Tissue plasminogen activator agents have better patency rates compared to streptokinase (Verrier & Deelstra, 2010). Early administration of fibrinolytic therapy remains key to improving outcomes, and several clinical trials have demonstrated decreased mortality when fibrinolytic therapy was administered in the prehospital setting (Morrison, Verbeek, McDonald, Sawadsky, & Cook, 2000). Of course, prehospital administration of fibrinolytic therapy requires a well-trained and well-coordinated emergency medical system with the ability to perform and transmit the 12-lead electrocardiogram to a qualified physician trained in STEMI recognition.

Clinical Application

Because thrombolytics and fibrinolytics must be administered within a very short time frame and have specific indications and contraindications, it is important for emergency departments to have clearly written protocols and checklists to guide nurses through the rapid and accurate administration of these medications.

Anticoagulants

Unfractionated Heparin

Commercially produced heparin is derived from porcine or bovine tissue. Heparin was discovered in 1916 and approved by the FDA for use in 1936 (Gold Standard/Elsevier, 2010). Unfractionated heparin (UFH) is the anticoagulant of choice for many conditions, including acute MI, pulmonary embolism (PE), and deep vein thrombosis (DVT). In the pathophysiological processes of atherosclerosis and ACSs, endothelial injury results in thrombi, platelet aggregation, and vasoconstriction. Fibrinogen is ultimately converted to fibrin to produce a fibrin stable clot. The role of heparin in these conditions is to prevent thrombus formation.

Heparin is an antithrombotic agent but does not lyse existing clots. It works in the intrinsic and common pathways of the clotting cascade to prevent further development of thrombi. In higher doses, heparin also interferes with platelet aggregation. Heparin prevents the conversion of prothrombin to thrombin (factor IIa) by accelerating the action of antithrombin III. Antithrombin III naturally inhibits thrombin. The net result is the neutralization of the clotting capabilities of thrombin. However, heparin does not inactivate fibrin-bound thrombin. Heparin also inactivates clotting factors IXa and Xa. In addition to being an anticoagulant, heparin also indirectly inhibits platelets because thrombin is a potent platelet stimulator.

Heparin binds to plasma proteins, blood cells, and endothelial cells. This nonspecific binding to plasma proteins and endothelial cells limits the bioavailability of UFH at low doses and also contributes to its variable response between patients. UFH is commonly administered intravenously, using a weight-based protocol to help control anticoagulation response. Weight-based heparin dosing reaches the therapeutic goal more consistently than standard therapy (Anderson et al., 2007). Heparin can also be administered subcutaneously. It is not absorbed from the GI tract, so it cannot be given orally.

The anticoagulation effects of IV heparin are almost instant. Activated partial thromboplastin time (aPTT) is used to monitor the therapeutic effectiveness and safety range of heparin. A baseline aPTT, prothrombin time (PT), International Normalized Ratio (INR), platelet count, hemoglobin level, and hematocrit should be drawn before UFH is started. The goal is to have aPTT at 1.5 times the control. A therapeutic aPTT should be reached within 24 hours of the initiation of therapy. Activated partial thromboplastin time results should be measured 6 hours after the dose is initiated and again 6 hours after any dose change. After two therapeutic aPTTs have been achieved, measurements can be obtained every 24 hours (Anderson et al., 2007).

In addition to weight, other patient variables affect aPTT. The aPTT response for a given dose of UFH increases with age and decreases in patients who have diabetes and in those who smoke (Anderson et al., 2007).

Bleeding is an obvious potential complication of heparin administration. Heparin is partially cleared via the kidneys and increased bleeding can occur in patients with renal dysfunction. The optimal period of time that heparin can be continued is not yet defined. Most clinical trials involving heparin have continued it for 2 to 5 days. An aPTT should be drawn with any change in patient condition, and heparin should be immediately discontinued when bleeding is the suspected cause. Patients should have baseline lab work drawn before therapy is initiated including aPTT, PT/INR, complete blood count, and platelets. Hemoglobin level, hematocrit, and platelet count are drawn on a daily basis. Heparin can cause mild to severe thrombocytopenia (platelet count less than 150,000/mm³) (Fischbach & Dunning, 2009). Heparin should be discontinued if platelets fall below 100,000/mm³. The half-life of UFH is very short. If reversal is needed, protamine is the antidote.

Mild thrombocytopenia occurs in 10% to 20% of patients, whereas more severe thrombocytopenia occurs in only 1% to 2% of patients (Anderson et al., 2007). Thrombocytopenia generally occurs 4 to 14 days after initiation of heparin therapy. A very rare, but very severe, form of thrombocytopenia, heparin-induced thrombocytopenia (HIT), can occur, resulting in thrombosis. Patients develop HIT due to an autoimmune response and should never receive heparin, not even the small doses of heparin used in solutions to flush invasive lines.

Low-molecular-weight Heparin

Low-molecular-weight heparin (LMWH) is smaller in size than UFH. It works by accelerating the activity of antithrombin III. LMWH has a more potent effect on factor Xa than on factor IIa, although both are inhibited. LMWH produces less inhibition of platelets than does UFH.

LMWH binds less to plasma proteins and endothelial cells than does UFH. It also has a longer half-life, which helps to produce a sustained and more predictable anticoagulation effect. For this reason, clotting times do not need to be monitored as they do with the use of UFH. If needed, antifactor Xa levels can be drawn 4 hours after a subcutaneous dose. At recommended doses, PT and aPTT are not greatly impacted. LMWH is also associated with a lower incidence of HIT, but a higher rate of minor bleeding than is UFH (Verrier & Deelstra, 2010). LMWH is renally cleared and special dosing is required for patients with chronic renal insufficiency. The half-life of LMWH is much longer than UFH at 4 to 6 hours. Protamine is effective in reversing 60% of the drug (Gold Standard/Elsevier, 2010).

LMWH is administered subcutaneously, either daily or twice a day, depending on the clinical indication. Patients can be taught self-administration. There are important teaching points regarding the administration of LMWH:

1. The full length of the ½ inch prepackaged needle should be injected.

2. The anterolateral or posterolateral walls of the abdomen should be used.

3. The skin fold should be held until the needle is fully withdrawn.

4. Injection sites should be rotated frequently.

5. Injection sites should not be massaged.

Enoxaparin, a form of LMWH, was first approved by the FDA for DVT prevention in patients undergoing orthopedic surgery. In 1998, enoxaparin received approval for use in the treatment of unstable angina and non-STEMI. Some studies have demonstrated better outcomes in treating ACSs with enoxaparin than with UFH (Gold Standard/Elsevier, 2010). As of the 2007 updated guidelines for the care of patients with STEMI, LMWH is also an option for anticoagulation in the care of these patients, including those receiving primary percutaneous coronary intervention (PCI) (Kushner et al., 2009). The use of LMWH and UFH continues to be studied in the ACS population undergoing early invasive treatment.

Direct Thrombin Inhibitors

Direct thrombin inhibitors are indicated for the treatment of thrombosis in patients with HIT. Direct thrombin inhibitors also have an advantage over heparin because they have the ability to inactivate fibrin-bound thrombin, thereby improving the antithrombotic effect. These medications also bind less to plasma proteins and produce a more reliable anticoagulant effect. Direct thrombin inhibitors include lepirudin and desirudin, recombinant forms

of hirudin. Anaphylactic reactions have been observed with the use of lepirudin (Greinacher, Lubenow, & Eichler, 2003). Argatroban is a synthetic direct thrombin inhibitor indicated for the treatment and prevention of HIT and associated thromboembolic events (GlaxoSmithKline, 2005). Bivalirudin is a synthetic direct thrombin inhibitor indicated in ACS for non-STEMI and STEMI (Anderson et al., 2007; Kushner et al., 2009). This medication is indicated as an alternative to heparin in all patients, not just patients with, or at risk for, HIT (The Medicines Company, 2009). As with all anticoagulants, direct thrombin inhibitors are contraindicated with major active bleeding.

Dabigatran (Pradaxa) is a recently approved oral direct thrombin inhibitor agent and may be used in select patients with atrial fibrillation as an alternative to warfarin. This new agent is only approved for use in non-valvular atrial fibrillation in patients with at least one other risk factor for stroke. A therapeutic effect is achieved in one hour. The half life is approximately 13 hours, and for this reason it is dosed twice daily. Dabigatran is out of the system in one to two days if renal function is normal. Dosing is adjusted to a low dose in patients with renal dysfunction. Patients who are taking dabigatran do not have to have routine monitoring for clotting times.

Factor Xa Inhibitors

Factor Xa inhibitors are a new class of anticoagulants. Fondaparinux was the first FDA-approved medication in this class. Fondaparinux is approved for DVT and PE prophylaxis in patients undergoing hip or abdominal surgery. It is also approved for the treatment of DVT or PE in conjunction with warfarin (Gold Standard/Elsevier, 2010). Fondaparinux was most recently approved as an anticoagulant alternative in patients with non-STEMI (Anderson et al., 2007). Fondaparinux is not approved as the sole anticoagulant in patients undergoing PCI because it does not exhibit potent enough antithrombin activity.

Factor Xa inhibitors produce antithrombotic action by neutralizing factor Xa and interrupting the clotting cascade that leads to thrombin formation. This class of medications does not inhibit thrombin (factor IIa). Administration is via once daily subcutaneous injection and there is no need for laboratory monitoring because bleeding time is not greatly altered. One dose can cover a wide range of body weights. There have been no reports of HIT. Because of renal clearance, fondaparinux is contraindicated in severe renal dysfunction. There is no antidote available for factor Xa inhibitors (Gold Standard/Elsevier, 2010). Recombinant factor VIIa may be used to help reverse the anticoagulation effect if life-threatening bleeding occurs.

Warfarin

Warfarin (Coumadin) is an oral anticoagulant agent. Like heparin, warfarin does not affect existing clots. One of the important actions of warfarin is the inhibition of the synthesis of factor II (prothrombin). Warfarin acts indirectly through the liver by altering the synthesis of other vitamin K-dependent factors in the extrinsic pathway. These vitamin K-dependent factors are left biologically inactive. Vitamin K is essential for the liver to manufacture several clotting factors, including factors II, VII, IX, and X.

Warfarin is primarily bound to albumin in the blood; very little of it circulates freely. It is, however, the freely circulating amount that produces a therapeutic value. The number of potential drug interactions is high because of the large amount of protein-bound warfarin.

There is a lag time of anywhere from 2 to 5 days, most typically 3 to 4 days, to reach a therapeutic level. The reason for this lag time is gradual disappearance of the clotting factors involved. At full therapeutic doses, vitamin K-dependent clotting factors decrease by 30% to 50% (Gold Standard/Elsevier, 2010). PT and INR should be monitored to evaluate effectiveness and safety. INR was developed to correct problems with standardization of anticoagulation intensity. INR relates the patient's PT to the intensity of actual coagulation. Hemorrhagic complications of warfarin use have decreased with the use of INR as the standard to monitor PT and guide dosing. Baseline PT and INR should be drawn prior to initiation of therapy.

Dosing usually starts at 5 mg per day. Loading doses are not recommended because time is required to gradually deplete existing clotting factors. Bolus dosing initially may result in excessive anticoagulation after clotting factors are depleted. PT and INR are monitored daily until a therapeutic level is reached. The dosage may need adjustment after 4 to 6 days because of individual sensitivity. After a therapeutic response (INR of 2.0 to 3.0 in most situations) is achieved, PT and INR are usually drawn twice weekly during the first 2 weeks of therapy. They are then drawn on a weekly basis for the remaining first 2 months of therapy and are monitored every 4 to 6 weeks on an ongoing basis for the duration of therapy. Patients with mechanical prosthetic valves need INRs of 2.5 to 3.5. It takes approximately 4 days to return to normal coagulation after the drug is discontinued.

Chronic conditions such as atrial fibrillation require lifelong therapy. Warfarin reduces the risk of embolic stroke in patients with atrial fibrillation by 65% to 70% (Gold Standard/Elsevier, 2010). Acute conditions, such as PE and DVT, usually require at least 6 months of therapy. A patient who had an acute MI with a resultant left ventricular thrombus also needs to be on warfarin for at least 6 months.

Patients who have malignant hypertension, coagulopathies, or history of bleeding are not candidates for warfarin therapy. Those who abuse alcohol or engage in activities with a high risk of trauma also are not candidates. Many drugs interact with warfarin to alter clotting time. Patients need to be instructed to inform every physician they see, including their dentists, that they are taking warfarin. They also need to be instructed to avoid the use of over-the-counter medications, unless approved by a physician. Over-the-counter medications containing aspirin, ibuprofen, or naprosyn should always be avoided by those taking warfarin.

Patients taking warfarin should include this information in their personal identification. Consistency in diet is important, especially with foods that are known to be high in vitamin K. For example, if a patient likes certain foods high in vitamin K it is important that his or her diet consistently contain these foods while warfarin dosing is being adjusted. Sudden or sporadic intake of high vitamin K foods can alter clotting times. Foods with a moderate to high content of vitamin K are listed in Box 3-1. Patient education regarding warfarin use is very important, and patient compliance is critical. Patients who are not reliable with medication administration may not be acceptable candidates for warfarin therapy. Patients should be taught to recognize less-obvious signs and symptoms of bleeding, such as black, tarry stools. They should also be instructed to report any signs of bleeding, including bleeding gums, epistaxis, and increased bruising. Patients should also be instructed about necessary safety precautions to avoid bleeding. These include:

* using an electric shaver

* using a soft-bristle toothbrush

* wearing protective gear while working outside (full shoes and gardening gloves)

* avoiding contact sports.

BOX 3-1: FOODS WITH MODERATE TO HIGH CONTENT OF VITAMIN K

Brussels sprouts	Green onions	Certain peas
Lettuce	Liver	Soybean oil
Avocado	Collard greens	Certain beans
Kale	Cauliflower	Parsley
Cabbage	Soybeans	Turnip greens
Green tea	Mustard greens	Spinach
Broccoli		

(Gold Standard/Elsevier, 2010)

Warfarin should be stored in a cool, dry place away from light. It loses its potency when exposed to high heat. Warfarin does cross the placenta and is a known teratogen that can cause birth defects. Women of childbearing age should be counseled about effective birth control and potential risks to the unborn child if pregnancy should occur.

ANTIPLATELET THERAPY

Glycoprotein IIb/IIIa Inhibitors

The three GP IIb/IIIa inhibitors currently used include:

1. abciximab (ReoPro)

2. eptifibatide (Integrilin)

3. tirofiban (Aggrastat)

All three of these medications interfere with the final pathway of platelet aggregation. They inhibit GP IIb/IIIa receptors, where platelets and fibrinogen bind to form a fibrin mesh. GP IIb/IIIa receptors are abundant on platelet surfaces; there are approximately 50,000 to 80,000 receptors per platelet (Gold Standard/Elsevier, 2010). When platelets are activated, a change occurs in their receptors that increases their affinity to bind to fibrinogen. Fibrinogen links to these receptors and simultaneously binds receptors on two separate platelets. Platelet cross-linking occurs, leading to platelet aggregation. These medications actually occupy the receptors and prevent fibrinogen binding, thereby inhibiting platelet aggregation.

GP IIb/IIIa inhibitors are administered intravenously and may be administered concomitantly with aspirin, clopidogrel, and heparin. UFH is typically used, and doses are reduced when given with GP IIb/IIIa inhibitors. GP IIb/IIIa inhibitors prevent platelet aggregation, regardless of the source of platelet stimulation (Anderson et al., 2007). For example, they are effective in blocking thrombin-induced platelet aggregation.

Abciximab (ReoPro) was the first FDA-approved GP IIb/IIIa inhibitor. It has a short half-life, which is balanced by a very strong affinity for receptors. Abciximab can block more than 80% of GP IIb/IIIa receptors. It also blocks other receptors and can produce an anticoagulation effect. Some of its receptor occupation can last for up to 10 days. Platelet aggregation gradually returns to normal 24 to 48 hours after the medication is discontinued (Anderson et al., 2007). Eptifibatide and tirofiban generally exhibit effects consistent with their plasma levels. Their half-lives are approximately 2 to 3 hours, and platelet aggregation returns to normal within 4 to 8 hours of stopping the medication. When given alone, eptifibatide and tirofiban have no effect on PT or aPTT (Anderson et al., 2007).

GP IIb/IIIa inhibitors increase the risk of bleeding, which typically occurs at the vascular access site. Platelet count and hemoglobin level should be monitored during the use of GP IIb/IIIa inhibitors. However, thrombocytopenia is not a common complication.

GP IIb/IIIa inhibitors are indicated in the treatment of unstable angina and non-STEMI because they reduce the incidence of ischemic complications (Anderson et al., 2007). Their use with PCIs has also improved the results and safety of these procedures. They are also effective in reducing the rate of reocclusion of reperfused vessels.

Adenosine Diphosphate Inhibitors

Clopidogrel (Plavix) is a thienopyridine derivative that is approved by the FDA for prevention of atherosclerotic events. It prevents adenosine diphosphate (ADP)-mediated activation of platelets. ADP activates the GP IIb/IIIa receptors. Clopidogrel irreversibly inhibits the binding of ADP to platelet receptors and thereby prevents ADP from activating the GP IIb/IIIa receptors (Fraker & Fihn, 2007). Clopidogrel causes platelet inhibition for the life of the platelet, which is approximately 10 days. Dose-dependent inhibition of platelet aggregation is seen 2 hours after a single oral dose. With repeated daily doses, maximal inhibition of platelet aggregation (up to 60%) occurs in 3 to 7 days (Gold Standard/Elsevier, 2010). Bleeding time gradually returns to normal approximately 5 days after the drug is discontinued.

Clopidogrel is indicated in the treatment of unstable angina and non-STEMI. Clopidogrel is also recommended after discharge for all patients with STEMI. Clopidogrel has important clinical implications for patients who receive intracoronary stenting with either bare metal or drug eluting stents. Clopidogrel in conjunction with aspirin is recommended for one year with either bare metal or drug eluting stents to decrease the risk of developing in-stent thrombosis. Longer therapy is sometimes indicated in high-risk patients. Details regarding the recommendations for antiplatelet therapy after intracoronary stenting are discussed in Chapter 6. The maintenance dose of clopidogrel is 75 mg per day. Clopidogrel is administered in conjunction with aspirin after discharge. In 2009, the FDA announced a warning that patients who take clopidogrel should avoid the use of omeprazole (Prilosec). When omeprazole is taken with clopiodgrel, the ability of clopidgrel to block platelet aggregation is cut in half. The reason for this effect is that clopidogrel does not become effective until it is metabolized into its active form by the liver enzyme CYP2C19. Omeprazole blocks this enzyme and therefore reduces the effectiveness of clopidogrel (U.S. Food and Drug Administration [FDA], 2009). Most recently, the FDA established a black box warning for clopidogrel because of the diminished effectiveness of the drug in patients who are poor metabolizers. The reason for poor metabolism in some patients is because of the genetic differences in the liver enzyme CYP2C19. Tests are available to identify patients who are poor metabolizers. After they are identified, alternate antiplatelet therapy or altered dosing may be indicated in these patients (FDA, 2010).

Prasugrel is a newer agent in the same class as clopidogrel and has recently been approved by the FDA. Prasugrel has been shown to reduce ischemic complications compared to clopidogrel; however, it is also associated with a higher risk of bleeding, particularly in patients with small body size (less than 60 kg) and in those 75 years of age and older. The usual maintenance dose of prasugrel is 10 mg, but lower doses should be considered in patients with a higher risk for bleeding. Prasugrel is contraindicated in patients with a history of stroke or transient ischemic attack (Gold Standard/Elsevier, 2010).

Clinical Application

Clopidogrel is substantially more expensive than aspirin. Because both medications interfere with platelet function, it is important for patients to understand the added benefit of clopidogrel in order to assure compliance. It is also important prior to discharge to assess for any financial barriers that may limit the patient's ability to comply with treatment. Financial assistance may be available through Partnership for Prescription Assistance (www.pparx.org)

Aspirin

Aspirin was first introduced in medicine in 1899 (Gold Standard/Elsevier, 2010). Since then, it has been widely used for its many therapeutic benefits, including its anti-inflammatory, analgesic, antipyretic, and antithrombotic effects. Aspirin 81 mg to 325 mg is prescribed routinely in all patients with acute and chronic ischemic heart disease. Aspirin therapy should be prescribed, regardless of symptoms. Aspirin reduces risk in both primary and secondary prevention of cardiovascular disease and reduces adverse cardiovascular events by an average of 33% (Anderson et al., 2007). In patients with unstable angina, aspirin decreases short-term and long-term risks of fatal and nonfatal MI (Fraker & Fihn, 2007).

Aspirin works by inhibiting cyclooxygenase and inhibiting the synthesis of thromboxane A_2.

Thromboxane A_2 is a potent vasoconstrictor and platelet agonist that is released as a result of vascular injury. Aspirin produces a rapid antiplatelet and vasodilative effect by the immediate inhibition of thromboxane A_2 production. Aspirin also inhibits endothelial production of prostaglandin I_2. Prostaglandin I_2 produces vasodilatation and inhibits platelet aggregation. However, the effects of inhibiting thromboxane A_2 dominate over the effects of prostaglandin I_2 inhibition. Aspirin appears to affect platelet function for the life of the platelet and results in prolonged bleeding time. Aspirin may also protect LDL-C from the oxidation process and improve endothelial dysfunction.

Chewing of aspirin can accelerate absorption into the blood during an acute cardiac event. Contraindications to aspirin administration include allergy, history of GI bleeding, and coagulation disorders. Clopidogrel is used in patients who are allergic to aspirin.

Aspirin is specifically indicated after coronary artery bypass graft surgery for multiple reasons. It prevents early saphenous vein graft closure and is also effective in reducing postoperative MI, stroke, renal failure, and bowel infarction. Aspirin also reduces subsequent mortality. To achieve the maximal benefit of postoperative aspirin use, aspirin must be given within 48 hours of surgery. Aspirin is continued indefinitely postoperatively.

Decreased prostaglandin synthesis with aspirin is responsible for the GI side effects. Aspirin also causes direct irritation of the GI tract. Enteric-coated aspirin can help minimize this common side effect.

CONCLUSION

Many of the medications discussed in this chapter are administered indefinitely; therefore, patients throughout the continuum of healthcare are actively taking them. Nurses in all settings play an important role in patient education and assessment of therapeutic and adverse effects.

Nurses in the cardiovascular setting play a critical role in the accurate administration of potentially dangerous medications, such as IV anticoagulant and antiplatelet therapies. Nurses in the emergency department setting also may play a role in administration of potentially life-saving therapies involving thrombolytic and fibrinolytic agents. The agents that increase myocardial oxygen supply play a major role in the reduction of risk for cardiovascular disease and the mortality associated with it.

EXAM QUESTIONS

CHAPTER 3
Questions 21-26

Note: Choose the one option that BEST answers each question.

21. The class of medications most effective in lowering LDL-C is

    a. bile acid sequestrants.

    b. nicotinic acid.

    c. fibrates.

    d. HMG-CoA reductase inhibitors.

22. The two classes of medications most effective in lowering triglycerides are

    a. nicotinic acid and fibrates.

    b. fibrates and bile acid sequestrants.

    c. HMG-CoA reductase inhibitors and bile acid sequestrants.

    d. nicotinic acid and HMG-CoA reductase inhibitors.

23. Patients taking HMG-CoA reductase inhibitors should receive which of the following instructions?

    a. Do not take the medication if you are also taking beta-blockers or angiotensin-converting enzyme inhibitors.

    b. Immediately report any muscle weakness to a physician.

    c. Always take the medication with grapefruit juice.

    d. Have a cholesterol level drawn after the second day of therapy so that the dose can be adjusted, if necessary.

24. Patients who receive thrombolytics or fibrinolytics as reperfusion therapy should have the medication administered within what time frame from initial presentation?

    a. 90 minutes

    b. 60 minutes

    c. 30 minutes

    d. 15 minutes

25. Advantages to the use of LMWH include

    a. ability for the patient to self-administer subcutaneously at home if needed.

    b. use of bedside activated clotting time monitoring to measure drug effectiveness.

    c. ability to take the oral form after initial IV loading.

    d. shorter half-life than UFH, so it can be continued until right before surgery or another invasive procedure.

26. Patients with cardiovascular disease may be treated with various types of antiplatelet therapy, including

    a. streptokinase, glycoprotein IIb/IIa inhibitors, and aspirin.

    b. aspirin, glycoprotein IIb/IIIa inhibitors, and clopidogrel (Plavix).

    c. streptokinase, clopidogrel (Plavix), and aspirin.

    d. LMWH, warfarin, and bivalirudin.

CHAPTER 4

RISK FACTORS FOR AND PREVENTION OF CORONARY HEART DISEASE

CHAPTER OBJECTIVE

After completing this chapter, the learner will be able to discuss the impact of risk factors on the development of coronary heart disease.

LEARNING OBJECTIVES

After completing this chapter, the learner will be able to

1. define a risk equivalent for coronary artery disease.

2. list the nonmodifiable and modifiable risk factors for coronary artery disease.

3. discuss the five A's all healthcare practitioners can use in providing smoking-cessation counseling.

4. define blood pressure goals for people with hypertension and diabetes, renal disease, coronary heart disease, or cardiac risk equivalent.

5. describe the steps of lifestyle modification used in the reduction of cholesterol for primary prevention.

6. identify the current low-density lipoprotein cholesterol treatment goals for those with a coronary heart disease risk equivalent.

7. describe the difference between type II diabetes and metabolic syndrome.

8. describe differences between women and men in heart disease risk and presentation.

INTRODUCTION

A *risk factor* is a characteristic found in a healthy person that is independently related to the future development of a disease such as coronary heart disease (CHD). A risk factor can be a lifestyle habit, an environmental factor, or an inherited characteristic. Risk factors are classified as modifiable (can be changed) or nonmodifiable (cannot be changed).

Prevention has historically been differentiated as *primary* or *secondary*. For CHD, primary prevention is defined as reducing risk in people without known CHD to prevent the development of the disease in the future. Secondary prevention is defined as reducing risk in people with known CHD to prevent a future cardiac event. However, with the increased understanding of the development and progression of coronary atherosclerosis, the lines between primary and secondary prevention are merging. The overall goals in both primary and secondary prevention are to reduce the risk of complications and death associated with the development of CHD. Atherosclerosis, the underlying cause of most heart attacks, begins early in life, often before the age of 20. There is strong evidence that CHD is largely preventable and, therefore, the topics of risk assessment and reduction are vitally important in cardiovascular nursing. Approximately 90% of those who present with CHD have at least one major risk factor from among hyperlipidemia, hypertension, cigarette smoking, or diabetes (Lloyd-Jones et al., 2009). In addition, reduction in mortality from CHD is attributable to advances in treatment as well as to changes in cardiovascular risk factors (Lloyd-Jones et al., 2009).

Those at greatest risk for experiencing a future coronary event are people with a history of CHD. The term *risk equivalent* is used to define people without existing CHD who have the same risk of a future coronary event as those already diagnosed with CHD.

There are four CHD risk equivalent groups:

1. people with other forms of atherosclerotic vascular disease (peripheral vascular disease, abdominal aortic aneurysm, or symptomatic carotid disease)

2. people with type 2 diabetes

3. people with chronic kidney disease

4. people with two or more CHD risk factors who score at the equivalent risk on the Framingham Risk Tool (a mathematical health risk appraisal model in which points are assigned to each risk factor in order to calculate the probability of developing CHD in a 10-year period).

(Anderson et al., 2007)

NONMODIFIABLE RISK FACTORS

Previous Cardiac Event

History of past CHD is the most powerful risk factor for a future event. People with known CHD, or a CHD risk equivalent, are among the highest risk people for having a future cardiac event.

Family History

Family history refers to the presence of CHD in a first-degree relative. From a cardiac standpoint, a first-degree relative is defined as a mother, father, brother, or sister. Development of CHD in people younger than 55 years of age for men and younger than 65 years of age for women is considered pre-

mature. A history of myocardial infarction (MI) in a first-degree relative doubles the risk for CHD (Kramer, Newton, & Froelicher, 2010). The risk is greater when the MI occurs at a premature age.

Age

Cardiovascular disease is a disease of the aged. Approximately 82% of people who die of CHD are older than 65 years of age. The lifetime risk of developing CHD after 40 years of age is 49% for men and 32% for women. The average age for first MI in men is 64.5 years and 70.3 years in women (Lloyd-Jones et al., 2009).

Gender

Men are generally considered to be at a higher risk for CHD than women until women reach menopause. For this reason, historically, many women have not believed that they are vulnerable to heart disease. The incidence of CHD in women generally lags behind men by about 10 years (Lloyd-Jones et al., 2009). In addition, women commonly present with different symptoms (more nausea and fatigue) and have less documented disease on cardiac catheterization (angiography) than men. For these reasons, women have historically been misdiagnosed and under treated. In recent years, however, a major initiative has been underway to educate healthcare providers and women about the realities of women and heart disease. This educational movement is getting important messages out to women, including these facts:

• CHD kills more women than all cancers combined.

• More women than men die each year from cardiovascular disease.

• Women have a higher mortality rate than men after a heart attack.

(Lloyd-Jones et al., 2009)

Despite the information known today about women and heart disease, misconceptions still exist, leading people to believe heart disease is not a real problem for women.

Clinical Application

Women commonly exhibit what some providers call "atypical" symptoms of CHD, including nausea, fatigue, shortness of breath, and abdominal discomfort. However, these symptoms are not necessarily atypical for women. Any woman with discomfort from the nose to the navel, especially if she has risk factors for CHD, should be carefully evaluated for CHD.

MODIFIABLE RISK FACTORS

Tobacco Use

Cigarette smoking is the leading avoidable cause of death in the United States (Fiore et al., 2008). Smoking is also the single most important modifiable cardiovascular risk factor. Approximately 21% of adult Americans smoke, resulting in approximately 45 million adult American smokers (Fiore et al., 2008). Overall, persons who smoke have a two- to four-fold increased risk for CHD (Sohn, Hawk, Martin, & Froelicher 2010). The risk associated with smoking increases with the number of cigarettes smoked per day, the duration of smoking in years, and the younger the age at onset of smoking. Smoking

low-tar, low-nicotine, or filtered cigarettes does not decrease the risk of CHD. In addition to increasing the risk of CHD, smoking also increases the risk of cancer and lung disease. Tobacco use should be approached as a chronic disease itself, as opposed to a mere risk factor (Fiore et al., 2008).

Cigarettes are the delivery system for nicotine. Nicotine and carbon monoxide are the two most important chemicals in cigarette smoke. Nicotine is the physically addictive substance in tobacco; therefore, smoking cessation can lead to nicotine withdrawal. Nicotine withdrawal can cause irritability, anxiety, depression, anger, inability to focus, insomnia, and increased appetite (Fiore et al., 2008). These symptoms are commonly observed in smokers who are admitted for acute coronary events.

To provide effective patient counseling, it is important to understand the effects of tobacco, nicotine, and carbon monoxide on cardiovascular health. Box 4-1 outlines these effects.

Smoking Cessation Interventions

Smoking cessation is a safe and cost-effective risk factor intervention for all patients. Smoking cessation counseling, including minimal interventions of less than 3 minutes by a wide variety of clinicians, has been proven effective in reducing tobacco use. Physician advice to stop smoking adds to the success of cessation efforts. Intensive

---

BOX 4-1: CARDIOVASCULAR EFFECTS OF TOBACCO, NICOTINE, AND CARBON MONOXIDE

- Endothelial dysfunction: increased arterial wall stiffness with increased coronary vasoconstriction
- Increased catecholamine release: increased incidence of cardiac dysrhythmias
- Enhanced oxidation of low-density lipoprotein cholesterol (LDL-C)
- Lowered high-density lipoprotein cholesterol (HDL-C) level
- Enhanced hypercoagulability and thrombosis formation: increased C-reactive protein and fibrinogen levels and increased platelet aggregation
- Increased blood viscosity: increased hematocrit
- Decreased oxygen-carrying capacity of the blood

Net effect: accelerated development of atherosclerosis and increased risk of acute cardiac events

(Martin & Froelicher, 2005)

interventions are more effective than minimal interventions and should be used whenever possible. Interventions including four or more sessions are particularly effective and the forum can include individual counseling, group counseling, or telephone follow up. Therapies with the highest success include those that offer practical counseling coupled with support (Fiore et al., 2008). Structured programs can also be part of a comprehensive cardiac rehabilitation program. Referral to a formal nurse-led smoking cessation program can improve the effectiveness of smoking cessation counseling by up to 61% (Gibbons et al., 2002).

Improvements have been seen in the number of patients who receive smoking cessation counseling, with more than 70% receiving some form of counseling as of 2005 (Fiore et al., 2008). However, although smoking cessation counseling is effective, safe, and cost effective, it remains underutilized. In particular, the use of smoking cessation medications is highly under utilized as a strategy to improve success with cessation.

The use of nicotine-replacement therapy can substantially improve smoking cessation success rates (Fiore et al., 2008). Historically, there has been concern about the use of nicotine replacement therapy in any patient with cardiovascular disease. Although nicotine replacement therapy should be used with caution in patients with very recent MI (within 2 weeks), worsening angina, or serious dysrhythmias, its effects on the cardiovascular system are less dangerous than that of cigarette smoking (Sohn et al., 2010).

Nicotine replacement therapy comes in several forms, including a patch, gum, inhaler, nasal spray, or lozenge. The nasal spray and inhaler are available by prescription only. The lozenge and gum can be purchased over the counter. The patch can be prescribed or purchased over the counter. A prescription nicotine patch is beneficial when insurance coverage applies to prescription medication only.

Nicotine replacement therapy works by supplying the patient with either a bolus or continuous dose of nicotine. Some patients who are highly addicted to nicotine may require higher doses or two forms of replacement therapy. Two combinations of nicotine replacement therapy have been found to be effective: a) the long-term patch with the use of either gum or nasal spray and b) the patch with the inhaler (Fiore et al., 2008). Nicotine replacement therapy is not recommended for people who smoke less than 10 cigarettes per day, those who use smokeless tobacco, pregnant women, and adolescents.

Another pharmacotherapy used in smoking cessation is the oral agent bupropion, which has been used for many years in the treatment of depression. Bupropion's exact mechanism of action in achieving smoking cessation is not fully understood but there are two proposed mechanisms of action: a) neuronal blockade of the re-uptake of norepinephrine and dopamine and b) blockade of the nicotinic acetylcholinergic receptors. Like nicotine replacement therapy, the use of bupropion can substantially improve the rate of cessation success (Fiore et al., 2008). Unlike nicotine replacement therapy, bupropion is initiated while the patient is still smoking. Therapeutic blood levels are achieved in approximately 1 week. Patients are usually instructed to pick a quit date during the second week of therapy. Therapy is generally continued for 6 to 12 weeks, but can be continued for up to 6 months or longer based on the individual risks and benefits (Sohn et al., 2010). Bupropion may also be used in conjunction with a nicotine patch (Fiore et al., 2008).

The most recently released pharmacotherapy agent approved for the use in smoking cessation is varenicline (Chantix), which is a non-nicotine medication approved by the U.S. Food and Drug Administration (FDA) in 2006. Its actions consist of a partial nicotine receptor agonist effect as well as an antagonist effect. Varenicline is a medication that is titrated up to the maintenance dose of 1 mg twice daily. At this recommended dose, the patient's chance of long-term success triples. There is also evidence that with a lower dose of only 1 mg daily there is double the chance of long-term abstinence (Fiore et al., 2008).

Varenicline is renally cleared and must be used with caution with any renal insufficiency. Due to reports of depression, agitation, behavior changes, suicidal ideation, and even suicide, the FDA recommends that patients disclose any psychiatric history to their provider before starting the medication, and that providers monitor for any behavior or mood changes after starting a patient on the medication (Fiore et al., 2008). Varenicline is not used in conjunction with nicotine replacement therapy.

Cessation of smoking after an initial MI reduces CHD mortality rates by 50% (Sohn et al., 2010). Therefore, cessation counseling is an imperative nursing intervention. A rapid and substantial reduction in coronary risk occurs when smoking cessation is achieved. After 15 years of smoking cessation, the CHD risk of a former smoker approaches that of a nonsmoker (Sohn et al., 2010).

Although structured group-cessation programs can be very effective, the majority of smokers prefer to quit on their own or with individual counseling. In addition, the majority of people who have achieved cessation have done so on their own. Most smokers who successfully quit have had several previous unsuccessful attempts. It is crucial for nurses not to underestimate the importance of individualized education and support in the success of smoking cessation. A failed attempt at cessation should be viewed as practice for future successful cessation.

Because the rate of relapse in smoking cessation efforts is high, especially early in cessation efforts, relapse prevention is an important aspect of smoking cessation counseling and education. Relapse prevention counseling includes helping patients identify high-risk situations and providing coping skills to deal with those high-risk situations. When patients achieve smoking cessation, healthcare providers should congratulate them and encourage them during each visit to remain nonsmokers.

Issues that negatively affect cessation include depression and weight-management concerns. The average weight gain associated with smoking cessation is 6 to 10 lb (Sohn et al., 2010). Weight gain is caused by the metabolic changes associated with smoking cessation. If depression is associated with smoking cessation, then weight gain can increase. Weight gain is particularly a concern among female smokers. Premenstrual stress can also play a role in the smoking-cessation efforts of women. Planning a smoking-cessation date to avoid the peak of premenstrual stress is an important consideration.

Summary of factors critical to achieving smoking cessation are:

- brief counseling sessions by every healthcare provider during every patient encounter

- referral to structured follow-up programs or telephone QUIT lines

- use of medications in addition to counseling to increase effectiveness

- motivational interviewing techniques for those smokers currently not willing to make a quit attempt

- integration of relapse prevention into counseling techniques.

(Fiore et al., 2008; Gibbons et al., 2002)

Clinical Application

Listed here are practical guidelines (five A's) for smoking cessation counseling in any setting by any provider:

1. **Ask** *the patient if he or she uses tobacco.*

2. **Advise** *the patient about the importance of quitting.*

3. **Assess** *the patient's interest in quitting.*

4. **Assist** *the patient by helping him or her pick a quit date. Also assist by linking the*

patient to resources that can provide coun-
seling and pharmacotherapy.

5. ***Arrange*** *a follow-up phone call with the*
patient. Inform patient of available quit
line support 1-800-QUITNOW for access
to all state quit lines (Fiore et al., 2008).

Additional on-line resources available for
patients can be found at http://smokefree.gov

Hypertension

Hypertension is another major risk factor for CHD, including MI and sudden cardiac death. Those with hypertension have double the risk of developing CHD than those who have normal blood pressure (Dennison, Miller, & Cunningham, 2010). Hypertension is also an independent risk factor for the development of stroke and renal failure (Rosendorff et al., 2007). Each increase in 20 mm Hg for systolic blood pressure (SBP) or 10 mm Hg diastolic blood pressure (DBP) doubles the risk of a fatal coronary event (Rosendorff et al., 2007).

Hypertension can cause direct vascular injury and increases myocardial oxygen demand. Hypertension increases the work of the left ventricle, causing hypertrophy and increased left ventricular wall thickness, which puts patients at risk for subendocardial ischemia and diastolic dysfunction. Left ventricular hypertrophy can lead to left ventricular dilatation and, eventually, systolic dysfunction and heart failure.

The definition of hypertension is SBP greater than 140 mm Hg or DBP greater than 90 mm Hg. In addition, patients who are being treated for elevated blood pressure are considered to have hypertension even when their blood pressures are at goal. Blood pressure is considered normal only if it is less than 120 mm Hg systolic and less than 80 mm Hg diastolic. People who are considered prehypertensive (systolic pressure between 120 and 139 mm Hg and diastolic pressure between 80 and 89 mm Hg) require lifestyle modification to prevent cardiovas-

cular disease. There are now two stages of hypertension rather than three:

Stage 1: Systolic 140 to159 mm Hg or diastolic 90 to 99 mm Hg

Stage 2: Systolic 160 mm Hg or greater or diastolic of 100 mm Hg or greater.

(U.S. Department of Health and Human Services [USDHHS], 2004)

According to American Heart Association (AHA) statistics, 1 in every 3 adults has hypertension (Lloyd-Jones et al., 2009). Great strides have been made in increasing awareness of hypertension, but there is still much opportunity for improvement, including increasing the number of patients who achieve treatment goals among adults who have hypertension:

- Almost 79% are aware that they have high blood pressure.

- About 69% are under active treatment.

- Only 45% have their blood pressure under control.

(Lloyd-Jones et al., 2009)

The incidence of hypertension rises with age. The 20-year risk of developing hypertension in middle-aged men and women who are not yet hypertensive is greater than 90% (Rosendorff et al., 2007). Hypertension is more prevalent in men younger than 45 years of age. Between 45 and 64 years of age, men and women are equally affected by hypertension, and after 64 years of age a higher percentage of women than men have hypertension (Lloyd-Jones et al., 2009). The prevalence of hypertension in Blacks is substantially higher than in Whites and Blacks develop high blood pressure earlier in life and have higher average blood pressures (Lloyd-Jones et al., 2009). Women who take oral contraceptives have a higher prevalence of hypertension than women of childbearing age who do not take oral contraceptives. Other risk factors for the development of hypertension include family history, genetics, lower socioeconomic status, obesity, physical inactivity, psychological stress, dietary factors of high fat and sodium, high alcohol intake, and sleep apnea (Lloyd-Jones et al., 2009).

For people younger than 50 years of age, DBP is very important. As a person ages, however, SBP becomes a more important indicator of cardiovascular risk. In people older than 50 years of age, an SBP greater than 140 mm Hg is a more important indicator of cardiovascular risk than is diastolic hypertension (USDHHS, 2004). Although SBP continues to rise with age, DBP begins to decline at 60 years of age. This rise in SBP with associated decrease in DBP results in a widening of the pulse pressure. There is also an increased risk of cardiovascular events associated with a widened pulse pressure (Rosendorff et al., 2007).

Isolated systolic hypertension is defined as an SBP greater than 160 mm Hg with a normal DBP. Isolated systolic hypertension increases the risk of nonfatal MI and cardiovascular death in low-risk patients and the general population. Isolated systolic hypertension accounts for 70% of cases of hypertension in older adults (USDHHS, 2004). Systolic hypertension is often more difficult to control than diastolic hypertension. As antihypertensive medication is used to bring down SBP, there is concern that the DBP may drop too low in those with isolated systolic hypertension, especially in very old adults.

Clinical Application

The coronary arteries are perfused during diastole so it is important to maintain an adequate DBP.

In adults, 90% to 95% of hypertension is known as *primary,* or *essential,* hypertension. Essential hypertension is characterized by the existence of hypertension with no known cause. *Secondary hypertension* refers to hypertension with an identifiable cause that can be corrected. The vast majority of hypertension in children is secondary. The exact pathophysiology involved in essential hypertension is not fully understood. Possible contributing factors in essential hypertension include:

- excessive salt and water retention from impaired ability of the kidneys to excrete sodium and water

- dysfunction of the autonomic nervous system, with increased sympathetic nervous system stimulation and higher levels of circulating norepinephrine, resulting in increased vasoconstriction

- impaired endothelial dysfunction with decreased production of nitric oxide

- dysfunction of the renin-angiotensin-aldosterone system (RAAS).

Coexisting risk factors are also associated with essential hypertension, including hyperlipidemia, diabetes, and obesity. Although the majority of hypertension in adults is essential, healthcare providers should always assess for identifiable causes of secondary hypertension. An unidentified secondary cause is often the reason for resistant hypertension. The most common causes of secondary hypertension in adults include:

- chronic kidney disease

- renal artery stenosis

- primary aldosteronism

- sleep apnea.

Other possible causes of secondary hypertension include a variety of renal, endocrine, neurologic, and cardiac disorders. These possible causes will be discussed in the section on resistant hypertension.

Treatment of Hypertension

The Joint National Committee on Prevention, Detection, Evaluation, and Treatment of High Blood Pressure, a coalition of leaders from 46 healthcare agencies, established guidelines for treating hypertension that were released in 2003. Since that time, the AHA released a scientific statement in 2007: Treatment of Hypertension in the Prevention and Management of Ischemic Heart

Disease. Key points from these two documents include:

1. The ability to reduce blood pressure effectively is generally considered more important than the use of a specific agent.

2. First line agents typically include thiazide diuretics, angiotensin-converting enzyme (ACE) inhibitors (or angiotensin II receptor blockers), or calcium channel blockers.

3. Beta blockers may be used as the first line agent in patients who are post-MI or have coronary artery disease (CAD) with angina.

4. Two or more medications are usually required to effectively treat hypertension in the majority of patients. When initial blood pressure assessment is greater than 20 mm Hg systolic or 10 mm Hg diastolic above the blood pressure goal, then initiation of therapy with two medications should be considered. One of the two medications should be a thiazide diuretic.

5. Blood pressure lowering should achieve the goal of less than 140 mm Hg systolic and less than 90 mm Hg diastolic in patients without any co-existing conditions that increase risk.

6. Blood pressure lowering should achieve the goal of less than 130 mm Hg systolic and less than 80 mm Hg diastolic in patients with diabetes, chronic kidney disease, CHD, or any CHD risk equivalent.

7. DBP should be lowered slowly in any patient with evidence of myocardial ischemia. Caution should be used to avoid DBPs below 60 mm Hg in patients with CAD, or diabetes, or who are older than 60 years of age.

8. Patient motivation is critical in the effective treatment of hypertension. Empathy is a powerful motivator, and motivation improves when patients have positive relationships with their healthcare providers.

(Rosendorff et al., 2007; USDHHS, 2004)

Effective antihypertensive therapy greatly reduces CHD risk. Goals of hypertension management include the prevention of target organ damage:

- *Heart:* Hypertension is associated with the development of left ventricular hypertrophy, CAD, MI, and heart failure.

- *Brain:* Hypertension increases the risk of transient ischemic attacks and ischemic or hemorrhagic stroke. Malignant hypertension can also cause cerebral encephalopathy when blood pressure is so high that the brain can no longer maintain autoregulation.

- *Kidneys:* Hypertension causes nephropathy through the production of atherosclerotic renal lesions. Chronic renal disease causes hypertension, and hypertension accelerates the progression of chronic renal disease to end-stage disease.

- *Peripheral arteries:* Hypertension produces vascular damage that impairs endothelial vasodilatation and accelerates atherosclerosis in the peripheral arteries as well as in the coronary and cerebral arteries.

- *Eyes:* Vessel damage to the retina caused by hypertension is called *hypertensive retinopathy.*

Four lifestyle interventions have been shown in clinical trials to delay or prevent the onset of hypertension:

1. weight reduction
2. increased physical activity
3. sodium reduction
4. the DASH diet.

(USDHHS, 2004)

Weight reduction is the most effective lifestyle modification. Weight reduction can reduce blood pressure by 5 to 20 mm Hg per 5 lb of weight loss. For effective blood pressure management, patients should engage in physical activity almost every day for 30 to 45 minutes.

Some individuals are salt sensitive and others are not; therefore, sodium reduction impacts blood pressure for some patients and not others. All patients with high blood pressure should evaluate the effects of a sodium-restricted diet.

Clinical Application

It is important for patients with hypertension to understand that 75% of sodium intake comes from processed food, not from added salt.

After weight loss, the DASH diet is the second most effective lifestyle intervention. DASH stands for Dietary Approaches to Stop Hypertension. The DASH diet manipulates potassium, calcium, and magnesium, while holding sodium constant. Low calcium consumption is associated with hypertension and high potassium consumption is associated with lower blood pressure in people with hypertension.

The DASH diet is high in fruits, vegetables, and low-fat dairy products. It is low in saturated fat and total fat and rich in potassium and calcium. This diet has been found to reduce both systolic and diastolic blood pressure. The DASH diet can reduce blood pressure by 8 to 14 mm Hg (USDHHS, 2004). Unlike weight reduction, smoking cessation has not been shown to decrease blood pressure.

Pharmacological treatment of blood pressure has been shown to protect against stroke, coronary events, heart failure, and progression of renal disease and to reduce all-cause mortality. Thiazide diuretics are commonly used as first-line agents in the treatment of hypertension. Thiazide diuretics are cost effective and have a relatively low risk of side effects. The one concern about thiazide diuretics is the impact of thiazide-induced hyperglycemia and diabetes mellitus on long-term CHD risk (Rosendorff et al., 2007).

If a patient's blood pressure is greater than 20 mm Hg above systolic goal or 10 mm Hg above diastolic goal, then therapy can be started with two medications, one of which is typically a thiazide diuretic. Stage two hypertension treatment is started with two initial medications. All patients with hypertension should have their blood pres-

sures aggressively controlled to less than 140/90 mm Hg. Patients with diabetes, chronic kidney disease, CHD, or CHD risk equivalents have lower blood pressure targets of less than 130/80 mm Hg.

Special Considerations for Older Adults

Target blood pressure goals are the same for older adults as for younger adults. Older adults can show substantial benefits when hypertension is adequately treated. Systolic pressure, rather than diastolic, is a better predictor of events among this group of patients. Pseudohypertension may occur in older adults due to excessive vascular stiffness. Thiazide diuretics are also the preferred first-line treatment in older adults. Long-acting dihydropyridine calcium channel blockers (for example, amlodipine) can also be used.

Clinical Application

Assessment for orthostatic hypotension is particularly important in older adult patients being treated for hypertension. Their risk of orthostatic hypotension is greater because the percentage of water as body weight declines with age.

Special Considerations for African-Americans

African-Americans have the highest prevalence and severity of hypertension (Lloyd-Jones et al., 2009). Hypertension also develops earlier in life among this population. African-Americans produce less renin and, therefore, are not as receptive to beta-blockers or medications that block the RAAS. For this reason, pharmacological agents other than beta-blockers and ACE inhibitors (or angiotensin II receptor blockers) may be required to achieve blood pressure goals (USDHHS, 2004).

Special Considerations for Patients with Diabetes

An ACE inhibitor or angiotensin II receptor blocker is usually the first-line agent in patients with diabetes. Medications that interrupt the RAAS reduce microvascular and macrovascular complications in both type I and type II diabetes. ACE inhibitors reduce end-organ damage in patients with diabetes, even without the presence of hypertension. The blood pressure goal for effective management of hypertension in patients with diabetes is less than 130/80 mm Hg. Patients with diabetes commonly require two or more medications to keep their blood pressures within this limit (Rosendorff et al., 2007; USDHHS, 2004).

Special Considerations for Patients with Renal Disease

Three or more medications are generally needed to keep blood pressure below 130/80 mm Hg and reduce the decline of renal function in patients with renal disease (USDHHS, 2004). Medications that interrupt the RAAS are effective in decreasing renal disease in patients with diabetic and non-diabetic renal disease. Most patients with renal disease also need to be on loop diuretics in addition to antihypertensives.

Resistant Hypertension

Before the diagnosis of resistant hypertension is made, pseudo-resistance must be ruled out. Common causes of pseudo-resistance include the white coat effect, poor technique in taking blood pressure, or poor adherence by the patient to the prescribed regime. A patient is considered to have resistant hypertension if he or she is on 3 or more medications at full-dose therapy, including a diuretic, and still unable to achieve target blood pressure. A patient is also considered to have resistant hypertension if it takes 4 medications to achieve goal (Calhoun et al., 2008). Reasons for resistant hypertension, classified by lifestyle factors, contributing medications, and the presence of an underlying secondary diagnosis are listed in Box 4-2.

Strategies to treat resistant hypertension include:

1. Exclude the existence of pseudo-resistance.

2. Focus on lifestyle interventions, as appropriate, to reduce sodium intake, alcohol intake, and reduce body weight.

BOX 4-2: CAUSES OF RESISTANT HYPERTENSION

Lifestyle Related
- High dietary sodium
- Obesity
- Heavy alcohol intake

Medication Related
- Nonnarcotic analgesics, especially non-steroidal anti-inflammatory drugs (NSAIDs)
- Sympathomimetics (decongestants/diet pills)
- Stimulants
- Oral contraceptives
- Glucocorticoids and mineralcorticoids
- Herbals (ephedra/ma huang)
- Natural licorice (found in smokeless tobacco)

Secondary Diagnoses (Most Common)
- Obstructive sleep apnea
- Chronic kidney disease
- Primary aldosteronism
- Renal artery stenosis

Secondary Diagnoses (Less Common)
- Pheochromocytoma
- Cushing's disease
- Hyperparathyroidism
- Coarctation of the aorta
- Intracranial tumor

(Calhoun et al., 2008)

---

3. Discontinue or decrease doses of drugs that are contributing to hypertension. Nonsteroidal anti-inflammatory drugs (NSAIDS) are one of the more common culprits. Although acetaminophen can also cause an increase in blood pressure, its effects are less pronounced. Whenever possible, acetaminophen should be used for nonnarcotic pain relief. However, this may not be possible if anti-inflammatory effects are important. If required, the lowest dose of NSAIDs possible should be used.

4. Screen for secondary diagnoses. Certain clinical findings provide clues to the cause of secondary hypertension:

   • Abdominal or renal bruits are associated with renovascular disease. Bilateral renal artery stenosis should be suspected in patients with flash pulmonary edema, especially in the presence of normal ventricular function.

   • Unexplained hypokalemia can be associated with primary aldosteronism. However, hypokalemia may be a late sign and resistant hypertension can occur in this diagnosis without hypokalemia. Approximately 20% of those with resistant hypertension have primary aldosteronism.

   • Lower blood pressure in the legs than in the arms is associated with aortic coarctation.

   • Pheochromocytoma should be expected in patients with episodes of headache, palpitations, and sweating.

5. Maximize pharmacological therapy:

   • Maximize diuretic therapy with a long-acting thiazide diuretic. Chlorthalidone is the preferred agent in resistance.

   • Consider the possible addition of a mineral corticoid antagonist, such as spironolactone or eplerenone.

   • Use a loop diuretic if chronic kidney disease is present.

   • Combine medications that have different modes of actions. Recent research has shown favorable results when an ACE inhibitor or angiotensin receptor blocker is combined with a calcium channel blocker.

   • Consider giving at least one antihypertensive at bedtime to achieve better overall control.

(Calhoun et al., 2008)

Patients with resistant hypertension should be referred to a hypertension specialist if the cause of resistance cannot be determined or if control cannot be obtained within 6 months.

Clinical Application

Proper technique for blood pressure assessment includes using a proper sized cuff. Use of a cuff that is too small is one of the most common causes of inaccurate readings, resulting in a recorded measurement that is falsely high. An adult sized cuff should be used for upper arm circumferences of 27 to 34 cm. Arm circumferences larger or smaller require different size cuffs for accurate assessment (Pickering et al., 2005).

Patient Education and Long-term Management Issues

Patient adherence is an important part of therapy. The costs and side effects of medication should be carefully considered and discussed with the patient. Self-monitoring of blood pressure by patients has been shown to improve adherence because patients receive timely feedback from their therapy.

Patients need to be instructed to avoid over-the-counter medications, such as decongestants. They also need to receive information regarding the risk of untreated hypertension. Aggressive risk-factor modification is also indicated in any patient with coexisting risk factors. Patients should have monthly follow-up blood pressure checks with medication adjustments until target results are achieved. More frequent follow up is indicated for patients with stage 2 hypertension and for those with cardiovascular disease, renal disease, or diabetes.

After blood pressure goals are achieved, follow-up should continue at 3- to 6-month intervals. Serum potassium and creatinine levels should be evaluated twice annually to assess renal function. Dose reduction of medications should be attempted after 1 year of controlled therapy.

Clinical Application

Literacy, as well as healthcare literacy, is important to consider in providing patient education. Healthcare professionals often use terms that are not understood by patients. Illiteracy and healthcare illiteracy are often unrecognized because patients may be embarrassed and not disclose an inability to read or lack of understanding of instructions.

Dyslipidemia

Approximately 38% of the adult population and 10% of teenage children have abnormal lipid profiles (Lloyd-Jones et al., 2009). Elevated levels of cholesterol impact the function of the endothelium, resulting in impaired vasodilatation, increased platelet aggregation and monocyte adhesion, and increased thrombus formation.

Lipid levels may be affected by preexisting conditions, such as renal disease, hypothyroidism, and genetic lipoprotein disorders. Low-density lipoprotein cholesterol (LDL-C), high-density lipoprotein cholesterol (HDL-C), and triglycerides are all independent risk factors for cardiovascular disease. Hyperlipidemia includes elevated total cholesterol (hypercholesterolemia), elevated LDL-C, or elevated triglyceride levels. Dyslipidemia refers to hyperlipidemia or a low HDL-C level.

Hypercholesterolemia

There is a 20% to 30% increase in CHD risk for each 10% percent increase in serum cholesterol. There is also a corresponding 2% to 3% risk reduction for each 1% reduction in total cholesterol (Gibbons et al., 2002).

Elevated LDL-C

LDL-C levels should be less than 100 mg/dl for those with known CHD or a risk equivalent, according to the current published guidelines of the third Adult Treatment Panel (ATP-III) from the National Cholesterol Education Program (Grundy et al., 2002). Since the publication of these guidelines, however, new research has been published showing improved risk reduction when LDL-C goals of less than 70 mg/dl were met (Grundy et al., 2004). The most recent report of the National Cholesterol Education Program (Grundy et al., 2004) defines an LDL-C goal of less than 100 mg/dl as the minimal treatment goal for those with CAD. Setting an LDL-C goal of less than 70 mg/dl is a therapeutic option for high-risk patients. For primary prevention in healthy people, a LDL-C less than 130 mg/dl is considered optimal. Many experts believe the normal value should be lowered to less than 130 mg/dl for all people.

The size of LDL-C particles is also important. Smaller, denser particles are associated with a higher incidence and accelerated progression of CAD (Berra & Fair, 2010). Smaller particles might also be better able to enter the subendothelial space and be more prone to oxidation.

Hypertriglyceridemia

Borderline-high or high triglyceride levels are now considered independent risk factors for CHD. Borderline-high to high levels are 150 to 500 mg/dl. Alcohol and estrogen use can contribute to hypertriglyceridemia.

Low HDL-C

HDL-C facilitates the transport of excess cholesterol back to the liver. This role helps explain the protection HDL-C provides against the development of heart disease. The lower the concentration of HDL-C, the higher the risk of CHD:

- HDL-C less than 40 mg/dl = low HDL-C
- HDL-C greater than 60 mg/dl = high HDL-C

High levels of HDL-C are associated with a decreased risk of CHD. A 2% to 3% reduction in risk is associated with a 1 mg/dl increase in HDL-C (Kramer, Newton, & Froclicher, 2010). In general, women typically have higher HDL-C levels than do men. Estrogen tends to raise HDL-C levels and might explain why premenopausal women are usually protected from heart disease.

Treatment of Hyperlipidemia

The ATP-III guidelines of 2002 were the first updated management guidelines since 1993. With these new guidelines, the number of people eligible for cholesterol-lowering medications tripled. These guidelines recommend a screening with a fasting lipid profile once every 5 years beginning at 20 years of age. Table 4-1 defines cholesterol values according to the ATP-III guidelines.

LDL-C Treatment Goals

Approximately one third of treated patients are at their LDL-C treatment goals and less than 20% of those with CHD are at their LDL-C goals (Lloyd-Jones et al., 2009). For healthy people with high total cholesterol and high LDL-C, the following therapeutic lifestyle changes are recommended within the ATP-III guidelines:

- Reduce intake of saturated fats to less than 7% calories from saturated fat and less than 200 mg/day of cholesterol. Also reduce trans fats to less than 1% of calories (Gidding et al., 2009).

- Allow monounsaturated fats to be up to 20% of calories. Choose fats and oils with less than 2 g of saturated fat per tablespoon. Use canola oil or olive oil. Avoid tropical oils and hydrogenated vegetable oils.

- Increase soluble fiber to 20 to 30 g per day by eating oats, legumes, grains, vegetables, and fruits.

- Follow a healthy eating plan. Obtain carbohydrates primarily from whole grains, fruits, and vegetables. Include five servings of fruits and vegetables daily with six servings of whole grains. Low-fat dairy products should be included and proteins should come from fish, legumes, skinless poultry, and lean meats. Fish, especially oily fish, should be included in the diet at least twice weekly (Gidding et al., 2009). Avoid foods with partially hydrogenated oils. Foods high in calories and low in nutrition should be limited. These include candy and soft drinks containing high amounts of sugar. Limit alcohol intake to a moderate amount. Eat foods with little or no salt. These guidelines do not need to be applied to every meal but rather to an overall eating pattern over several days.

- Achieve a caloric balance between intake and expenditure, and increase physical activity to achieve weight loss if needed. To balance the number of calories consumed with the number expended each day, multiply the patient's weight by 15 calories. This is the typical number of calories used per day by a person who is moderately active. People who are less active require fewer calories.

- Increase physical activity and exercise.

- Use 2 g of plant sterols or stanols per day. Sterols are a group of compounds found in the cell membranes of plants and animals. Cholesterol is a sterol found in animal cells. Plant sterols, however, are poorly absorbed and

TABLE 4-1: CHOLESTEROL VALUES			
Total Cholesterol	**LDL-C**	**HDL-C**	**Triglycerides**
< 200 desirable	< 100 optimal and minimal goal for those with CHD *new research* < 70 optimal	< 40 low	< 150 normal
200-239 borderline	100-129 above optimal	≥ 60 desirable	150-499 borderline-high to high
≥ 240 high	130-159 borderline-high 160-189 high ≥ 190 very high		≥ 500 very high
(Grundy et al., 2002; Grundy et al., 2004)			

not synthesized by the human body and can be used to help lower cholesterol levels. Some sterols are saturated to form a stanol derivative. Spreads fortified with plant sterols or stanols are available commercially. Soybeans and sesame and sunflower seeds also contain plant sterols. Sterols or stanols are added to the diet after 6 weeks if total cholesterol and LDL-C goals are not met.

• Pharmacological agents are added to the treatment plan if target levels are not met at 12 weeks.

• Follow an interdisciplinary approach to lowering lipids, involving physicians, dietitians, nurse experts, exercise specialists, and pharmacists.

(Grundy et al., 2002)

If a person has CHD or a risk equivalent, then secondary prevention guidelines are used. These include obtaining a lipid profile within 24 hours of admission for hospital inpatients and initiating lipid-lowering therapy prior to discharge. Patients should continue lifestyle interventions while on medication therapy. In addition, the American College of Cardiology/American Heart Association (ACC/AHA) guidelines for secondary prevention recommend an increased consumption of omega-3 fatty acids.

Clinical trials have shown that reducing cholesterol reduces the risk of MI, stroke, and death for people with and without a history of CHD. A large meta-analysis evaluating 38 cholesterol-lowering trials demonstrated that for every 10% reduction in total cholesterol, there was a 15% reduction in death related to CHD (Grundy et al., 2002). Results have been shown to be effective regardless of age, sex, or diabetes status. Newer trials have shown that high-risk groups benefit from statins, even when they have normal LDL-C levels, and outcomes are improved when LDL-C levels are taken below the currently recommended guidelines (Grundy et al., 2004). For most patients with existing CAD, treatment is indicated (Gibbons et al., 2002). Patients with diabetes are considered to

have the same risk as those with known CHD and therefore should have the same target LDL-C goals as those patients with CAD. Most patients with diabetes are prescribed lipid-lowering drugs to achieve an LDL-C reduction of 30% to 40%, regardless of baseline LDL-C levels (Fonseca et al., 2005). As with all patients who are at high-risk for cardiovascular disease, an LDL-C goal of less than 70 mg/dl is a therapeutic option. The LDL-C goal is a primary treatment goal in secondary prevention. Table 4-2 outlines the effects of cholesterol-lowering medications on LDL-C levels.

TABLE 4-2: EFFECTS OF LIPID-LOWERING DRUGS ON LDL-C LEVELS	
Class of Drugs	**% Reduction**
HMG-CoA reductase inhibitors (standard doses)	↓ 30% to 40%
Bile acid resins	↓ 15% to 30%
Nicotinic acid	↓ 15% to 30%
Fibrates	↓ 5% to 20%
Intestinal absorption inhibitors	↓ 18%
(Berra & Fair, 2010; Grundy et al., 2002; Grundy et al., 2004)	

Decreasing triglycerides and normalizing insulin sensitivity can reduce small, dense LDL-C particles. Certain lipid-lowering medications also have a favorable impact on LDL-C particle size. These medications include bile acid sequestrants, nicotinic acid, and fibrates (Berra & Fair, 2010).

Secondary Treatment Goals

Treatment for triglycerides and HDL-C levels are considered secondary to treatment for LDL-C levels. The exception is when a patient's triglyceride levels are greater than 500 mg/dl; then, triglyceride reduction may be considered before LDL-C reduction. Table 4-3 outlines the effects of cholesterol-lowering medications on triglyceride levels and HDL-C.

Diabetes Mellitus

The American Diabetes Association has established the criteria for diagnosis of diabetes mellitus

TABLE 4-3: EFFECTS OF LIPID-LOWERING DRUGS ON HDL-C AND TRIGLYCERIDE LEVELS

Class of Drugs	HDL-C % Increase	Triglyceride % Reduction
Nicotinic acid	↑ 15% to 35%	↓ 20% to 50%
Fibrates	↑ 10% to 20%	↓ 20% to 50%
HMG-CoA reductase inhibitors	↑ 5% to 15%	↓ 7% to 37%
Bile acid sequestrants	↑ 3% to 5%	does not decrease, may even increase
Intestinal absorption inhibitors	↑ 1%	↓ 8%

(Berra & Fair, 2010; Grundy et al., 2002)

as a random glucose greater than 200 mg/dl, a fasting glucose greater than 126 mg/dl, or a hemoglobin (Hb) A1C greater than 6.5% (American Diabetes Association, 2010; Kramer et al., 2010). Type 1 and type 2 diabetes mellitus increase a person's risk for CHD because of the accelerated atheromatous process associated with diabetes. Approximately 246 million people world wide have diabetes mellitus (Thomassian, 2010), with an increasing number of cases being diagnosed each year. By the year 2030, it is predicted that over 30 million people in the United States will have the diagnoses of diabetes (Thomassian, 2010). Type 2 diabetes accounts for 90% to 95% of all diabetes; therefore, diabetes is considered a modifiable risk factor. Diabetes increases the risk of all forms of cardiovascular disease, including stroke and peripheral vascular disease. Diabetes doubles the CHD risk for men and increases it five to seven times for women (Kramer et al., 2010).

Underlying causes of type II diabetes include obesity, physical inactivity, and genetics. The onset of diabetes can be postponed or prevented with aggressive lifestyle modification, including weight loss and increased levels of physical activity. Long-term diabetes control is an important measurement of risk and is assessed using the Hb A1C level. An Hb A1C level greater than 7% indicates uncontrolled diabetes.

Diabetes is associated with both microvascular and macrovascular complications. Microvascular complications include retinopathy, nephropathy,

neuropathy, and amputation. Macrovascular complications include CHD and stroke. Eighty percent of all diabetes-related deaths result from atherosclerotic disease, with CHD accounting for 75% of those deaths (Gibbons et al., 2002). In addition to being at higher risk for developing cardiovascular disease, patients with diabetes who suffer MIs are also at risk for developing higher complications, including heart failure, postinfarction angina, and mortality (Kramer et al., 2010).

Many of the modifiable risk factors for CAD are also risk factors for the development of type 2 diabetes, including obesity, physical inactivity, hypertension, HDL-C level less than 35 mg/dl, and triglyceride level greater than 250 mg/dl. Low HDL-C and high triglyceride levels are the common pattern of dyslipidemia in people with type 2 diabetes. Weight loss and increased physical activity improve these parameters and also modestly lower LDL-C. The Heart Protection Study showed a 22% reduction in major cardiovascular events in patients with diabetes who were taking simvastatin (a statin lipid-lowering medication). This study also showed that patients with diabetes older than 40 years of age, with total cholesterol levels greater than or equal to 135 mg/dl, may benefit from statin therapy, regardless of baseline LDL-C (Fonseca et al., 2005; Grundy et al., 2004).

Glycemic control (Hb A1C less than 7) reduces the risk of microvascular complications of diabetes (Gibbons et al., 2002; Skyler et al., 2009). The Hb A1C goal for non-pregnant adults is less than 7%

to reduce the risk of microvascular complications in both type 1 and type 2 diabetes. Some subgroups of patients with diabetes may also receive some reduction in macrovascular risks from tight glycemic control. These subgroups include type 1 diabetes and those with recently diagnosed type 2 diabetes who have not yet developed atherosclerotic disease. A more liberal Hb A1C goal might be appropriate in select populations, including those with a history of significant hypoglycemia and those who already have advanced complications, co-morbidities, and limited life expectancy (Skyler et al., 2009).

In general, tight glycemic control alone has not been found to be the primary strategy for reducing macrovascular complications in patients with diabetes. To reduce the risk of macrovascular complications, patients with diabetes need a comprehensive plan for risk reduction, including lipid-lowering therapy with statins, hypertension control, and aspirin therapy (Skyler et al., 2009).

Clinical Application

Patients with diabetes (without CAD) may need special instructions regarding their goals for LDL-C and blood pressure. Diabetes is considered a risk equivalent for CHD; therefore, patients with diabetes should have an LDL-C level less than 100 mg/dl (or less than 70 mg/dl based on newest research) and blood pressure less than 130/80 mm Hg.

Obesity

Obesity in the United States has reached an epidemic level, with projections indicating that 40% of adults and 25% of children will be obese by the year 2015 (Kuminyika et al., 2008). The AHA has identified obesity as a major cardiovascular risk factor. In addition, obesity adversely affects most other risk factors for CHD, including hypertension, dyslipidemia, and type 2 diabetes mellitus. It also increases myocardial oxygen demand in patients with CHD due to left ventricular hypertrophy associated with obesity.

Body mass index (BMI) is commonly used to define overweight and obesity. Box 4-3 defines a method for estimating BMI and for evaluating the results. BMI less than 25 is considered healthy for all adults, regardless of age. A BMI of 25 relates to approximately 110% of ideal body weight. BMI measurement is limited because it does not take into account distribution of body fat. Distribution of fat tissue around the abdomen increases CHD risk more than the distribution of fat tissue around the hip and pelvic area. Waist-to-hip ratios provides information about the distribution of fat tissue. A waist-to-hip ratio less than 0.8 for women and less than 1.0 for men is considered normal. Waist circumference is another way to evaluate body fat distribution around the abdomen. Waist circumferences greater than 35 inches for women and greater than 40 inches for men are considered criteria for abdominal obesity (Kumanyika et al., 2008).

BOX 4-3: BODY MASS INDEX

Estimated BMI calculation:

$$\frac{\text{Weight in lb}}{\text{Height in inches}^2} \times 703$$

BMI measurements

Healthy = 18.5 to 24.9

Overweight = 25.0 to 29.9

Obese = > 30

Extreme obesity = > 40

BMI goal: < 25

(Centers for Disease Control and Prevention, 2009; Kumanyika et al., 2008)

A healthy diet and an exercise program designed for weight loss are recommended for people with BMIs of 25 to 30. The simple goal is that energy expenditure must exceed energy intake for weight loss to occur. A healthy diet and exercise program should strive for 1 lb per week of weight loss. A negative caloric balance of 400 calories per day produces a weight loss of 1 lb per week. Guidelines for healthy eating should be applied as a primary strategy for achieving weight loss. These guidelines were discussed in the section on dyslipidemia. Moderate intensity activity of 60 minutes per day is recommended for those trying to achieve a healthy weight (Kumanyika et al., 2008).

The achievement of weight loss is especially important for people with hyperlipidemia, hypertension, or elevated blood glucose levels. Achievement of weight loss has the following beneficial effects:

- improved lipid levels
- lowered blood pressure
- improved insulin resistance
- reduction in metabolic syndrome and type 2 diabetes.

Behavioral programs that incorporate self-monitoring, goal setting, and problem solving are the most effective in helping people achieve weight loss (Kumanyika et al., 2008). Pharmacological agents may be considered in high-risk patients with BMIs greater than 30.

Obesity is not only a risk factor for cardiovascular disease; it also increases the risk of other diseases and impacts the pathology of other chronic conditions (Kumanyika et al., 2008). Although the benefits of weight loss are clear and significant, weight loss goals are difficult to achieve. Most treatments for obesity have not demonstrated effective long-term results. Adequate treatment for obesity requires a long-term commitment of at least a year and treatment is not typically covered by insurers (Kumanyika et al., 2008). Obesity treatment is complex, involving hereditary and environmental factors that play a role in weight management. Even for those who are able to achieve weight loss, there is the challenge of successful maintenance because regaining of weight after successful loss is common.

Although challenging, clinicians can help increase the success of weight loss efforts by understanding that dietary counseling must involve more than providing information. Assessing the patient's readiness to change as well as assessing for barriers to success are two key components to effective weight loss counseling. To utilize these techniques effectively it is important for clinicians to be educated regarding behavior change and motivational interviewing.

Clinical Application

Prevention of obesity, especially in children, needs to be a high priority of healthcare providers because long-term weight loss is difficult to achieve after obesity occurs.

Clinical Application

Specific strategies that can be used in providing weight loss counseling include:

- *Instruct the patient to self-monitor eating by keeping a journal for several days (this strategy can be used throughout the change process).*
- *Set short-term goals such as a 10% initial weight loss.*
- *Encourage the patient to weigh him or herself regularly.*
- *Deliver simple positive messages such as*
  - *eat more fruits and vegetables.*
  - *drink water instead of soda with meals.*
  - *split meals when dining out.*

Metabolic Syndrome

Metabolic syndrome represents a grouping of lipid and nonlipid risk factors of metabolic origin. Metabolic syndrome is present in 20% to 25% of the population. This represents approximately 48 million people. Metabolic syndrome is closely linked to the generalized disorder of insulin resistance. Excess body fat and physical inactivity promote the development of insulin resistance. Metabolic syndrome abnormalities include:

- defective glucose uptake by skeletal muscle

- increased release of free fatty acids by adipose tissue

- overproduction of glucose by the liver

- hypersecretion of insulin by beta cells in the pancreas.

A diagnosis of metabolic syndrome is made when three or more of the following indicators are present:

- waist circumference greater than 40 inches for men and greater than 35 inches for women

- triglyceride level greater than 150 mg/dl

- HDL-C level less than 40 mg/dl for men and less than 45 mg/dl for women

- blood pressure greater than 135 mm Hg systolic or greater than 85 mm Hg diastolic

- elevated fasting glucose level greater than 100 mg/dl.

Physical Inactivity

Like obesity, physical inactivity is associated with other cardiovascular risk factors. Modest amounts of exercise can result in important health benefits. Higher levels of activity and fitness are associated with decreased risk of CHD (Kramer et al., 2010). Exercise is recommended for primary and secondary prevention of cardiovascular disease. Benefits of exercise include:

- lowered blood pressure

- decreased platelet aggregation

- increased HDL-C

- improved glucose metabolism

- reduction in bone loss

- improvement of weight loss

- decreased depression and anxiety

- decreased risk of chronic disease, including type 2 diabetes, cardiovascular disease, and certain types of cancer.

For primary prevention, healthy people should exercise aerobically at a moderate level (equivalent to a brisk walk) for a minimum of 30 minutes per day, 5 days a week, or at a vigorous level for a minimum of 20 minutes, 3 days a week. Shorter durations of activity can be counted toward the minimum requirements if the activity lasted a minimum of 10 minutes. Shorter periods of activity along with general activities of daily living cannot be counted toward the minimum requirements (Haskell et al., 2007).

In addition to aerobic activity, muscle strength training is recommended to be done on two nonconsecutive days of each week. Muscle strength training should include 8 to 10 exercises with enough weight to produce fatigue after 8 to 12 repetitions per exercise. Muscle strength training prevents bone loss during middle age and also promotes the development of lean muscle mass, which is more efficient in helping achieve weight loss. Any activity above the minimum recommendations will result in greater health benefits (Haskell et al., 2007).

Walking, as a component of secondary prevention, has been shown to increase survival, decrease reoccurrence rates, and also slow progression of CHD (Gibbons et al., 2002). In addition, walking improves quality of life and decreases hospitalization. For detailed information about cardiac rehabilitation and activity progression after an acute event, see Chapter 5.

Physical activity in the older patient population can be challenging but it is no less important. In addition to aerobic activity and muscle strength training, flexibility, and balance exercises are also important. In older patients, activity has the added benefit of decreasing disability, functional decline, and risk of falls. If an older adult can achieve the minimum recommended level of activity, it is important that the step approach be used to gradually increase activity and avoid the risk of a sedentary lifestyle (Nelson et al., 2007).

Stress and Other Psychosocial Risk Factors

The body has a physiologic response to psychological stress. Stress can cause coronary vasoconstriction. A release of catecholamines in response to stress also promotes alterations in thrombosis and coagulation to favor clot formation. The number of MIs in the early morning hours are higher than during other times of the day because of morning increases in levels of circulating catecholamines. Exposure to acute stress or highly stressful life events can also increase the risk of an acute cardiac event (Maden & Froelicher, 2010).

Depression, anxiety, anger, and hostility are other psychosocial risk factors associated with the development of CHD. Hostility is the most powerful of these risk factors (Gibbons et al., 2002). There are two theories used to explain the increased risk of CHD related to psychosocial factors. The first theory is based on the physiological neuroendocrine response to psychosocial stress. The second theory is related to poor health behaviors of people with these psychosocial risk factors (Maden & Froelicher, 2010).

Alcohol

Moderate alcohol intake can produce protective cardiovascular effects by increasing HDL-C, lowering platelets, and enhancing fibrinolysis. Light drinkers have lower blood pressures than nondrinkers and those who drink in excess. Excessive alcohol intake can lead to hypertension and increase the risk of sudden cardiac death, in addition to other adverse effects associated with high alcohol consumption.

The AHA recommends moderate alcohol consumption for appropriate individuals, including those with no contraindications to moderate alcohol consumption and those with no cultural or religious beliefs against alcohol use. Moderate alcohol consumption is defined as no more than one alcoholic beverage per day for women and no more than two alcoholic beverages per day for men.

EMERGING RISK FACTORS

In recent years, much information has developed on what have been termed "emerging risk factors." Despite the emergence of novel risk factors, their predictive value has not been found to be any more effective than a traditional risk score such as the Framingham Risk Score (Rosendorff et al., 2007).

Hyperhomocysteinemia

Increased homocysteine levels are independently associated with increased risk of cardiovascular disease. Elevated homocysteine levels are responsible for producing endothelial toxicity, accelerating the oxidation of LDL-C, impairing endothelial-derived relaxation factor, and impairing arterial vasodilatation (Kramer et al., 2010). Deficiencies in folate and vitamins B6 and B12 lead to elevated serum levels of homocysteine. Supplementation with folic acid and B vitamins decreases homocysteine levels. However, there is currently no evidence that lowering homocysteine levels decreases cardiovascular mortality and morbidity. Supplementation with folic acid, with or without vitamin B6 or B12, is not recommended as a secondary prevention strategy (Anderson et al., 2007).

Lipoprotein (a) Level

Lipoprotein (a) (Lp[a]) has been shown to be an independent factor in cardiovascular risk (Berra & Fair, 2010). Lp(a) is similar to LDL-C. There is currently a lack of standardization for Lp(a) testing, and more research is needed to fully understand its role. In clinical practice, reduction in LDL-C similarly reduces risks associated with Lp(a).

Oxidative Stress

Although much has been written about the harmful effects of oxidative stress, the AHA discourages the use of antioxidant vitamin supplements, such as vitamin E, vitamin C, beta carotene, and selenium, and instead recommends dietary changes to increase antioxidant intake. Increased consumption of fruits and vegetables increases antioxidant levels. Cruciferous vegetables and blueberries are particularly high in antioxidants.

Left Ventricular Hypertrophy

Left ventricular hypertrophy increases with age, obesity, and hypertension, and is independently associated with an increased risk of cardiovascular disease, including an increased risk for the development of MI, heart failure, and sudden cardiac death (Gibbons et al., 2002). When associated with a reduction in blood pressure, a decrease in left ventricular mass can reduce a person's risk of cardiovascular disease. Reduction of left ventricular mass can be achieved with effective treatment of hypertension.

Inflammation and Infection

Atherosclerosis is a diffuse inflammatory process. Extravascular sources of chronic infection are thought to be possible culprits in the inflammatory process. Chlamydia pneumoniae is one infectious agent that is associated with atherosclerotic plaque. Herpes simplex virus is another agent that has been proposed as a culprit (American Heart Association, n.d.).

High-sensitivity C-reactive protein (hs-CRP) is elevated during systemic inflammation and high blood levels represent a marker of cardiovascular risk. Those people with hs-CRP levels in the top one third have two times the risk of MI compared to those with levels in the lower one third. The value of hs-CRP as an independent marker of risk has not been completely established (American Heart Association, n.d.). Traditional risk factors of smoking, dyslipidemia, hypertension, and elevated glucose are also associated with the inflammatory response. Hs-CRP testing is not routinely done because those with traditional risk factors warrant aggressive treatment, regardless of hs-CRP levels. In addition, other noncardiovascular conditions that cause inflammation can cause an elevation is hs-CRP.

Special Recommendations Regarding Prevention in Women

Hormone replacement therapy was once thought to protect women from heart disease after menopause. However, the landmark Heart and Estrogen/Progestin Replacement Study concluded that hormone replacement therapy should not be initiated in women with heart disease (Grady, Herrington, Bittner et al., 2002).

In addition, the Women's Health Initiative Clinical Trial arm that examined the effects of continuous combined hormone replacement therapy (estrogen-progestin [Prempro]) was stopped in July 2002, when the risks associated with this therapy were shown to outweigh the benefits (Kramer et al., 2010). This large study demonstrated a substantial increase in cardiovascular risk among women taking this form of hormone replacement therapy. The study showed an increased risk of heart disease, stroke, breast cancer, and dementia in women older than 65 years of age. It also showed a relative risk reduction for hip fracture and colorectal cancer (Kramer et al., 2010).

The estrogen alone arm of the Women's Health Initiative was stopped in March 2004. Again, the risks of therapy were felt to exceed the benefits. The study showed a neutral impact on heart disease and breast cancer but an increased risk of stroke and dementia in women older than 65 years of age. There was also a decreased risk of hip fracture with this therapy (Kramer et al., 2010). The Women's Health Initiative demonstrated that hormone replacement therapy should not be used for the primary prevention of CHD in women. Evidence-based guidelines for cardiovascular disease prevention in women state that hormone therapy and selective estrogen receptor modulators should not be used for the primary or secondary prevention of CHD (Mosca et al., 2007). In addition, according to these guidelines, aspirin for primary prevention is generally not indicated in women younger than 65 years of age.

CONCLUSION

The burden of cardiovascular disease is great; thus, the opportunity for prevention is also great. Risk factors associated with CHD are on the rise in the United States. However, the majority of cardiovascular risk factors are considered modifiable, and even small changes in risk factors can have significant results. Risk factor reduction, including smoking cessation, reduction of LDL-C, and effective treatment of hypertension, has been proven to reduce the risk of cardiac events. It is also likely that control and reduction of other risk factors, including diabetes mellitus, HDL-C, triglycerides, obesity, depression, and physical inactivity, will also reduce the risk of cardiac events (Gibbons et al., 2002). Cardiovascular nurses must see risk factor modification as a primary goal for all patients, even healthy ones, in all settings. Through education, motivation, support, and referral, nurses can use their knowledge of cardiovascular risk and risk reduction to make an impact on this devastating disease.

EXAM QUESTIONS

CHAPTER 4
Questions 27-36

Note: Choose the one option that BEST answers each question.

27. Secondary prevention of CHD is best described as prevention of

    a. obesity in adolescents.

    b. subsequent cardiac events in people who have already had a cardiac event.

    c. disability from secondhand smoke.

    d. hypertension and hyperlipidemia.

28. One group of people considered to have a risk equivalent for CHD are those with

    a. type 2 diabetes.

    b. a history of tobacco use.

    c. hypertension.

    d. a type A personality and job stress.

29. Examples of nonmodifiable cardiac risk factors include

    a. smoking and hypertension.

    b. hyperlipidemia and type 2 diabetes.

    c. metabolic syndrome and obesity.

    d. age and family history.

30. One true statement concerning women and heart disease is

    a. women have better survival rates than men after a heart attack.

    b. heart disease is the second leading cause of death in women, after cancer.

    c. women commonly present with different symptoms of heart disease than do men.

    d. hormone replacement therapy has been shown to significantly reduce the risk of heart disease in women after menopause.

31. The single most important modifiable cardiovascular risk factor is

    a. smoking.

    b. physical inactivity.

    c. elevated homocysteine level.

    d. low HDL-C.

32. When providing smoking cessation counseling, it is important to

    a. inform the patient of the minimal risk reduction associated with smoking.

    b. instruct all patients with a cardiac history to avoid nicotine replacement therapy.

    c. include information about relapse prevention.

    d. only provide counseling one time to avoid offending the patient.

33. A true statement concerning lifestyle modifications and blood pressure is

    a. smoking cessation is the most effective lifestyle change for lowering blood pressure.

    b. weight loss and the DASH diet are the two most effective lifestyle interventions for lowering blood pressure.

    c. no lifestyle intervention has proven effective in reducing blood pressure.

    d. lowering cholesterol is the most effective lifestyle change for lowering blood pressure.

34. The ATP-III guidelines for lifestyle changes in cholesterol reduction include

    a. consuming less than 1% of all calories from fat.

    b. using herbal supplements before each meal.

    c. eating 20 to 30 g of fiber daily.

    d. avoiding the use of all monounsaturated fats.

35. The LDL-C goal for patients with CAD is

    a. less than 100 mg/dl, according to the ATP-III guidelines, and even lower according to recent research.

    b. less than one half of total cholesterol.

    c. less than 160 mg/dl if HDL-C is normal.

    d. dependent on the patient's triglyceride and total cholesterol levels.

36. Characteristics associated with metabolic syndrome include

    a. smoking, high circulating hormone levels, and hypertension.

    b. type 2 hypertension and type 2 diabetes.

    c. elevated catecholamines, severe obesity, and sleep apnea.

    d. high triglycerides, low HDL-C, and abdominal obesity.

CHAPTER 5

CORONARY HEART DISEASE AND ACUTE CORONARY SYNDROMES

CHAPTER OBJECTIVE

After completing this chapter, the learner will be able to discuss the scope of coronary heart disease management throughout the continuum of presentation, from stable angina through acute myocardial infarction.

LEARNING OBJECTIVES

After completing this chapter, the learner will be able to

1. describe the pathophysiology associated with vulnerable plaque and acute coronary syndromes.

2. define the difference between stable and unstable angina.

3. explain the goals of medical treatment of coronary heart disease.

4. describe the importance of aggressive risk factor management in the treatment of coronary heart disease.

5. contrast non-ST-segment elevation myocardial infarction with unstable angina.

6. define the primary treatment strategy for patients with ST-segment elevation myocardial infarction and those with non-ST-segment elevation myocardial infarction

7. discuss potential complications of myocardial infarction.

8. explain the benefits of participation in a formal cardiac rehabilitation program as part of a long-term management strategy after acute coronary syndrome.

INTRODUCTION

Coronary heart disease (CHD) is responsible for 1 in every 5 deaths in the United States and is the number one killer in both men and women. In the U.S., someone experiences a coronary event every 25 seconds (Lloyd-Jones et al., 2009). Although death rates have fallen from CHD over the last 40 years, someone still dies approximately each minute from a coronary event in the United States (Lloyd-Jones et al., 2009).

CHD is the presence of atherosclerosis or atherosclerotic plaque in the epicardial coronary arteries. As atherosclerotic plaque progresses, the lumen of the coronary artery can become narrowed and blood flow can be impaired. Reduced blood flow can lead to ischemia (a lack of oxygen to the myocardium). Prolonged ischemia can result in injury and, ultimately, necrosis of myocardial tissue. The presentation of CHD ranges from stable angina to acute myocardial infarction (MI). The term *acute coronary syndrome* (ACS) is used to describe the presentation of CHD in the form of unstable angina (UA), non-ST-segment elevation MI (non-STEMI), or ST-segment elevation MI (STEMI).

PATHOPHYSIOLOGY OF CORONARY HEART DISEASE

The development of CHD begins in adolescence and continues throughout life. CHD is considered a chronic condition. Cardiovascular risk factors (discussed in Chapter 4) accelerate the process. Atherosclerosis involves the deposit of lipids, calcium, fibrin, and other cellular substances within the lining of the arteries (Aouizerat, Gardner, & Altman, 2010). This deposit initiates a progressive inflammatory response in an effort to heal the endothelium. The end result of this inflammatory process is the production of a fibrous atherosclerotic plaque that can partially or totally occlude blood flow.

Although atherosclerosis begins early in life, it may not produce clinical symptoms for several decades. The first step in the development of atherosclerotic plaque is the accumulation of intimal macrophage foam cells that are rich in lipids. As time progresses, smooth muscle cells become more involved as they accumulate intracellular lipids, and fatty streaks form between the endothelium and the intima of the artery (Aouizerat et al., 2010; Rimmerman, 2010). In this early developmental phase, the inflammatory process is activated and immune cells, such as T lymphocytes and mast cells, begin to invade the lesion (Aouizerat et al., 2010). As progression continues, extracellular lipids are deposited among the layers of smooth muscle cells. These deposits begin to destroy the integrity of intimal smooth muscle cells.

As the lesion matures into one of clinical significance, an extracellular lipid core develops (Rimmerman, 2010). This core is sometimes called an *atheroma*. Calcium deposits may be contained within the lipid core. At this stage, foam cells also die and contribute their necrotic components to the growth of the lipid core. The lipid core thickens the artery wall, usually at the external edge, but does not greatly narrow the lumen. Eventually, fibrous tissue (mainly collagen) forms a fibrous cap that covers the lipid core (Aouizerat et al., 2010; Rimmerman, 2010). This lesion is sometimes referred to as a *fibrous atheroma* due to the accumulation of the fibrous connective tissue within the intima. These lesions cause more noticeable vessel narrowing and are clinically significant because they are prone to ulcerations and sudden rupture. Microscopic ulcerations of the vulnerable plaque initiate plaque rupture in most coronary events. Both mechanical and inflammatory vascular changes impact the vulnerability of plaque (Aouizerat et al., 2010).

The release of enzymes from immune response cells contributes to the vulnerability of rupture by weakening the collagen matrix of the fibrous cap. When a plaque ruptures, the core of the lipid is exposed to circulating blood (Rimmerman, 2010). This exposure results in platelet adherence, activation, and aggregation and activation of the coagulation pathway, with resultant thrombus formation. After rupture, reparative cells respond, and incorporate existing thrombi into the expanding lesion. New fibrous tissue is formed to repair the lesion, (Aouizerat et al., 2010) causing further narrowing of the lumen of the vessel. At this stage in the atherosclerosis process, the tunica media and tunica adventitia are also affected by the inflammatory response.

Stable plaques have thick fibrous caps that separate the lipid core from the endothelium. Stable plaques are less complicated than vulnerable plaques and tend to have smooth outlines. More vulnerable plaques have thinner caps. The edge of the fibrous cap, called the *shoulder,* is a particularly vulnerable area and is commonly the location of ruptured plaque (Rimmerman, 2010). Both mechanical features and inflammatory responses impact the vulnerability of a lesion. The role of the inflammatory response in ACSs has been the focus of new emerging risk factors that measure levels and risk of vascular inflammation. Biomarkers for this inflammation include high-sensitivity C-reactive protein, fibrinogen, homocysteine, lipoprotein A, serum amyloid A, and interleukin-6 (Aouizerat et al., 2010).

Rupture of a coronary plaque produces an acute coronary event and increases the short-term risk of cardiac death or nonfatal MI (Anderson et al., 2007). It is important to know that most vulnerable plaques identified during cardiac catheterization (angiography) are not found in tightly stenotic vessels. Patients can have plaque in the coronary arteries that does not cause lumen stenosis. This plaque can be visualized using intracoronary ultrasound. It is this plaque that is usually most vulnerable and the cause of ACSs. In most patients, MI results from atheromas that produce less than 50% narrowing of the vessel lumen (Aouizerat et al., 2010). Plaques that cause greater than 75% stenosis, and therefore angina, are usually more stable plaques and less likely to rupture. Figure 5-1 compares features of vulnerable and stable plaque.

FIGURE 5-1: VULNERABLE PLAQUE COMPARED TO STABLE PLAQUE

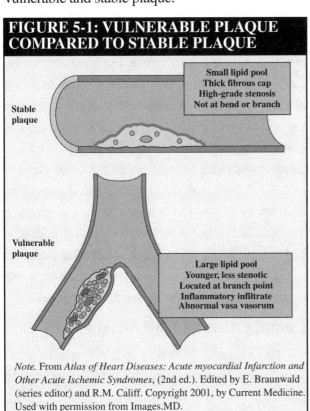

Note. From *Atlas of Heart Diseases: Acute myocardial Infarction and Other Acute Ischemic Syndromes*, (2nd ed.). Edited by E. Braunwald (series editor) and R.M. Califf. Copyright 2001, by Current Medicine. Used with permission from Images.MD.

Because vulnerable plaque typically does not produce symptomatic stenotic disease, stress testing has a limited ability to detect vulnerable plaque. Vulnerable plaque may not be visible as a stenotic lesion, but may be visualized using intracoronary ultrasound cardiac catheterization.

Clinical Application

When a patient with CHD risk factors has a cardiac catheterization that shows minimal stenotic disease, it is important to understand that this patient may still have a substantial plaque burden and may be at high risk for vulnerable plaque rupture. Aggressive risk factor modification is key in such patients as well as for patients with stenotic disease. Patients with significant risk factors are at the highest risk for progressive atherosclerosis. For this reason, all patients with risk factors should be aggressively treated with risk-reduction strategies, regardless of the results of diagnostic tests.

Clinical Signs and Symptoms of Coronary Heart Disease

Patients with CHD develop symptoms due to an imbalance between oxygen supply and demand. Angina pectoris is the clinical symptom that results from decreased blood flow to the myocardium. It usually occurs in patients with CHD involving 70% or more stenosis that also involves at least one major epicardial artery (Gibbons et al., 2002). Decreased blood flow results in ischemia, or a temporary lack of oxygen to the heart muscle. Although typically caused by CHD, angina can also be caused by other cardiac conditions, such as coronary artery spasm, valvular heart disease, uncontrolled hypertension, and hypertrophic cardiomyopathy (HCM).

Most patients describe angina as a sensation of pressure, tightness, heaviness, burning, or squeezing. This sensation can be felt behind the sternum and in the upper back, shoulder, arm, jaw, or epigastric area. Angina is rarely described as a sharp or stabbing pain, and it should not worsen with changes in position or respiration. Anginal pain usually does not occur in the middle to lower abdomen and does not usually radiate to the lower extremities. The duration of angina is typically defined in minutes, as opposed to seconds or hours.

Some patients do not experience any of the symptoms as described above. Instead, they may experience dyspnea, nausea, palpitations, or diaphoresis, alone or in combination. These additional symptoms also may be accompanied by discomfort of the chest, back, shoulder, arm, or jaw. Approximately 50% of patients with acute MI have had preceding angina (Gibbons et al., 2002).

When assessing a patient with angina, ask the following questions regarding symptoms:

- What is the quality of discomfort (pressure, squeezing, heaviness)?

- Where is the discomfort located? Does it radiate? If so, where?

- When did the discomfort start, and how long did it last?

- What came before the discomfort?

- What lessens or relieves the discomfort? What makes it worse?

Clinical Application

It is important to use the word "discomfort" when assessing patients with potential angina. Many patients with dyspnea or chest pressure deny the presence of pain.

FEATURES OF ANGINA

Angina pectoris can be classified as stable or unstable.

Stable Angina

Stable angina pectoris typically occurs with physical exertion or emotional stress and is relieved by rest or sublingual nitroglycerin. Angina is considered stable when its pattern is predictable over several weeks. To be considered predictable, angina should be triggered by the same amount of physical or emotional stress and should be easily relieved by rest or sublingual nitroglycerin.

Unstable Angina

Angina is considered unstable when it occurs with minimal exertion or when an increased dose of nitroglycerin is required to achieve relief. Rest angina is also considered unstable angina. Any angina that increases in severity or is very severe on first presentation is considered unstable. Unstable angina is caused by unstable or ruptured plaque that causes abrupt closure of a coronary artery. It is treated very differently than stable angina. This treatment will be discussed later in this chapter, in the section on non-STEMIs and UA.

Aggravating Factors

Patients with CHD develop symptoms due to an imbalance between oxygen supply and demand. Certain conditions can upset the balance between myocardial oxygen supply and demand. Conditions that can increase myocardial oxygen demand include hyperthermia, hypertension, tachycardia, and conditions that produce overstimulation of the sympathetic nervous system, such as cocaine use and hyperthyroidism. Certain coexisting cardiac conditions can also increase myocardial oxygen demand and reduce supply, including aortic stenosis and HCM. Noncardiac conditions that decrease the delivery of oxygen to tissues can also exacerbate angina. These include conditions that decrease hemoglobin levels (such as gastrointestinal bleeding) or conditions that decrease oxygen saturation levels (such as exacerbations of chronic lung disease).

Complications of Chronic Angina

The extent of ischemia and its impact on left ventricular function determine the outcomes in patients with angina (Gibbons et al., 2002). Complications of ischemia include the development of mitral regurgitation or left ventricular thrombi. These complications are a result of left ventricular dilation and dysfunction.

Angina in Women

The presentation of angina in women is often different than in men. Coronary spasm, mitral valve prolapse, and microvascular disease are more likely to be the cause of symptoms in women. Women presenting with anginal symptoms who proceed to cardiac catheterization have less documented stenotic disease of major epicardial coronary arteries. Women are also more likely to have UA than acute MIs (Anderson et al., 2007). Women are also older on presentation with ACSs and have a higher incidence of complications, including the development of heart failure (Anderson et al., 2007). Substernal chest pressure that radiates to the arm or jaw is less common in women than in men. Women may complain of more generalized epigastric discomfort or present with less specific complaints, such as dyspnea or fatigue. Women are also prescribed less intensive pharmacological regimes for CHD than men, including less frequent prescription of aspirin (Anderson et al., 2007).

Many women, and even some healthcare providers, do not consider heart disease a major health risk for women. For this reason, many women delay presenting with symptoms and may attribute their symptoms to other noncardiac causes. Although heart disease kills more women than all cancers combined, many women still consider breast cancer and other forms of cancer as their primary health risk.

Clinical Application

Women presenting with symptoms of discomfort from their nose to their navel should be evaluated for the presence of CHD. Women should be educated about the risk and specific manifestation of CHD in their gender.

Before menopause, women appear to have a protective mechanism in place against CHD. However, after menopause, the risk of CHD in women begins to approach that of men, but they lag behind men in their presentation of CHD by about 10 years. The protective effect of the premenopausal state has led to testing and use of hormone replacement therapy as a strategy to reduce the risk of heart disease in women. However, based on the results of the Women's Health Initiative, hormone replacement therapy is no longer a recommended strategy to reduce the risk of heart disease in postmenopausal women (Kramer et al., 2010).

Angina in Older Adults

Among older adults, angina is commonly described with more generalized symptoms, such as weakness, dyspnea, and confusion. These symptoms are often attributed to the aging process, and the possibility of angina is overlooked.

Older adults also face special challenges in the medical management of angina. In many cases, these patients have multiple factors that impact the effects of cardiovascular drugs. In addition, many medications need to be started at lower doses. Older adults are particularly sensitive to drugs with a hypotensive response. This population is also more likely to have coexisting conditions that complicate treatment.

Angina in People with Diabetes

Autonomic dysfunction occurs in about one third of patients with diabetes and can affect the symptoms they experience with angina and ACSs. Patients with diabetes may be less likely to experience pain. Up to 25% of all patients presenting with ACSs have diabetes (Anderson et al., 2007). Patients with diabetes have more severe multivessel disease and also have higher rates of complications after acute cardiac events.

DIAGNOSIS OF CORONARY HEART DISEASE

Initial diagnosis of CHD involves a thorough history and physical examination, including a 12-lead electrocardiogram (ECG). Lab studies, cardiac imaging studies, stress testing, and cardiac catheterization may be used as additional diagnostic tools. Assessment information also includes the presence of cardiovascular risk factors and a history of CHD, cerebrovascular disease, or peripheral vascular disease, which increases the likelihood that the presentation of symptoms is related to myocardial ischemia.

The 12-lead ECG can be normal in up to 50% of patients with chronic stable angina (Gibbons et al., 2002); therefore, a normal ECG does not exclude CHD. However, an abnormal ECG or the presence of a cardiac dysrhythmia increases the likelihood that CHD is the cause of the symptoms.

In addition to a 12-lead ECG, initial assessment parameters for evaluating a patient for CHD include blood pressure, ankle-brachial index, and laboratory testing, including hemoglobin level and hematocrit to rule out anemia, a fasting blood sugar level to rule out diabetes, and a fasting lipid profile to assess for hyperlipidemia.

When a patient presents with potential symptoms of angina, other cardiac and noncardiac conditions should be considered. Pulmonary disorders, gastrointestinal disorders, chest wall pain and, sometimes, psychiatric conditions can have symptoms similar to those of angina.

Stress Testing

Stress testing, with or without myocardial imaging, is a common tool used in the diagnosis of CHD. Stress testing can be done using exercise or chemicals. Treadmills or bicycles are used for exercise stress tests. Certain patients are not candidates for exercise stress testing without accompanying myocardial imaging because the ECG alone may not provide adequate diagnostic information. These patients include those with left bundle branch block, greater than 1 mm ST-segment depression at rest, paced ventricular rhythm, or Wolff-Parkinson-White syndrome (Gibbons et al., 2002).

When patients exercise, myocardial oxygen demand increases and coronary arteries dilate in response to this increased demand. In a patient with CHD, the coronary arteries are not able to adequately dilate to meet the needs of the increased myocardial oxygen demand, and abnormalities occur on the 12-lead ECG or associated imaging studies. The most common protocol for exercise stress testing is the Bruce protocol. Table 5-1 describes the key features of the Bruce and modified Bruce protocols.

Four pharmacological agents are used in chemical stress testing: dobutamine, dipyridamole, adenosine, and regadenoson. Dobutamine works differently from the other 3 agents. Dipyridamole, adenosine, and regadenoson cause coronary microvascular dilatation similar to the coronary artery vasodilation that occurs with exercise. The coronary vasodilation caused by these three medications is related to interaction with the adenosine A2a receptor, which is responsible for coronary vasodilation. In addition to stimulation of this adenosine receptor, dipyridamole and adenosine are non-selective adenosine receptor stimulators and also stimulate the A1, A2b, and A3 receptors. Stimulation of these other receptors is what causes the unwanted side effect of atrioventricular (AV) block (A1 receptor) and bronchospasm (A2b and A3 receptors). Due to the vasodilation effect, all three medications commonly cause chest pain because vasodilation pulls blood away from compromised areas of the myocardium. Another common side effect caused by vasodilation is flushing. Because of the risk of bronchospasm, any patient with reactive airway disease or active wheezing prior to stress testing is not a candidate for dipyridamole or adenosine. Because of the selectivity to

TABLE 5-1: COMMON EXERCISE STRESS TEST PROTOCOLS

Type of Protocol	Stage 1 Starting Point	Key Features
Bruce Protocol	1.7 mph 10% grade 5 metabolic equivalents (METs)	• Stage 2: 2.5 mph, 12% grade, 7 METs • Stage 3: 3.4 mph, 14% grade, 9 METs • There are a maximum of 10 potential stages • 3 minute stages to allow for achievement of steady state • Increase in MET level between stages is more pronouned than in other protocols
Modified Bruce Protocol	1.7 mph 0 grade	• Two warm up stages of 3 minutes each • 2nd stage: 1.7 mph and 5% grade • 3rd stage corresponds to stage 1 of standard Bruce protocol • Used in elderly and those with decreased exercise capacity due to cardiac function

(Akinpelu & Gonzalez, 2009)

the A2a receptor, regadenoson does not have the side effects of AV block or bronchoconstriction. Another advantage of regadenoson over dipyridamole and adenosine is that it can be given via a rapid 10-second infusion and does not need to be weight-based. Dipyridamole and adenosine are weight-based infusions given over 4 minutes. Aminophylline can be given as an antidote to all three medications but is seldom needed with adenosine because of its short half-life or with regadenoson because of its limited side effects.

All pharmacological stress testing is done in conjunction with myocardial imaging. In the United States today, more than one third of stress tests done with myocardial perfusion imaging are done with chemicals (O'Donnell, Mehta, Faulhaber, 2008).

Clinical Application

Patients scheduled for chemical stress testing involving adenosine or dipyridamole should be assessed for the presence of lung disease and wheezing prior to the test. Patients who are currently taking aminophylline-containing medications should not undergo chemical stress testing involving dipyrdamole, adenosine, or regadenoson because aminophylline coun-teracts the medications being administered for the stress test.

Dobutamine stress testing more closely mimics exercise stress testing. During a dobutamine stress test, high-dose dobutamine is used to increase contractility and heart rate, thereby increasing myocardial oxygen demand. In response to this increased myocardial oxygen demand, the coronary arteries dilate. They do not, however, dilate to the extent they do with agents that produce more direct coronary vasodilation. A potential side effect of dobutamine that is not present with dipyridamole, adenosine, or regadenoson is cardiac tachydysrhythmias.

Exercise or chemical stress testing is combined with pretest cardiac imaging, such as cardiac echocardiography or radionuclide imaging; pretest and posttest cardiac images are compared. When echocardiography is used, CHD is suspected when echocardiography images show a new wall motion abnormality after exercise or after the administration of high-dose dobutamine. Echocardiography is not used as the imaging modality with dipyridamole, adenosine, or regadenoson stress testing. When radionuclide imaging is used, the peak stress images are compared to the resting images. An area of relative hypoperfusion on the peak stress images is suspicious for CHD.

The imaging portion of a stress test provides information about the extent, severity, and location of ischemia. The exercise portion of a stress test (excluding dipyridamole and adenosine testing) can provide prognostic information (Gibbons et al., 2002). One example of prognostic information obtained from exercise stress testing is the heart rate recovery score. This score is calculated by taking the heart rate at peak exercise and subtracting the heart rate at 1-minute after exercise. A normal score is a heart rate greater than 12 beats per minute; this is associated with a low risk of death. A low score is considered less than 8 beats per minute and is associated with a high risk of death. A score of 8 to 12 is considered an intermediate risk (Gibbons et al., 2002). When patients are able to exercise on a treadmill for 6 to 12 minutes, exercise stress testing is generally performed instead of chemical stress testing. Patients on beta-blockers who are scheduled to undergo exercise stress testing should have these medications held for approximately 48 hours prior to testing. If these medications are not held, an adequate heart rate may be difficult to achieve. Exercise stress testing is less sensitive in women than in men (Gibbons et al., 2002).

There are certain absolute contraindications to stress testing in high-risk patients, including those with:

- acute MI less than or equal to 2 days old
- acute myocarditis or pericarditis
- acute pulmonary embolism
- acute aortic dissection
- symptomatic heart failure
- severe aortic stenosis
- symptomatic dysrhythmias
- high-risk unstable angina.

(Gibbons et al., 2002)

Coronary Computed Tomography Angiogram

Coronary computed tomography angiogram (CTA) can be used to assess for calcium deposits or soft fatty plaque in coronary arteries. The utilization of this technology in the diagnosis of coronary artery disease (CAD) is rapidly evolving. The procedure involves the administration of an iodine-based contrast agent and the patient does receive an exposure to radiation. As the technology evolves and technique improves, radiation doses are being lowered. The administration of an intravenous (IV) beta-blocker is used to slow the heart rate and capture the best images. Although coronary CTA is less invasive than cardiac catheterization, the latter remains the gold standard in the diagnosis of CAD. Currently, coronary CTA demonstrates the most diagnostic value in the following patient subgroups: a) patients who are asymptomatic and have a high risk for CHD, b) patients with low to intermediate risk who have atypical symptoms, c) patients with low to intermediate risk who have symptoms with negative biomarkers and a nondiagnostic ECG, and d) patients who have a stress test with equivocal results (Anderson et al., 2007; Cleveland Clinic, n.d.).

Cardiac Catheterization

Cardiac catheterization, or angiography, is currently the gold standard for determining the presence, location, and extent of obstructive CHD. Cardiac catheterization is an invasive procedure that has a small but serious risk of adverse outcomes, including stroke, MI, and death. For this reason, patients are carefully chosen and must meet certain criteria. The American Heart Association and American College of Cardiology have very specific guidelines stating indications for cardiac catheterization. Patients for whom cardiac catheterization is an indication include:

- patients with disabling angina, despite medical treatment

- patients with high-risk criteria for CHD on noninvasive testing

- patients who have survived sudden cardiac death

- patients with angina and clinical signs of CHD

- patients with low ejection fractions and ischemia on noninvasive testing

- patients with inadequate information obtained from noninvasive testing.

(Gibbons et al., 2002)

In addition to determining the location and severity of lesions, cardiac catheterization can evaluate intracardiac pressures and left ventricular function. Cardiac catheterization is also done to evaluate patients with possible vasospastic angina who have chest pain at rest. Provocative testing can be done in the cardiac catheterization laboratory using ergonovine maleate. If needed, intracoronary vasodilators can be given to treat the induced spasm.

Patients can receive diagnostic cardiac catheterization and return home the same day if no further treatment is done. Cardiac catheterization is performed by inserting a catheter through the femoral artery and guiding it to the heart. If femoral artery access cannot be used, then radial or brachial access can be used. Care of the insertion site (usually the groin) after the procedure is a major nursing focus. A period of bed rest in an observation unit is indicated after the procedure. The amount of bed rest required prior to discharge depends on the type of closure used for the femoral artery insertion site. If the traditional method of sheath removal is used, the patient typically remains on bed rest for 4 to 8 hours. If a closure device is used, then a much shorter period of bed rest and an earlier discharge are possible. Nursing care after cardiac catheterization involves frequent assessment of the insertion site for external bleeding and hematoma development. Distal pulses are also assessed to assure adequate circulation.

Clinical Application

The development of bleeding or a hematoma at the insertion site is treated by applying firm manual pressure. Patients and families must be instructed to activate the Emergency Medical Services (EMS) and apply firm manual pressure to the site if bleeding occurs after discharge.

TREATMENT OPTIONS FOR STABLE ANGINA

Stable patients who are diagnosed with greater than 70% stenosis during cardiac catheterization have three primary treatment options: medical treatment, primary (percutaneous) coronary intervention (PCI), or coronary artery bypass grafting (CABG). PCI most often includes balloon angioplasty with either a bare metal or drug-eluting stent. Lifestyle modification and aggressive risk factor reduction is included in all three treatment arms. The goal of medical treatment in CHD is to improve quality of life by reducing symptoms and preventing complications that include disease progression, MI, and death. The highest priority of treatment is to prevent death. When treatment decisions are made, first preference is given to those treatments proven to reduce the risk of death (Gibbons et al., 2002).

Pharmacological Management

Treatment of angina usually begins with medical therapy. Medical management of patients with CHD includes the use of a combination of medications:

- antiplatelet therapy

- antianginal therapy

- lipid-lowering therapy (discussed in Chapter 3).

Antiplatelet Therapy

Antiplatelet therapy is prescribed for all patients. Aspirin is the primary antiplatelet agent used for patients with known CHD or those with symptoms suggestive of CHD. For patients with known CHD, peripheral vascular disease, or stroke, aspirin in doses from 75 to 325 mg has been shown to reduce the risk of MI, stroke, and vascular death by approximately 33% (Gibbons et al., 2002).

Clopidogrel was found to be more effective than aspirin in reducing the risk of MI, stroke, and death in patients with atherosclerotic vascular disease (Hirsch & Bhatt, 2004). However, there is a dramatic cost difference between aspirin and clopidogrel that prevents clopidogrel from being more widely used as a primary antiplatelet agent. Clopidogrel is used as an alternative for patients who are aspirin sensitive (Rimmerman, 2010). Prasugrel, a newer antiplatelet agent, is not indicated in the treatment of stable angina. It is indicated to prevent thromboembolic complications in patients with ACS who are treated with PCI (Gold Standard/Elsevier, 2010).

Antianginal Agents

Patients with CHD are also prescribed antianginal agents. These agents include beta-blockers, nitrates, and calcium channel blockers. The goals of antianginal therapy are to reduce symptoms and improve activity tolerance, thereby improving quality of life.

Beta-blockers

Beta-blockers are the first-line agents in the treatment of stable angina. Beta-blockers are very effective in controlling angina brought on by physical exertion. The initial target heart rate goal is 55 to 60 beats per minute at rest for patients with stable angina (Gibbons et al., 2002). Resting heart rate may need to be lowered if angina cannot be controlled. Patients can experience side effects with beta-blockers that limit dosing and they are not used to treat vasospastic angina. Beta-blockers are the one class of antianginal medications that have survival benefits in certain groups of patients, such as those patients who have had a recent MI (Antman et al., 2004; Kushner et al., 2009).

Nitrates

Nitrates improve exercise tolerance and prolong the time to onset of angina. For nitrates to remain effective, patients need to have an 8- to 10-hour nitrate-free period each day. Headache is the most common side effect of nitrate use. Headaches usually subside over time in patients taking long-acting nitrates. Patients with a history of angina should always carry sublingual nitroglycerin.

Clinical Application

Headaches associated with nitroglycerin administration should be treated because pain activates the sympathetic nervous system, which increases myocardial oxygen demand and, potentially, myocardial ischemia.

Calcium channel blockers

Calcium channel blockers or long-acting nitrates are used as first-line agents for vasospastic angina because they are direct coronary vasodilators. These medications can also be added to beta-blocker therapy when angina is not controlled. Calcium channel blockers must be used very cautiously in patients with impaired systolic left ventricular dysfunction. Amlodipine and felodipine (newer dihydropyridine calcium channel blockers) are more selective coronary arterial vasodilators and are better tolerated than other calcium channel blockers in patients with left ventricular dysfunction (Gibbons et al., 2002).

Ranolazine

In 2006 the FDA approved ranolazine for the treatment of angina. The exact mechanism of action is not fully understood, but it is thought that ranolazine works on the cardiac ion channels to reduce the amount of intracellular sodium. Increased intracellular sodium can result in an increase in intracellular calcium due to the sodium-calcium exchange pump. By lowering intracellular sodium, ranolazine can reduce intracellular calcium overload and improve ventricular function. Because of impact on the cardiac action potential, ranolazine can also prevent dysrhythmias induced by ischemia. Unlike other antianginal agents, the effects of ranolazine are not dependent on changes in heart rate or blood pressure. Ranolazine is not used as a first-line antianginal medication because of its ability to prolong the QT interval. Ranolazine is used in combination with other antianginal agents including amlodipine, beta-blockers, and nitrates (Mayo Clinic, 2010).

For a more detailed discussion of pharmacological agents, see Chapters 2 and 3.

Nonpharmacological Treatment Options

PCI and CABG are the two nonpharmacological treatment options for patients with CHD. These two forms of cardiac revascularization are discussed, along with transmyocardial revascularization, in Chapter 6.

External counterpulsation is another nonpharmacological treatment option that is used for patients with debilitating angina on maximal medical therapy and those who are not candidates for revascularization. During this therapy, a series of cuffs are wrapped around the patient's legs. Compressed air is used to apply pressure in the cuffs in synchronization with the cardiac cycle. The cuff pressure results in an increased arterial pressure that is used to increase retrograde aortic blood flow into the coronary arteries during diastole. Patients receive 35 hours of treatment over a 4- to 7-week period (Gibbons et al., 2002).

Long-Term Management

For patients with stable angina, it is important to evaluate the effectiveness of risk factor reduction with each follow up. An assessment of the patient's anginal symptoms, functional capacity, and tolerance to medications is also important. The patient should know to report worsening angina or rest angina. Follow-up office visits are usually scheduled every 4 to 6 months during the first year after initiation of antianginal therapy. Long-term follow up is generally based on the patient's other existing medical conditions but should occur at least annually. Patients with conditions that exacerbate angina require more frequent follow-up. Follow up visits can be alternated between the primary care physician and cardiologist.

Clinical Application

Patients who alternate follow-up visits between a cardiologist, a primary care physician, and perhaps another specialist need to be instructed on the importance of always carrying a current medication list to alert all involved physicians of any medication changes between office visits.

ACUTE CORONARY SYNDROME OVERVIEW

CHD presents in a continuum, as seen in Figure 5-2. Patients presenting with an ACS are treated differently from patients presenting with stable angina. During an ACS, there is urgency

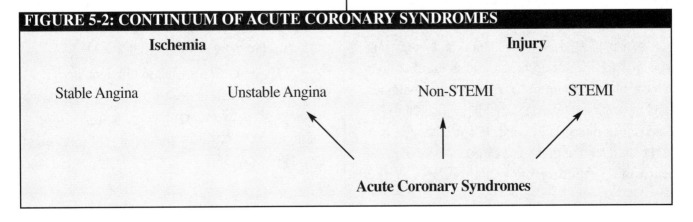

FIGURE 5-2: CONTINUUM OF ACUTE CORONARY SYNDROMES

Ischemia　　　　　　　　　　　　　　　　　　　　　　Injury

Stable Angina　　　　　Unstable Angina　　　　　Non-STEMI　　　　　STEMI

Acute Coronary Syndromes

for treatment to preserve myocardial function. Acute myocardial ischemia develops when oxygen supply is insufficient to meet the metabolic demands of cardiac cells. When cells are deprived of oxygen, ischemia occurs within 10 seconds. Myocardial function is affected after 1 minute of ischemia, and cells begin to swell after just a few minutes. After 20 minutes of oxygen deprivation, irreversible cellular injury begins to occur (Aouizerat et al., 2010).

Clinical Application

All patients should be taught the importance of immediately seeking medical attention for any symptoms that could suggest a heart attack. Patients need to understand the physiological importance of early treatment in preserving myocardial function.

ACSs include UA, non-STEMI, and STEMI. The rupturing of unstable vulnerable plaques is a frequent cause of ACS. When vulnerable plaques rupture, thrombi form at the site of injury, blocking blood flow and causing ischemia or injury to myocardial cells. Patients with a longer history of ischemic heart disease may have collateral circulation that provides protection during the occlusion of a coronary vessel. Collateral vessels are those that connect major branches of coronary arteries. As luminal narrowing gradually occurs, pressure changes promote the development and use of these collateral vessels to supply oxygen to ischemic areas. New capillaries can grow in response to ischemia. Younger patients without collateral circulation are more vulnerable to extensive damage from an occluded coronary artery.

When an ACS begins, the endocardial region is the first to become ischemic and is the first area where tissues begin to die. As ischemia continues and the injury extends, the middle myocardium (or subendocardium) is affected. If left untreated and MI continues, the injury can extend toward the epicardium, affecting the full thickness of the

myocardium. A full-thickness MI is commonly referred to as a transmural MI.

Differentiating ST-Segment Elevation MI and non-ST-Segment Elevation MI

MIs are now classified by their initial presentation as either STEMI or non-STEMI. Figure 5-3 compares a normal ST-segment with two examples of ST-segment elevation. Patients presenting with STEMI are candidates for reperfusion therapy.

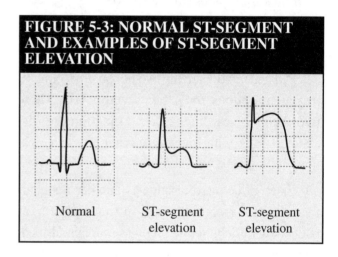

FIGURE 5-3: NORMAL ST-SEGMENT AND EXAMPLES OF ST-SEGMENT ELEVATION

Normal   ST-segment   ST-segment
                elevation   elevation

STEMI and non-STEMI can both produce either a Q-wave or non-Q-wave MI. Non-Q-wave MIs are usually associated with damage that has not extended through the full thickness of the myocardium. A Q-wave MI is diagnosed by the presence of a pathological Q-wave in the leads of infarction on a 12-lead ECG. This type of MI is usually associated with full thickness damage of the myocardium. Q-waves are the first negative deflection of the QRS complex. When they are too large, they represent altered depolarization due to necrotic tissue. Figure 5-4 shows an example of a Q-wave that is considered pathological. Pathological Q-waves are more common with STEMI.

A 12-lead ECG is used to differentiate STEMI from non-STEMI. However, a 12-lead ECG cannot distinguish between non-STEMI and UA. Cardiac biomarkers help differentiate between these two conditions.

ST-SEGMENT ELEVATION MYOCARDIAL INFARCTION

An estimated 500,000 STEMIs occur each year (Antman et al., 2004; Kushner et al., 2009). Complete occlusion of a vessel by a thrombus produces STEMI. Figure 5-5 shows an occlusive clot responsible for STEMI. Patients with STEMIs are classified more specifically by the portion of the left ventricle suffering injury.

Primary Treatment Strategy in STEMI

Reperfusion is the primary treatment strategy in STEMI because the underlying pathophysiology is a fibrin stable clot. However, adjunctive supportive pharmacological treatment can be administered while the patient is prepared for a reperfusion strategy. The administration of supportive pharmacological therapy should not delay the time to reperfusion. Supportive pharmacology is discussed later in this chapter.

Patients with STEMI need to receive reperfusion therapy as quickly as possible. Reperfusion is defined as the restoration of oxygen to ischemic tissue. Two methods of reperfusion are available: administration of fibrinolytics or PCI. If a patient is receiving a fibrinolytic, the drug should be administered within 30 minutes of arrival in the emergency department (ED) or on first contact with the paramedics. If a patient is receiving PCI, balloon inflation should occur within 90 minutes of arrival in the ED or at first contact with the paramedics.

PCI is the preferred method of reperfusion if patients can be promptly treated within the 90-minute time frame by an experienced operator in an experienced cardiac catheterization laboratory. Fibrinolysis is the preferred method of reperfusion when there is a delay to PCI or if PCI is not an option. If any contraindications to fibrinolytic therapy exist, the patient should be transferred directly to a facility capable of performing PCI. PCI is also the

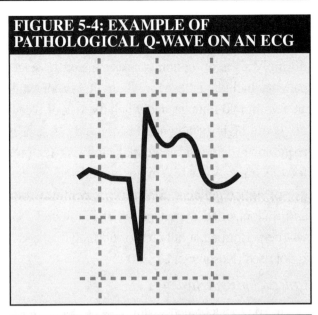

FIGURE 5-4: EXAMPLE OF PATHOLOGICAL Q-WAVE ON AN ECG

FIGURE 5-5: OCCLUSIVE CLOT PRODUCING STEMI

Platelet-rich

First diagonal

Note. From *Atlas of Heart Diseases: Acute Myocardial Infarction and Other Acute Ischemic Syndromes* (2nd Ed.) Edited by E. Braunwald (series editor) and R.M. Califf. Copyright 2001, by Current Medicine. Used with permission from Images.MD.

preferred option for safety reasons if the onset of symptoms is longer than 3 hours, if there is any question as to the diagnosis of STEMI, and in patients in shock or with severe congestive heart failure (Antman et al., 2004; Kushner et al., 2009). A planned facilitated PCI (after administration of a fibrinolytic) is an option for reperfusion in select patients, including those for whom PCI is not available within 90 minutes and when the risk of bleeding is not high. A thorough history and physical is required to determine potential high-risk features for bleeding. A few examples would include the use of anticoagulants, a history of peptic ulcers, and uncontrolled hypertension. If facilitated PCI will be performed, a full dose of fibrinolytic therapy is not used (Kushner et al., 2009).

Criteria for Reperfusion

In addition to patients with ST-segment elevation on a 12-lead ECG, patients with a new (or presumably new) left bundle branch block and those with evidence of posterior wall MI are also candidates for immediate reperfusion therapy. An initial ECG should be completed within 10 minutes of arrival to the hospital, if not already completed in route by EMS. If the initial ECG is not diagnostic of ST-segment elevation and the patient remains symptomatic, then serial ECGs should be done at 5- to 10-minute intervals until a diagnosis is made or until symptoms resolve (Antman et al., 2004; Kushner et al., 2009). Imaging studies such as echocardiography can also be done in the ED if the patient's symptoms suggest acute MI but the ECG is not clearly demonstrating ST-segment elevation. An echocardiogram shows wall motion abnormality of the affected wall during an acute MI.

ST-segment elevation may be difficult to determine in the presence of left bundle branch block because a normal degree of ST-segment elevation exists with left bundle branch block. In posterior wall MI, ST-segment elevation does not show on a standard 12-lead ECG, but an echocardiogram may show poor function of the posterior wall, helping to confirm the diagnosis. Reperfusion with PCI is discussed in detail in Chapter 6.

Fibrinolytic Therapy

There are inclusion and exclusion criteria for the administration of fibrinolytics. Criteria necessary to administer fibrinolytics include:

- symptom onset within 12 hours of administration (ideally within 3 hours)
- ST-segment elevation greater than 1 mm in two leads evaluating the same wall of the myocardium or the presence of a new left bundle branch block
- ECG and other findings consistent with a true isolated posterior wall MI.

Contraindications to the administration of fibrinolytics include:

- prior intracranial hemorrhage
- known structural cerebrovascular lesion
- malignant intracranial neoplasm
- significant closed head injury within the last 3 months
- ischemic stroke within the last 3 months (unless within the last 3 hours)
- suspected aortic dissection
- active bleeding or bleeding diathesis (excluding menses)
- symptoms older than 24 hours
- ST-segment depression (unless indicative of a true posterior wall MI).

(Antman et al., 2004; Kushner et al., 2009)

Several fibrinolytic agents are available. Some are fibrin selective and, therefore, clot specific; others are nonfibrin selective and, therefore, create more systemic effects. Fibrinolytics were discussed in more detail in Chapter 3.

Intracranial hemorrhage is a potential complication of fibrinolytic therapy, and any STEMI patient at substantial risk for intracranial hemorrhage should be treated with PCI rather than fibrinolytic therapy. Any change in neurological status within 24 hours of administration of a fibrinolytic is considered an intracranial hemorrhage until proven otherwise. All fibrinolytic, anticoagulation, and antiplatelet therapy should be immediately discontinued when a change in neurological status occurs until intracranial hemorrhage is ruled out. Signs of successful reperfusion with fibrinolytics include relief of presenting symptoms, reduction of at least 50% of initial ST-segment elevation on repeat ECG, and hemodynamic and electrical stability.

Clinical Application

The pain of aortic dissection can mimic the pain of MI. ECG changes associated with pericarditis can also mimic the ECG changes seen in acute MI. It is key in both of these circumstances to differentiate these diagnoses from acute MI because treatment with fibrinolytic therapy could be devastating in either case.

Specific Types of STEMIs

Inferior Wall Myocardial Infarction

On a 12-lead ECG, inferior wall MIs show ST-segment elevation in the inferior leads, leads II, III, and aV_F. Figure 5-6 shows a 12-lead ECG representation of an inferior wall MI. The inferior wall of the left ventricle is fed by the right coronary artery (RCA); therefore, an occlusion of the RCA is suspected in patients with inferior wall MI.

Inferior wall MIs are sometimes associated with additional involvement of the posterior wall of the left ventricle or the right ventricle. A right-sided ECG using right-sided chest leads should be performed with all patients with inferior wall MIs to assess for involvement of the right ventricle. Patients with right ventricular involvement are treated differently, as discussed later in this chapter. The more proximal the occlusion of the RCA, the greater the amount of myocardium involved in the infarction.

Complications of Inferior Wall Myocardial Infarction

Because the RCA also feeds the sinoatrial (SA) and AV nodes in the majority of people, bradycardia and first- and second-degree heart block are common complications of inferior wall MI. Patients with inferior wall MIs have increased parasympathetic activity, which causes nausea and vomiting (Bene & Vaughan, 2005). Patients with inferior-posterior MIs are also at risk for the development of papillary muscle rupture, which results in acute mitral regurgitation and is an emergent situation.

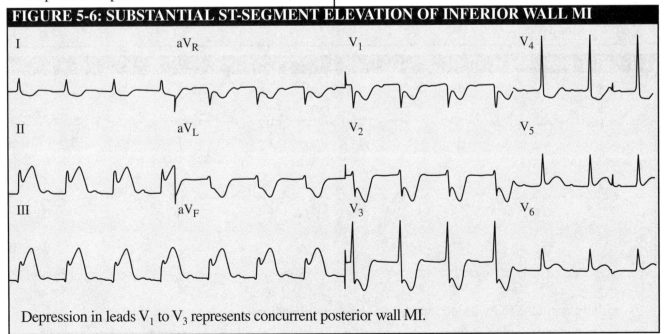

FIGURE 5-6: SUBSTANTIAL ST-SEGMENT ELEVATION OF INFERIOR WALL MI

Depression in leads V_1 to V_3 represents concurrent posterior wall MI.

<u>*Clinical Application*</u>

First- and second-degree heart block seen in inferior MI usually does not progress to complete heart block because the bundle of His and bundle branches are not fed by the RCA.

Anterior Wall Myocardial Infarction

The left anterior descending artery (LAD) supplies blood to the anterior portion of the septum and the anterior wall of the left ventricle. An occlusion of the LAD produces an infarct of the anterior wall of the left ventricle, producing ST-segment elevation in leads V_3 and V_4 on a 12-lead ECG. If the lesion is proximal and the septum is involved, ST-segment elevation occurs in leads V_1 through V_4. Figure 5-7 shows a 12-lead ECG representation of an anterior septal MI. Both Figures 5-6 and 5-7 can be compared to the normal ECG in Figure 5-8.

FIGURE 5-7: ST-SEGMENT ELEVATION OF ANTERIOR SEPTAL MI IN LEADS V_1 TO V_4

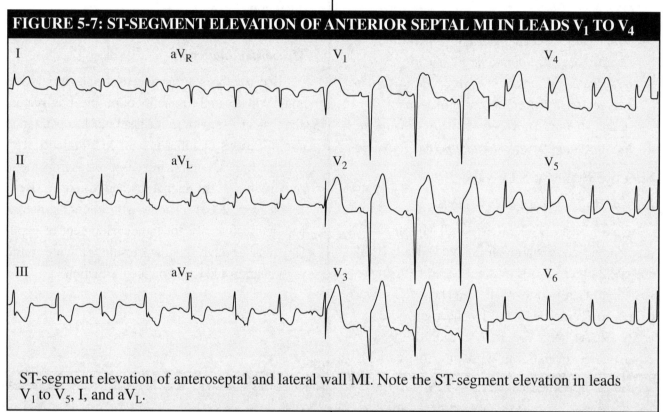

ST-segment elevation of anteroseptal and lateral wall MI. Note the ST-segment elevation in leads V_1 to V_5, I, and aV_L.

FIGURE 5-8: NORMAL ECG

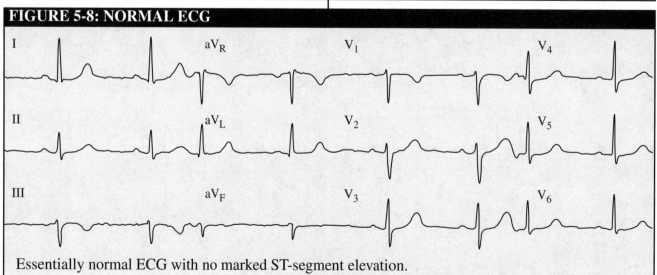

Essentially normal ECG with no marked ST-segment elevation.

Complications of Anterior Wall Myocardial Infarction

Because the bundle branches of the conduction system run through the septum, patients with occlusion of the LAD are at risk for the development of bundle branch blocks and complete heart blocks. Patients with septal infarcts are also at risk for ventricular septal rupture. Patients with anterior wall MIs have a worse prognosis than those with inferior wall MIs (Smith, Zvosec, Sharkey, & Henry, 2002). A large anterior wall MI can result in profound left ventricular dysfunction, leading to heart failure and cardiogenic shock.

Clinical Application

The assessment of a new holosystolic murmur in an unstable patient with an anteroseptal MI can indicate a ventricular septal rupture. This condition is a medical emergency requiring emergency surgery to repair the rupture.

Lateral Wall Myocardial Infarction

The circumflex artery, off the left main coronary artery, supplies blood to the lateral wall of the left ventricle. Other coronary branches also supply portions of the lateral wall. The leads on a 12-lead ECG that look at the lateral wall of the myocardium are leads I and aV_L (high lateral leads) and V_5 and V_6 (low lateral leads). The myocardium supplied by the circumflex artery is less represented on a 12-lead ECG than the myocardium supplied by the RCA or LAD. For this reason, occlusions of the circumflex artery may be less visible on a 12-lead ECG than occlusions of the LAD and RCA. A large portion of the myocardium is supplied by the circumflex artery, and a stand-alone lateral wall MI should be treated as aggressively as other forms of MI.

Complications of Lateral Wall Mydocardial Infarction

The circumflex artery supplies the AV node, bundle of His, and papillary muscles in about 10% of people. Therefore, conduction abnormalities and papillary muscle dysfunction, with resultant mitral regurgitation, are potential complications of lateral wall MIs.

Posterior Wall Myocardial Infarction

Posterior wall MIs are caused by obstruction of the posterior descending artery (PDA), usually originating from the RCA. They commonly occur in conjunction with inferior wall MIs. The PDA in some patients can originate from the circumflex artery; in these patients, a posterior MI may occur in conjunction with lateral wall MI. A true isolated posterior MI does not produce ST-segment elevation on a standard 12-lead ECG because no electrodes are placed directly over the posterior wall of the left ventricle. A posterior wall MI may show ST-segment depression in the leads reciprocal to the posterior wall, including leads V_1 to V_3.

Right Ventricular Myocardial Infarction

All of the previously described MIs refer to an infarction of the left ventricle. Infarction of the right ventricle occurs in one third to one half of inferior wall MIs (Bene & Vaughan, 2005). The presence of a right ventricular MI is important because mortality is increased when the right ventricle is involved (Bene & Vaughan, 2005). In most people, the marginal branch of the RCA feeds the right ventricle; therefore, an occlusion proximal to this branch infarcts the right ventricle. An ECG with right precordial leads should be done on all patients with inferior MIs to assess for the presence of a right ventricular infarct. ST-segment elevation can be seen in the right precordial leads if the ECG is performed early during the MI.

Patients with right ventricular infarctions and hemodynamic alterations need special treatment. The right ventricle supplies the left ventricle with its preload. When the right ventricle fails, the left side of the heart does not receive adequate preload; therefore, cardiac output decreases. Patients with right ventricular infarctions may show clinical signs of right-sided heart failure (such as increased jugular venous pressure); however, their lungs remain clear because left-sided preload is low. IV fluids are indicated in the treatment of these patients to help assure adequate preload. Venous vasodilators and diuretics are avoided because they decrease preload. If fluid administration is ineffective in supplying adequate preload to the left side of the heart, inotropic medications such as dobutamine may be needed to support the failing right ventricle.

Patients with right ventricular infarctions are at higher risk for the development of atrial fibrillation. They also have an increased risk of atrial fibrillation because the right atrium can stretch from volume overload due to right ventricular failure and infarct. The presence of atrial fibrillation can further complicate a right ventricular infarct because the loss of atrial kick further decreases right ventricular preload. Loss of atrial kick can decrease cardiac output by up to 25% (Bond, 2010). Patients who are hemodynamically unstable require emergency cardioversion.

Key Nursing Care in the Acute Treatment of STEMI

Patients with STEMI are initially admitted to a coronary care or critical care unit. Listed here are key coronary care nursing interventions in the care of patients with STEMI:

- On admission, assure that aspirin was already administered in the pre-hospital setting or ED.

- Assess that response to beta-blocker therapy is adequate enough to control heart rate and dysrhythmias without causing hypotension.

- Assess for the presence of angina and need for additional antianginal medications.

Clinical Application

In patients for whom there is concern for the development of hypotension, treatments with proven mortality benefits, such as beta-blocker and angiotensin-converting enzyme (ACE) inhibitor administration, need to have priority over the administration of IV nitroglycerin in the management of continuing ischemia.

- Reassess oxygen saturation after 6 hours of supplemental oxygen and discontinue if saturation is more than 90%.

- Administer anxiolytics as needed to reduce anxiety.

Clinical Application

Control of pain and anxiety is key for patient comfort and also to reduce myocardial oxygen demand. Pain and anxiety activate the sympathetic nervous system and increase myocardial oxygen demand.

- Assess heart sounds for new holosystolic murmurs.

- Restrict activity for at least the first 12 hours, and then begin a step approach to activity progression (phase I cardiac rehabilitation exercises).

- Utilize cardiac monitoring and ST-segment monitoring to assess for recurrent ischemia and the presence of dysrhythmias.

- Insulin therapy may be used to achieve blood glucose levels less than 180 mg/dL in STEMI patients. Care should be taken to avoid hypoglycemia (Kushner et al., 2009).

- Observe for signs of left ventricular dysfunction, including hypotension or clinical signs of heart failure.

- Include the family. Family visits do not have a negative impact on vital signs or cardiac rhythm.

(Antman et al., 2004; Kushner et al., 2009)

When hemodynamic stability is achieved, patients can be transferred to a step-down or progressive care unit. With successful reperfusion, some patients can transfer to a step-down unit within 24 hours. Post-PCI care is discussed in Chapter 6.

NON-ST-SEGMENT ELEVATION MYOCARDIAL INFARCTION AND UNSTABLE ANGINA

Non-STEMI and UA are usually caused by a ruptured plaque that causes a partially occluded vessel. The partial occlusion is generally caused by incomplete thrombosis. This incomplete thrombosis is often referred to as a soft clot or platelet plug. A non-STEMI cannot be differentiated from UA at the time of presentation because the 12-lead ECG findings, such as ST-segment depression and T-wave inversion, may be similar. In UA, these ECG changes are usually more transient; in non-STEMI, they are usually more persistent. Any transient ST-segment or T-wave change more than 0.5 mm during a symptomatic episode that occurs at rest is a sign of ischemia related to CAD (Anderson et al., 2007). Patients who present with either ST-segment depression or T-wave inversion can be having either a non-STEMI or UA. Cardiac biomarkers are used to differentiate between non-STEMI and UA. Approximately 40% of all MIs are non-STEMIs (Bene & Vaughan, 2005). Patients in this category are at an increased risk for recurrent ischemia, MI, and death. The risk is highest during the first 2 months after the acute event (Anderson et al., 2007).

Clinical Application

0.5 mm of change in an ST segment is a subtle change. Therefore, clinicians must be skilled to detect even the most subtle changes in order to recognize injury or ischemia on the 12-lead ECG.

Clinical Application

It is important for the nurse to recognize that although the patient with a non-STEMI may not receive urgent reperfusion nor have an ECG as impressive as the patient with a STEMI, the risk of complications and death is high after a non-STEMI and treatment with evidence-based practice recommendations is important to reduce complications in this group of patients.

Cardiac Biomarkers

Cardiac biomarkers are released into the blood when necrosis occurs as a result of membrane rupture of the myocytes. Cardiac biomarkers used in the evaluation of ACSs include myoglobin, creatine kinase (CK), CK-MB, and troponins I and T.

Myoglobin is the biomarker that rises the earliest, within 2 hours after myocardial damage (Anderson et al., 2007). Although it is a very sensitive biomarker, is it not specific to myocardial damage.

CK is an enzyme present in the heart, brain, and skeletal muscle, so elevations are not specific to myocardial damage. CK-MB is more specific to the heart. Therefore, CK-MB measurements are helpful in identifying more than minor amounts of myocardial damage. CK-MB rapidly rises in the presence of myocardial damage.

Troponins I and T are found only in cardiac muscle. They are the most sensitive biomarkers for myocardial damage. Because troponin levels remain elevated for a long period, with a gradual return to normal, they are beneficial in patients presenting late after symptom onset. Troponin levels are capable of diagnosing small amounts of myocardial necrosis not measured by rises in CK-MB levels (Anderson et al., 2007). Elevated cardiac troponin levels identify myocardial necrosis but do not particularly identify ischemia or infarction as the cause of necrosis. A positive troponin level in the presence of ECG changes that are consistent with injury or ischemia confirm the diagnosis of myocardial infarction. In addition, an elevated troponin level after a PCI procedure is also consistent with a myocardial infarction. Cardiac troponins I and T are generally considered equal in their diagnostic values, except in patients with renal dysfunction, who may have a nonspecific elevation in cardiac troponin T that is not related to myocardial injury.

In patients with renal dysfunction, cardiac troponin I is more specific for myocardial injury than cardiac troponin T and is the preferred cardiac biomarker in this population (Anderson, et al., 2007).

New markers as well as new combinations of markers to assess cardiac risk are being investigated. B-type natiuretic peptide (BNP) is one marker that is known to add additional prognostic value in the patient's overall risk assessment. In addition, there are newer methods of assessing for changes in troponin levels while the levels are still within the normal range. This method of assessing the delta values allows for the detection of changes early on, before the troponin levels are expected to rise above normal (Anderson et al., 2007).

Table 5-2 summarizes the cardiac biomarkers. Biomarker results are not needed to proceed with reperfusion in a STEMI. Cardiac biomarkers are also not used to diagnose reinfarction within 18 hours after the onset of STEMI because initial biomarker elevation can still exist.

Primary Treatment Strategies for Non-STEMI and UA

Because the underlying pathophysiology of Non-STEMI and UA is a soft clot or platelet plug, the primary treatment strategy is focused heavily on antiplatelet therapy. In addition to aspirin, clopidogrel and glycoprotein IIb/IIIa inhibitors are used as antiplatelet therapy. Anticoagulation therapy is also required in conjunction with antiplatet therapy in these patients.

In addition to a focus on antiplatelet therapy, treatment of patients with UA and non-STEMI involves a decision between an early invasive strategy or an initial conservative strategy. The early

invasive treatment arm involves cardiac catheterization and revascularization within the first 4 to 24 hours of admission. The potential advantage of an early invasive strategy is that approximately 60% to 70% of patients will be able to have a PCI to the culprit lesion. In addition there are approximately 20% of patients who will be identified as having left main CAD or triple vessel disease with left ventricular dysfunction. The remainder of patients will not have significant obstructive CAD (Anderson et al., 2007). Early invasive treatment is recommended for high-risk patients, but can also be used in other patient groups. Due to the potential higher rate of complications in women who have PCI, an early invasive strategy is not recommended for women who present with low-risk features (Anderson et al., 2007). High-risk patients include those with the following features:

- recent PCI or history of CABG
- recurrent ischemia
- depressed left ventricular function or clinical signs of heart failure
- sustained ventricular dysrhythmias or hemodynamic instability
- significant ST-segment changes on a 12-lead ECG or high-risk findings on other noninvasive testing
- positive troponins.

(Anderson et al., 2007)

The specifics of antiplatelet and anticoagulation therapy are driven by the invasive or conservative strategy as well as the patient's risk status.

The specific use of antiplatelet medications in patients with non-STEMI or UA depends on several factors, including patient risk and decision for ini-

TABLE 5-2: SUMMARY OF CARDIAC BIOMARKERS				
Cardiac Biomarker	**Specificity/Sensitivity**	**Rise**	**Peak**	**Duration**
Myoglobin	Sensitive but not specific	Within 2 hours	4 to 10 hours	< 24 hours
CK-MB	Highly specific	4 to 6 hours	18 to 24 hours	2 to 3 days
Troponin I or T	Highly specific and sensitive	4 to 6 hours	18 to 24 hours	10 or more days

tial invasive or conservative treatment strategy. A loading dose of clopidogrel or prasugrel as soon as possible is recommended for all patients receiving either initial invasive or conservative treatment. When patients are receiving an early invasive strategy, the clopidogrel is to be administered before angiography. If prasugrel is used, it is not administered until the time of the procedure. High-risk patients receiving an early invasive strategy should receive a glycoprotein IIb/IIIa inhibitor. The addition of glycoprotein IIb/IIIa inhibitors may also be considered in patients who are being managed conservatively. The anticoagulant that is used in non-STEMI is dependent on patient risk (including risk of bleeding), treatment strategy, hospital/physician preferences, and duration of therapy, including the concern for developing heparin induced thrombocytopenia. There are four potential types of anticoagulants that can be used in patients with non-STEMI or UA. These types of anticoagulants include: unfractionated heparin (UFH), low-molecular-weight heparin (LMWH), factor Xa inhibitors, and direct thrombin inhibitors. Specifics related to antiplatelet and anticoagulant medications are discussed in Chapter 3.

Supportive Medical Therapy Used in All Patients with ACS

All patients with ACSs, including STEMI, non-STEMI, and UA will receive supportive medical management in addition to their primary treatment strategies.

Oxygen

Oxygen is used in patients with an arterial oxygen saturation less than 90%. Oxygen can also be administered to patients with STEMI or non-STEMI presentation during the first 6 hours. After the first 6 hours, oxygen is not indicated unless the patient's oxygen saturation is low (Kushner et al., 2009).

Aspirin

Initial treatment of all patients presenting with ACSs includes aspirin immediately on arrival, if not already taken at home or given by EMS. Non-enteric-coated aspirin, in the dose range of 162 to 325 mg, should be chewed by the patient. A targeted history and physical should be completed, focusing on the goal of early reperfusion for STEMI patients. Special attention should be paid to contraindications to fibrinolytic therapy and assessment of possible myocardial mimics, such as aortic dissection (pain mimic) and pericarditis (ECG mimic). There is an increasing focus on prehospital care of STEMI patients, including the ability of advanced life support providers to identify STEMI on a 12-lead ECG and complete a reperfusion checklist prior to arrival in the hospital.

Clopidogrel/Prasugrel

As discussed previously, additional antiplatelet therapy with clopidogrel (or prasugrel) is a primary strategy in the treatment of non-STEMI and UA. Clopidogrel or prasugrel is also used in the treatment of STEMI patients, regardless of whether they receive reperfusion. Specifics regarding administration are dependent on the type of immediate reperfusion strategy as well as any additional revascularization procedures. Antiplatelet therapy specific to revascularization procedures is discussed in Chapter 7.

Anticoagulants

Anticoagulant therapy is a key component in patients with STEMI, non-STEMI and UA. Four types of anticoagulants are used in patients with ACS, UFH, LMWH, direct thrombin inhibitor, and factor Xa inhibitor. The decision regarding which anticoagulant to use can be quite complex, taking into account many different factors. Patients with STEMI who have PCI as their reperfusion strategy will have anticoagulation as part of their PCI procedure. Patients with STEMI who receive fibrinolytic therapy as their reperfusion strategy should receive an anticoagulant for a minimum of 48 hours and ideally for the duration of the hospital stay up to 8 days (Kushner et al., 2009). Patients with non-STEMI/UA patients will also receive anticoagulation with either an early invasive or early conservative treatment strategy. The factor Xa inhibitor fondaparinux cannot be used as the sole anticoagulation in patients undergoing PCI in any setting because of the higher risk of catheter-associated thrombosis. Fondaparinux is most commonly used in patients with non-STEMI being managed conservatively who have a higher risk of bleeding (Anderson et al., 2007; Kushner et al., 2009).

Nitroglycerin

Up to three doses of sublingual nitroglycerin, 0.4 mg, can be given every 5 minutes. If ischemic discomfort continues after sublingual nitroglycerin and beta-blocker administration, an IV nitroglycerin drip can be started at 10 mcg/min and titrated in increments of 10 mcg every 3 to 5 minutes until symptoms are relieved or until the patient's blood pressure does not allow further titration. The effective dose range is 5 to 100 mcg/min, but doses of 200 mcg/min have been used (Gold Standard/Elsevier, 2010). Sublingual nitroglycerin and high-dose IV nitroglycerin dilate arteries and veins. In addition to managing ischemic symptoms, IV nitroglycerin can be used in treating patients who are hypertensive or who have signs of pulmonary congestion. Nitroglycerin should not be used in patients who are hypotensive, bradycardic, or tachycardic; those who have taken sildenafil within 24 hours or taldalafil within 48 hours; and those with right ventricular infarct. If blood pressure is a limiting factor, beta-blockers should be given priority administration over nitrates (Anderson et al., 2007).

Clinical Application

Sildenafil, tadalafil, and other similar vasodilators are used in the treatment of erectile dysfunction. Administration of nitrates in patients who have recently taken these medications can result in dangerous hypotension. Not all patients will disclose the use of these medications on initial interviewing, so careful questioning is needed. Patients need to under-stand there is a risk of dangerously low blood pressure if nitrates are given within a certain time frame of taking these medications. In addition, similar vasodilators are used in the treatment of pulmonary hypertension and women should also be assessed for taking these medications. Consult a pharmacist if there is any question regarding the safe length of time between a vasodilator medication and the administration of a nitrate.

Morphine Sulfate

Morphine sulfate is the pain reliever of choice for ischemic cardiac pain associated with STEMI. The initial dose is usually 2 to 4 mg IV. Morphine can be repeated at 5-minute intervals in increments of 2 to 8 mg (Kushner et al., 2009). In patients with non-STEMI or UA, morphine is typically given in doses of 1 to 5 mg when ischemic symptoms are not responsive to sublingual nitroglycerin and beta-blocker therapy (Anderson et al., 2007). Morphine is a preload reducer and also reduces anxiety and limits activity of the sympathetic nervous system.

Beta-Blockers

Oral beta-blockers should be administered within 24 hours in patients with STEMI, non-STEMI, or UA if no contraindications exist. Beta-blockers may also be given IV initially in patients with STEMI who present with hypertension. IV beta-blockers should be used in caution in those patients presenting with non-STEMI or UA. Although beta blockers can reduce the incidence of reinfarction and ventricular fibrillation during the inpatient stay, they can also increase the incidence of cardiogenic shock (Anderson et al., 2007; Kushner et al., 2009). Beta-blockers are contraindicated in patients with low cardiac output, signs of heart failure, and in those identified as high risk for cardiogenic shock. Relative contraindications for beta-blockers include advanced first degree AV block, second or third degree AV block, active asthma, or reactive airway disease (Anderson et al., 2007).

ACE Inhibitors

ACE inhibitors are given within the first 24 hours of an acute MI (STEMI or non-STEMI) in patients with most of the following characteristics: anterior wall MI, presence of pulmonary congestion, left ventricular ejection fraction less than 40%, hypertension, diabetes, and chronic kidney disease (Anderson et al., 2007; Kushner et al., 2009).

COMPLICATIONS OF MYOCARDIAL INFARCTION

Hemodynamic Alterations

When myocardial function is impaired as a result of MI, stroke volume decreases. To compensate for decreased stroke volume, heart rate increases. If myocardial function is impaired to the point that adequate stroke volume cannot be maintained, diastolic filling pressures increase and pulmonary edema results.

Clinical Application

Tachycardia is a poor prognostic sign in the presence of an acute MI because it is a compensatory mechanism for decreasing stroke volume due to a failing left ventricle.

Hemodynamic alterations depend on the size and location of the infarction. A large MI affecting more than 40% of the myocardium can result in circulatory collapse and cardiogenic shock. The prognosis of patients in cardiac shock remains very poor unless successful revascularization can occur in a timely fashion. Long-term hemodynamic alterations from left ventricular dysfunction result in chronic heart failure. With current reperfusion technology, many patients with MIs are left with no clinical evidence of left ventricular dysfunction.

Ventricular Dysrhythmias

Ventricular fibrillation is a major cause of preventable death in the early period after MI. Many episodes of prehospital sudden death are caused by untreated ventricular fibrillation. During MI, dysrhythmias are caused by ischemia to the electrical conduction system, catecholamine release, and electrolyte imbalances. Hypokalemia and hypomagnesemia increase the risk of ventricular fibrillation. Routine magnesium sulfate is not administered in STEMI; however, any magnesium deficiency should be corrected. Any episodes of torsades de pointes (a special ventricular tachycardia associated with a prolonged QT interval) should be treated with IV magnesium sulfate.

Clinical Application

Patients presenting with signs of MI need to be connected to a cardiac monitor immediately and observed in an area with trained personnel who have immediate access to a defibrillator and other emergency cardiac equipment and medications.

Mechanical Complications

Septal Rupture

Septal rupture is most common with a large anteroseptal infarction. It most commonly occurs 3 to 7 days after an infarct (Verrier & Deelstra, 2010). The patient experiences sudden and severe left ventricular failure. Blood is shunted from the left side of the heart back to the right side through the ruptured area. This shunting of blood results in poor systemic perfusion. The rupture also produces a very loud holosystolic murmur. Emergency measures to reduce afterload are indicated while the patient is prepared for surgical repair.

Papillary Muscle Dysfunction or Rupture

Papillary muscle dysfunction and rupture result in acute mitral valve regurgitation. This complication occurs most frequently with inferior-posterior wall MIs and usually occurs within the first week after infarction (Verrier & Deelstra, 2010). As with septal ruptures, emergency measures to reduce afterload are indicated while preparing the patient for emergency surgery.

Pericarditis

Pericarditis, caused by inflammation of the pericardial sac, can occur immediately after an MI or several weeks later. When pericarditis occurs several weeks after an infarction, it is called *Dressler's syndrome*. When it occurs acutely, it is usually caused by a transmural infarct extending to the epicardium and causing an inflammatory response. Pain associated with pericarditis is sharp and severe. It is worse with inspiration and is relieved by leaning forward. A pericardial friction rub may be heard during auscultation of the heart. As with many complications of MI, the incidence of pericarditis has decreased significantly due to reperfusion therapy (Verrier & Deelstra, 2010).

Left Ventricular Aneurysm

Left ventricular aneurysm is a potential complication of MI. Ventricular aneurysms are classified as true or false, based on whether they are associated with myocardial rupture. A ventricular aneurysm classified as a true aneurysm is a local out-pouching of the ventricular wall that results in dysfunction of that portion of the left ventricle. One danger of a true ventricular aneurysm is that the bulging area can house thrombus, which can later embolize. Another potential complication of a true aneurysm is that it can be the source of ventricular arrhythmias. Aneurysms that are classified as true aneurysms, however, are not likely to rupture. True aneurysms are most associated with anterolateral and apical MI.

An aneurysm is classed as a false or pseudo-aneurysm when there is actual rupture into the pericardial sac. Adhesions in the pericardial sac contain the rupture. This type of aneurysm is most often associated with infarction to the thinner portion of the left ventricle, the posterior lateral wall. This type of aneurysm needs to be closely monitored for an increase in size, which requires immediate surgical repair to prevent further bleeding. (Bene & Vaughan, 2005).

Ventricular Remodeling

During an MI, cellular edema produces an inflammatory response, which leads to the recruitment of some stem cells and can lead to some tissue regeneration. Catecholamines are also released from myocardial cells during the acute phase of injury, increasing the risk of dysrhythmias during this vulnerable time.

Clinical Application

Beta-blockers are particularly important in suppressing cardiac dysrhythmias in ischemic tissue because they suppress catecholamine release.

Initially, damaged tissue is bruised and cyanotic. During this period, the cardiac biomarkers are released. By the second to third day, white blood cells invade the necrotic tissue. Scavenger cells release enzymes to break down necrotic tissue. The necrotic wall can become very thin during this phase, and cardiac rupture is most likely to occur at this time (Aouizerat et al., 2010). By the second week, a weak collagen matrix has formed, but the myocardium is still vulnerable to reinjury. By the third week, scar formation has started, and at 6 weeks, the necrotic area is completely replaced with scar tissue (Aouizerat et al., 2010). Although this scar tissue is very strong, it does not contribute to the contractile function of the myocardium.

In addition to post-infarction changes in necrotic tissue, the non-infarcted surrounding areas can also be affected. Surviving myocytes hypertrophy in an attempt to compensate for damaged tissue. Excessive non-contractile collagen is present in the newly hypertrophied myocardium, leading to a ventricle that is stiff and noncompliant. A stiff, non-compliant ventricle is unable to fill properly during the cardiac cycle, and cardiac output is impaired.

SPECIAL CONSIDERATIONS

Treatment of Cocaine-Induced Chest Pain

Cocaine use leads to sympathetic nervous system activation and direct stimulation of vascular smooth muscle, resulting in spasm and vasoconstriction. Cocaine also promotes platelet aggregation and thrombus formation. Chronic cocaine use accelerates the process of atherosclerosis. Cocaine-induced ischemic chest discomfort cannot be distinguished from UA or non-STEMI caused by CHD. Cocaine use has become widespread, so this etiology of symptoms and ECG changes must be considered. Nitroglycerin or calcium channel blockers are used to treat cocaine-induced chest pain. If ST-segment elevation is present, then calcium channel blockers are administered IV. If ST-segment elevation does not resolve with medical treatment, then reperfusion with PCI is indicated (Anderson et al., 2007). After successful medical treatment, it is recommended that patients with cocaine-induced chest pain and ECG changes be observed for 9 to 24 hours (Anderson et al., 2007).

Variant (Vasospastic or Prinzmetal's) Angina

Variant angina is caused by spasm of the coronary arteries. This type of angina usually occurs spontaneously but can be triggered by exercise, hyperventilation, and cold. The only associated risk factor for variant angina is smoking. Patients can have long asymptomatic periods between episodes. The pathophysiology of variant angina is not fully understood. One possible explanation is that endothelial dysfunction causes an imbalance between local vasodilative and local vasoconstrictive factors.

Transient ST-segment elevation usually occurs with variant angina but usually does not result in MI if the spasm occurs in a nonstenotic vessel. However, if the patient has spasms in vessels that are already stenosed, MI can occur. This type of angina is treated with nitroglycerin and calcium channel blockers.

Cardiac Syndrome X

Cardiac syndrome X is the term used to describe the condition when the patient has anginal symptoms and ECG or stress testing objective evidence of ischemia, but there is nonobstructive CAD on cardiac catheterization. This syndrome occurs in women more often than in men. One possible explanation involves microvascular dysfunction. In some patients who have severe symptoms, an abnormal pain perception is also thought to be involved (Anderson et al., 2007). Exercise and statin therapy can be used to improve endothelial function. Risk factor reduction is appropriate because some patients will later present with MI. Antianginal medications are used to control symptoms. In severe cases that are not responsive to medications, transcutaneous electrical nerve stimulation or spinal cord stimulation has been used for pain control (Anderson et al., 2007).

LONG-TERM MANAGEMENT OF ALL ACUTE CORONARY SYNDROMES

After an acute event, most patients resume a medical management course similar to patients with stable angina. Patients who have experienced an ACS continue a daily dose of aspirin indefinitely. The long-term maintenance dose of aspirin is generally 81 to 162 mg daily. Clopidogrel or prasugrel may be used if a patient is unable to take aspirin. Clopidogrel or prasugrel is also continued for a short time in all patients with STEMI or non-STEMI regardless of revascularization (Anderson et al., 2007; Kushner et al., 2009). Antiplatelet therapy after a revascularization procedure is discussed in Chapter 7.

Beta-blockers are initiated within 24 hours in all patients with ACS and continued indefinitely after discharge. ACE inhibitors are given within the first 24 hours to patients meeting specific criteria and are continued indefinitely. An angiotensin II receptor blocker may be used as an alternative for patients unable to tolerate ACE inhibitors. Beta-blockers and ACE inhibitors help alter ventricular remodeling that occurs after MI. Aldosterone blockers are given after MI to patients with ejection fractions less than 40%, those who have clinical heart failure, and those who have diabetes. Aldosterone blockers are added to therapy for patients who are already on ACE inhibitor therapy. Aldosterone blockers cannot be added to therapy for patients with renal dysfunction or hyperkalemia.

Discharge medications also include a lipid-lowering agent (preferably a statin) that should be initiated 24 to 96 hours after admission (Anderson et al., 2007; Kushner et al., 2009).

Discharge medical management includes three main objectives:

- Medications to improve prognosis
  - Aspirin
  - Clopidogrel (or prasugrel)
  - Beta-blockers
  - Lipid-lowering drugs (statins)
  - ACE inhibitors or angiotensin II receptor blockers
  - Aldosterone antagonists
- Medications to control ischemia (if revascularization is not done or if above medications are not effective)
  - Beta-blockers (increased doses)
  - Nitrates (all patients should be given sublingual nitroglycerin)
  - Calcium channel blockers
- Secondary prevention through risk factor reduction

  - Smoking cessation
  - Reduction of hyperlipidemia
  - Hypertension control
  - Diabetes control
  - Weight management
  - Increased physical activity
  - Annual influenza vaccine

Patients should not take nonsteroidal anti-inflammatory drugs (NSAIDs) for pain after STEMI or non-STEMI because of their association with increased risk of mortality and also with increased risk of complications, including hypertension, reinfarction, heart failure, and myocardial rupture. Acetaminophen, aspirin, small doses of narcotic, or nonacetylated salicylates are recommended as pain relievers over NSAIDs. If not effective, a nonselective COX-2 NSAID such as naproxen may be used (Kushner et al., 2009).

Patient Education

Medical Follow Up

Patients should be instructed on the importance of physician follow up. High-risk patients should be seen within 2 weeks after discharge and low-risk patients within 6 weeks. The patient should be instructed to notify the physician anytime there is a change in condition, such as a change in activity tolerance or perceived medication side effects.

Risk Factor Reduction

A major focus of patient education for any patient with CHD is secondary prevention by aggressive reduction of cardiac risk factors to reduce the risk of future events (discussed in detail in Chapter 4).

Recognition of Signs and Symptoms and Emergency Response

Another focus is the recognition of and response to symptoms of an acute coronary event. Patients should know how to activate the EMS and should know the location of the nearest hospital with 24-hour cardiac care. Patients should be instructed on the use of sublingual nitroglycerin or nitroglycerin spray and should be instructed to activate the EMS if symptoms do not improve after 5 minutes or after one sublingual nitroglycerin. The goal in earlier activation of the EMS is to reduce the time to reperfusion. Patients with signs and symptoms of ACS should also be instructed to chew aspirin (162 to 325 mg – if not already taken) while awaiting the arrival of EMS. It is important to instruct patients that they should never drive themselves or let a family member drive them to the hospital if they think they are having a heart attack. It is important to be transported by trained emergency personnel who can respond immediately to any complications.

Patients with a history of stable angina should be instructed to rest with the onset of angina and to take up to three sublingual nitroglycerin. Patients should notify the EMS if pain persists after the use of three sublingual nitroglycerin. Family members who are appropriate candidates may be given resources to learn about cardiopulmonary resuscitation and the use of automated external defibrillators.

Clinical Application

It is important to understand the patient's potential need for nitroglycerin when giving instructions on sublingual use after discharge. A patient who has no known coronary disease or who has been successfully revascularized should not need to take nitroglycerin and needs to activate the EMS after one nitroglycerin if substantial relief has not occurred. In contrast, a patient with chronic stable angina may expect predictable bouts of angina that require treatment with up to 3 sublingual nitroglycerin.

Medications

Education regarding prescribed medications is a key intervention for nurses, pharmacists, dietitians, and other members of the interdisciplinary team. Education occurs prior to discharge and continues in the office and cardiac rehabilitation settings. Patients with chronic cardiac disease are commonly prescribed multiple medications and the risk for noncompliance is high. Patients who have had revascularization and are experiencing an improvement in symptoms might not understand the importance of continued medical treatment. Noncompliance with medications is associated with increased adverse outcomes in patients with cardiac conditions. Those patients with fixed or low incomes might also have financial concerns regarding their medication regimes.

Activity

Patients should be instructed on special postdischarge activity restrictions, including driving restrictions, weight-lifting restrictions, and instructions regarding sexual activity. These decisions are usually individualized based on the patient's clinical condition. Driving regulations may also vary between states. Most patients with an uncomplicated hospital course can drive about 1 week after discharge (Kushner et al., 2009). Patients may be uncomfortable asking about resuming sexual relationships, so instructions regarding sexual activity should be included as a routine part of all discharge instructions. Patients with a history of angina during sexual relationships may be instructed by their physician to take nitroglycerin prior to engaging in sexual activities.

Daily walking is the exercise of choice after an acute cardiac event. After the initial recovery period, stable patients should walk a minimum of 30 minutes daily. Patients should walk preferably every day, but at least 3 to 4 days per week. The daily walking regime should be supplemented by an increase in activities of daily living (ADLs). Special considerations for the initial recovery period are discussed later in this chapter. All patients with STEMI should be referred to formal, comprehensive, multidisciplinary cardiac rehabilitation programs. All patients with ACS at moderate to high risk, and with multiple risk factors, should also be referred to formal cardiac rehabilitation programs, where supervised exercise and continued patient education can be provided. Additional information about exercise and cardiac rehabilitation is provided in the next section.

Anxiety and Stress

Anxiety is common during and immediately after the acute phase of a cardiac event. Nurses can help reduce anxiety by helping the patient gain accurate perceptions of the recovery process. Teaching the patient about relaxation techniques and methods of worry control can help reduce anxiety. An example of a worry-control technique is to schedule 5-minute periods twice a day to worry. At other times of the day, worries are set aside. Nurses can use the expertise of clinical nurse specialists to develop a comprehensive plan of care that includes the psychosocial needs of the cardiac patient.

Patient and family education is a very important tool in relieving stress when the patient and family are ready to receive information. If the patient and family are not ready, providing information can actually increase stress.

Teaching Principles

The key to effective patient education is to individualize the approach, based on the patient's preferred method of learning, and take advantage of every patient encounter. Nurses should be prepared to utilize all teachable moments. Many patients are afraid or have anxiety or depression after an acute cardiac event. Patients must be allowed to express concerns and have questions answered before they are able to accept new information. Patients should be active participants in the education process. Adult patients need to be in control of their learning; therefore, it is critical to assess the patient's readiness and desire for information.

In many cases, sharing scientific information about the value of the treatment or risk factor plan increases motivation. Patients who are engaged should be encouraged to seek out additional infor-

mation and resources from the library or on the internet. Family, as defined by the patient, should be included in education. When providing patient education, it is helpful to individualize the information to the patient. For example, discuss the patient's individual risk factors, type of CHD, area of infarction, and specific ejection fraction. This allows the patient to assimilate and take ownership of the information being provided.

Effective patient education requires a great deal of time and is often neglected. However, the rewards of effective patient education can be tremendous. Patients can benefit in the form of improved physical functioning and quality of life and, possibly, improved survival from increased adherence to the medical regime.

Clinical Application

It is important for nurses to assist patients in finding accurate sources of information, especially when using internet-based resources. The American College of Cardiology has a CardioSmart website that contains consumer and patient information approved by cardiologists (http://www.cardio smart.org).

Cardiac Rehabilitation

Exercise in the Early Recovery Period

Initiation of activity early in the recovery period after an acute cardiac event is important because 3% of total body muscle mass deconditions per day of bed rest (Levine, 2002). Patients also develop altered distribution of body fluids with bed rest and can develop orthostatic intolerance. The goal of rehabilitation in the early recovery period is to counteract the negative effects of deconditioning. Complications after an acute event are not increased with early activity progression in stable patients. Phase I cardiac rehabilitation exercises are initiated in a patient after an MI as soon as the patient is medically stable and after evaluation for orthostatic hypotension. Phase I exercises usually begin on day 1 or 2 for a patient after an acute

MI, depending on the size of the MI. Cardiac rehabilitation is typically initiated on postoperative day 1 for patients with CABG. Cardiac contraindications to beginning or continuing exercise include unstable angina, complete heart block, uncontrolled tachydysrhythmias, uncontrolled hypertension, and decompensated heart failure (Myers, 2010). The development of thrombophlebitis or another complicating illness may also restrict the ability to begin exercise.

In the early recovery period, patients should walk 5 to 10 minutes at a time. Only non-resistive range-of-motion (ROM) exercises should be performed because resistive exercises increase afterload and, therefore, the workload of the ventricles. The majority of patients begin with a 1.5 to 2.0 metabolic equivalent (MET) level of exercise (using a bedside commode, transferring to a chair, feeding self, washing face and hands), progressing to 2 to 3 METs of activity (sitting up longer, walking to bathroom, showering). The goal is for patients to be at a level of activity equivalent with ADLs by the time of discharge. With shorter hospital stays, the steps involved in inpatient rehabilitation programs have been modified to allow for more rapid progression. During early recovery, an increase of 20 beats per minute above resting heart rate, or a heart rate more than 110 beats per minute, may be used as a guideline for assessment of activity intolerance. These signs demonstrate an inappropriate chronotropic response to activity. Another sign of activity intolerance includes failure of systolic blood pressure to increase.

Exercise in the Late Recovery Period

Most patients should be at a 3 to 4 MET level of activity by the time of discharge. When a steady state of activity is well tolerated at home, the duration may be increased in 5-minute increments each week, up to 30 minutes per session. Activity should be performed at least three to four times, and may be performed up to six times, per week (Levine, 2002). Intensity may also be increased as activity is progressed. Exercises should involve large muscle groups and include a warm-up and cool-down. The warm-up should be active, such as slow walking, and the cool-down should include stretching. Isometric activities should be limited because of their potential to increase afterload. Isometric exercises involve the contraction of a muscle with no movement of the joint. Driving requires only 1.5 to 3.0 METs; however many patients do not drive after an MI until they return to work.

Patients need to be instructed to balance myocardial oxygen supply and demand by monitoring their response to activity. Shortness of breath means overexertion. Patients should lower activity if breathing and heart rate do not return to normal within 10 minutes of stopping exercise. Activity that is well tolerated is accompanied by no adverse symptoms, dysrhythmias, or excessive tachycardia. The same heart rate guidelines are used as with activity progression early in the recovery period.

Walking and secondary prevention have been shown to increase survival, decrease reoccurence rates, and possibly slow progression of CHD (Gibbons et al., 2002). In addition, a regular walking program after an acute cardiac event improves the patient's perception of quality of life. Exercise, as part of cardiac rehabilitation, limits disability and improves the physical function of participants (Myers, 2010). The hemodynamic benefits of exercise include reduction of heart rate and blood pressure. Exercise stress testing is recommended before starting an exercise program after an acute cardiac event. Exercise later in recovery should be guided by a symptom-limited stress test.

Low-risk patients can implement an exercise prescription at home or in a community setting. Low-risk patients include those with absence of ischemia or dysrhythmias on a stress test. High-risk patients, defined as those with ischemia or serious dysrhythmias on a stress test, should be in medically supervised exercise programs. The majority of patients exercising for secondary prevention are classified as low risk.

Formal Cardiac Rehabilitation

A formal cardiac rehabilitation program involves medically supervised exercise after an acute cardiac event. It usually begins 1 to 2 weeks after discharge and involves exercise three times weekly for a period of 4 to 12 weeks. The program is multidisciplinary and requires physician referral. Patients enrolled in a formal cardiac rehabilitation program must have baseline exercise testing and annual follow up. Exercise prescription is guided by exercise physiologists, and the patient's plan of care is directed by a registered nurse. Aerobic exercise and resistive training are components of the exercise program. Risk factor counseling, patient education regarding signs and symptoms and medications, and psychosocial support are also components of a comprehensive program.

Health insurance generally covers formal cardiac rehabilitation programs during the immediate recovery period after admission for MI, percutaneous transluminal coronary angioplasty (PTCA), and CABG for those with chronic stable angina. A patient copayment may be required. Many cardiac rehabilitation programs have sliding-scale fee structures to allow participation by those with financial limitations. Cardiac rehabilitation services have also been expanded to include patients with chronic heart failure and those who have undergone valve surgery or implantable cardioverter-defibrillator implantation.

Pooled data from a meta-analysis of studies involving cardiac rehabilitation in secondary prevention show a benefit of reduced cardiovascular mortality of approximately 25% at 1 and 3 years (Gibbons et al., 2002; Myers, 2010). Less benefits may be seen in patients with uncomplicated non-STEMI or UA who have successful revascularization compared to patients with more complicated non-STEMI or UA or those with STEMI (Anderson et al., 2007). Participation in formal exercise training is safe and patients benefit from increased functional capacity and exercise tolerance (Gibbons et al., 2002). However, exercise training needs to continue to show sustained improvement.

Patients who exercise experience a decrease in low-density lipoprotein cholesterol and triglyceride levels (Gibbons et al., 2002). Some patients experience a reduced need for oral hypoglycemic agents or insulin. Symptom reduction has been demonstrated in patients with angina and heart failure. Patients also experience improved psychosocial well-being and stress reduction. Patients who benefit from cardiac rehabilitation include those with angina, compensated heart failure, and decreased ejection fractions. Those with decreased exercise tolerance at baseline can benefit the most from participation, but are often among those not referred. Cardiac rehabilitation exercises are safe and beneficial in clinically stable patients with cardiac conditions. Unfortunately, only 10% to 20% of appropriate cardiac candidates participate in outpatient cardiac rehabilitation (Myers, 2010).

Psychosocial Issues

During hospitalization, post-discharge follow up, or cardiac rehabilitation, the patient's psychosocial status should be evaluated. Many patients with left ventricular dysfunction as a result of acute MI will experience role identity crisis after their acute events. Many patients miss large amounts of work and many have to alter their work roles if high levels of physical exertion and stress are involved. Altered work roles may add family and financial stresses. Patients may also experience anxiety and sleep disorders. An assessment of the patient's support system is an important part of the psychosocial assessment. Social isolation is a predictor of worse outcomes after an acute cardiac event such as MI (Maden & Froelicher, 2010). Social workers, pastoral care, and cardiac clinical nurse specialists are interdisciplinary resources for the management of psychosocial issues in the cardiac patient.

Depression is not uncommon after an acute cardiac event. Depression after an acute MI occurs approximately three times more often than in the general population, but only about 50% of cardiologists treat depression in their patients (Lichtman et al., 2008). Patients with depression are three to four times more likely to die within the first year following an MI (Maden & Froelicher, 2010). Depression also impacts participation in exercise, medication compliance, seeking attention for symptoms, and return to work. Minor depression may respond to increased accomplishment and association with others. Exercise can also improve minor depression, so patients should be referred to formal cardiac rehabilitation programs for the social support as well as exercise component. Mended Hearts is an organization for those who have survived a cardiac event. Referral to Mended Hearts is another option for social support for those who are depressed and those with limited social support. Nurses can impact depression through referrals to programs that increase social support and through the implementation of family centered care to increase family support. Another effective nursing strategy is to help clarify the reality of any negative perceptions the patient has about his or her recovery (Maden & Froelicher, 2010).

Up to 20% of patients will meet the criteria for major depression after acute MI. After an acute MI, a two-point Patient Health Questionnaire (PHQ-2) is recommended as the minimal screening. If the patient answers yes to either question, then a full nine-point questionnaire (PHQ-9) can be administered (Lichtman et al., 2008). The minimum two questions to be asked are: Over the past 2 weeks have either of the following been a concern:

1. little interest or pleasure in doing things

2. feeling down, depressed, or hopeless.

Selective serotonin reuptake inhibitors (SSRIs) can be useful in treating depression during the first year after an acute MI or in patients who have cardiac conditions with co-existing depression. This group of medications is generally considered safer than other antidepressant medications for use in patients with cardiac conditions because they have less cardiotoxic side effects (Maden & Froelicher, 2010). There are two SSRIs (sertraline and citalopram) that are considered first-line agents in treating patients with CHD because of their safety and effectiveness in this population (Lichtman et al., 2008).

CONCLUSION

Nurses who specialize in the care of patients with cardiac conditions have made a tremendous impact on patient outcomes, beginning with the introduction of coronary care units in the 1960s. From the original focus of dysrhythmia detection and treatment, to hemodynamic monitoring and aggressive intervention for all aspects of the disease process, these nurses continue to play an important role in impacting patient outcomes.

CHD is a chronic, progressive, and systemic process. The systemic disease – not just the symptomatic stenosis – must be treated. Medical advances in the treatment of CHD and ACS offer hope in altering the course of disease progression. Nurses in all settings care for patients with cardiovascular disease at some stage on the continuum. Nursing knowledge linked to clinical practice can make a difference in the care of patients with CHD.

EXAM QUESTIONS

CHAPTER 5
Questions 37-46

Note: Choose the one option that BEST answers each question.

37. Stable angina is best defined as angina that

    a. increases in severity.

    b. is new.

    c. occurs at rest.

    d. has a predictable pattern over time.

38. The gold standard diagnostic procedure to definitively diagnose the presence, location, and severity of CHD is

    a. stress testing with nuclear imaging.

    b. stress echocardiography.

    c. cardiac catheterization.

    d. spinal computed tomography.

39. Goals of medical treatment for CHD include

    a. providing surgical revascularization for all patients.

    b. reducing symptoms, preventing complications, and reducing the risk of death.

    c. placing all patients on antiarrhythmic drugs to prevent sudden cardiac death.

    d. placing all patients on warfarin to reduce the risk of stroke.

40. How are vulnerable plaque and ACS related?

    a. The rupture of vulnerable plaque is the most frequent cause of ACS

    b. They are not related in any way

    c. The episode of an ACS causes plaque to become vulnerable

    d. They are only related in men with ACS

41. Which of the following patients is a candidate for reperfusion therapy?

    a. A patient with a 5-year history of stable angina who develops chest pain with extreme exertion

    b. A patient with a history of CHD who develops shortness of breath with exertion after he stops taking his cardiac medications

    c. A patient with no history of CHD who presents with STEMI

    d. A patient who underwent CABG who presents for the second time with a non-STEMI

42. A non-STEMI is differentiated from an episode of UA by

    a. location of chest pain.

    b. cardiac biomarkers.

    c. ECG changes.

    d. extent of cardiac history.

43. Based on the underlying pathophysiology of non-STEMI, which medications are considered part of the *primary* treatment strategy?

    a. Aspirin, beta-blocker, and fibrinolytic

    b. Asprin, clopidogrel, and an anticoagulant

    c. Beta-blocker, ACE inhibitor, and statin

    d. Anticoagulant, calcium channel blocker, and ACE inhibitor

44. A potential mechanical complication of acute MI that requires surgical repair is

    a. reinfarction.

    b. death.

    c. pericarditis.

    d. papillary muscle rupture.

45. Risk factor reduction is important for all patients with CHD because

    a. it can eliminate all possible chances of developing CHD.

    b. CHD only occurs in patients with three or more risk factors.

    c. although it does not benefit patients with CHD, risk factor modification sets a good example for their children.

    d. CHD is a systemic and progressive disease and risk factor modification reduces the risk of future events.

46. Proven benefits of participating in formal exercise training (cardiac rehabilitation) include

    a. increased functional capacity and exercise tolerance.

    b. ability to eliminate all cardiac medications.

    c. increase in earning potential after return to work.

    d. access to a cardiac rehabilitation nurse in the home environment at all times.

CHAPTER 6

CARDIAC REVASCULARIZATION

CHAPTER OBJECTIVE

After completing this chapter, the learner will be able to discuss the indications for, and the benefits and potential complications of, cardiac revascularization.

LEARNING OBJECTIVES

After completing this chapter, the learner will be able to

1. define the indications for revascularization with coronary artery bypass graft surgery.

2. discuss advances in coronary artery bypass grafting that make the procedure less invasive.

3. describe complications and related nursing interventions associated with coronary artery bypass grafting.

4. explain the expected differences in the postoperative course of patients being fast tracked after coronary artery bypass grafting.

5. define the historical limitations of using percutaneous coronary intervention as a revascularization option in the treatment of coronary artery disease.

6. define advances in percutaneous coronary intervention in recent years and the impact of those advances on patient outcomes.

7. explain key nursing interventions in the care of a patient receiving percutaneous coronary intervention.

INTRODUCTION

There are two types of cardiac revascularization: surgical and percutaneous. Surgical revascularization is performed by coronary artery bypass grafting (CABG) and percutaneous revascularization is performed by percutaneous coronary intervention (PCI). CABG involves the use of graft material from the patient's arteries or veins to reroute blood around areas of long stenosis in coronary arteries. PCI is a catheter-based procedure in which mechanical devices are used to open shorter areas of stenosis in the coronary arteries.

CABG was first introduced in 1967; PCI followed 10 years later (Gibbons et al., 2002) with the introduction of percutaneous transluminal coronary angioplasty (PTCA), sometimes referred to today as *plain old balloon angioplasty,* or *POBA.*

Cardiac revascularization is performed to achieve several goals:

- improve survival
- minimize complications of ischemia
- relieve symptoms of ischemia
- improve functional capacity.

(Eagle et al., 2004)

In patients who do not have symptoms, revascularization is only performed if there is an expected survival advantage. Several factors must be considered in making a decision about cardiac revascularization. These factors include suitable coronary anatomy for the procedure, left ventricular function and amount of viable myocardium, symptoms of disease and impact on functional capacity, and other comorbid conditions and factors influencing life expectancy. Patients who have coronary anatomy unsuitable for revascularization are not candidates. Other conditions that limit the option for revascularization include advanced or metastatic cancer with a life expectancy of less than 1 year, end-stage cirrhosis with severe portal hypertension, and intracranial disorders that limit the ability to anticoagulate or substantially limit cognitive function (Anderson et al., 2007).

It is often difficult to adequately compare CABG and PCI today because there have been so many advances with both procedures as well as with medical therapy used in conjunction with these revascularization techniques. There has not been sufficient time to evaluate the long-term effects of these many recent advances. In addition, because of the length of time needed to obtain long-term results, published research studies often do not reflect the most current practices in either type of revascularization and many early studies that evaluated revascularization did not include large numbers of women, older adults, or patients presenting for repeat revascularization. However, although there are limitations, the most recent research has shown comparable survival outcomes with either type of revascularization. Because of durability and the need for repeat revascularization procedures, CABG remains the preferred reperfusion strategy for most patients with multivessel disease, especially if the proximal left anterior descending (LAD) coronary artery is involved, the patient has diabetes, or if left ventricular dysfunction is present. Today, it is reasonable for a patient with diabetes who has less severe coronary disease to be treated with PCI (Anderson et al., 2007; Eagle et al., 2004).

CORONARY ARTERY BYPASS GRAFTING

Indications for Coronary Artery Bypass Grafting

CABG surgery has an average initial hospital cost of approximately $30,000 per patient. When applied to the annual number of patients who are treated with the procedure in the United States, CABG costs approximately 10 billion dollars annually (Eagle et al., 2004). For this reason, CABG is performed only in patients whose survival and symptomatic benefit have been proven. When performed in this group of patients, CABG is considered a cost-effective intervention. With the increasing use of less-invasive strategies for CABG, and with the increasing use of drug-eluting stents, the initial hospital cost difference between CABG and PCI is narrowing.

Patients with left main disease or multivessel disease with decreased left ventricular function are definite candidates for CABG (Anderson et al., 2007; Antman et al., 2004; Eagle et al., 2004; Gibbons et al., 2002). Other indications for CABG include:

- left main equivalent disease with a significant LAD and left circumflex blockage.

- proximal LAD disease with greater than 75% occlusion, plus another vessel, plus a very positive stress test and an abnormal electrocardiogram (ECG).

- coronary heart disease (CHD) in patients who have survived sudden cardiac death.

(Eagle et al., 2004)

CABG increases the chance of survival in patients with reduced left ventricular function, severe ischemia, or potential for severe ischemia (Anderson et al., 2007). The poorer the left ventricular function, the greater the potential mortality benefit with CABG (Eagle et al., 2004). Reduced left ventricular function can be a result of chronic hypoperfusion, in addition to past myocardial infarction (MI). Areas with chronic hypoperfusion can be assessed for viability using noninvasive cardiac testing. Patients with large areas of viable myocardium can benefit from revascularization. Compared to high-risk patients, lower-risk patients receive only a modest survival benefit with CABG. Low-risk patients are generally only considered for CABG when their symptoms have been unresponsive to medical treatment and are limiting their quality of life or functional capacity. CABG has the greatest survival benefit for patients who are at greatest risk of death without surgery (Gibbons et al., 2002).

In addition to increasing survival, CABG is indicated to relieve symptoms and improve other outcomes. Angina is initially relieved in more than 90% of patients who undergo CABG (Ledoux & Luikart, 2010); however, angina can gradually reoccur over time due to either graft stenosis or progression of the patient's underlying CHD. Approximately 80% of patients remain free from angina after 5 years (Gibbons et al., 2002). These results are superior to medical treatment alone. The indications for CABG are very similar for patients with stable angina and unstable angina (UA). However, there is a greater sense of urgency for those with UA.

Traditional CABG

The traditional approach to CABG involves a median sternotomy and the use of a cardiopulmonary (heart and lung) bypass machine (see Figure 6-1). The cardiopulmonary bypass machine allows the surgeon to operate on a still and bloodless heart, while at the same time providing perfusion via a nonpulsatile flow to the other organs of the body. When the patient goes on the cardiopulmonary bypass circuit, venous blood is drained from the right side of the heart. The blood then passes through a pump, which mimics the heart, and then an oxygenator, which mimics the lungs. Blood then travels through a filter before it is returned to systemic circulation via an arterial cannula in the

FIGURE 6-1: HEART AND LUNG BYPASS MACHINE

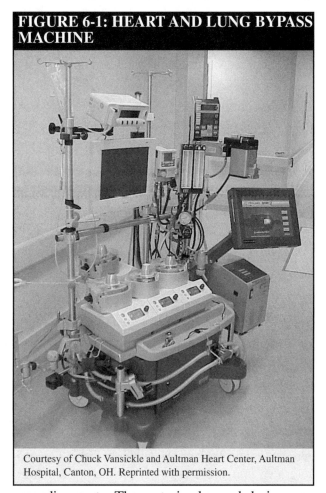

Courtesy of Chuck Vansickle and Aultman Heart Center, Aultman Hospital, Canton, OH. Reprinted with permission.

ascending aorta. The aorta is clamped during surgery to prevent coronary blood flow. The cardiopulmonary bypass machine also allows the temperature of the patient's blood to be controlled and has a vent to decompress the left ventricle when the aorta is cross-clamped. A perfusionist is responsible for the complex management of the cardiopulmonary bypass circuit.

Myocardial protection is required when the aorta is clamped to prevent myocardial ischemia and injury. Myocardial protection is accomplished by the use of cardioplegia to arrest the heart. A cardioplegic solution is typically infused antegrade throught the coronary arteries and retrograde through the coronary veins. Solutions for cardioplegia can be either crystalloid or crystalloid and blood mixtures, and are typically infused at hypothermic temperatures to aide in myocardial protection. Cardioplegia involving the use of blood is commonly used and is definitely recommended in emergent and urgent cases as well as in patients with depressed left ventricular function (Bojar, 2005; Ledoux & Luikart, 2010). Cardioplegic solutions containing blood help provide additional cardiac protection because of the increased oxygen-carrying capacity of blood. Blood can be mixed with a cardioplegic solution through the cardiopulmonary bypass machine. Cardioplegic solutions contain a variety of substances, such as potassium and magnesium and procainamide, to produce cardiac arrest (Bojar, 2005; Ledoux & Luikart, 2010).

Prophylactic use of an intra-aortic balloon pump (IABP) 2 or more hours before cardiopulmonary bypass can also increase myocardial protection in high-risk patients. IABP counterpulsation involves the placement of a balloon catheter in the descending aorta. The balloon is inflated during diastole and deflated during systole, delivering counterpulsation therapy. During balloon inflation (during diastole), myocardial perfusion is increased. During balloon deflation, just before systole, a vacuum is created to reduce afterload, thereby reducing the work of the left ventricle. IABP counterpulsation can also be used to help support left ventricular function in patients who have a difficult time being weaned from the cardiopulmonary bypass circuit.

Graft Material

One of the historical limiting factors of CABG has been the failure of saphenous vein grafts. Up to one half of all vein grafts close within 10 years after surgery (Eagle et al., 2004). Vein grafts are not as durable as arterial grafts. Antiplatelet therapy with aspirin and lipid-lowering therapy with statins improve the short- and long-term patency of saphenous vein grafts. Aspirin is given in the early postoperative period and continued indefinitely after discharge. Aspirin, 325 mg daily, is recommended post operatively for a minimum of one year, and usually indefinitely in patients who have had a saphenous vein used as a graft during CABG (Ferraris et al., 2005).

When CABG surgery began, vein grafts were the only graft material used. The most common vein graft is taken from the greater saphenous vein of the leg. Vein grafts can be harvested using standard incisions or endoscopically. Today, most saphenous veins are harvested endoscopically, which results in an improved cosmetic effect as well as a decreased risk of infection (Bojar, 2005). After harvest, the vein graft is turned inside out because veins have one way valves. It is then attached at one end to the ascending aorta and at the other end to the coronary artery distal to the blockage. Flow through vein grafts depends on pressure. Figure 6-2 shows a saphenous vein graft sutured to the aorta and the coronary artery. The saphenous vein graft is the graft on the left.

Clinical Application

Patients with hypotension or poor left ventricular function are at increased risk for acute vein graft closure due to low pressures and resultant poor flow through the vein graft.

A very important surgical advancement has been the success of internal mammary artery grafts. These grafts have shown major improvement in late patency rates, with more than 90% patency at 10 years (Eagle et al., 2004). Internal mammary artery grafts have also improved long-term survival rates and reduced postoperative mortality (Eagle et al., 2004). Harvesting of the internal mammary arteries is technically more difficult than harvesting of saphenous vein grafts (Ledoux & Luikart, 2010). The left internal mammary artery (LIMA) is most commonly used to bypass the LAD and has become standard practice. When the LAD is bypassed using an internal mammary artery, patients have improved long-term outcomes (Antman et al., 2004; Eagle et al., 2004).

When used as a pedicle graft (a graft left attached to the original site), the proximal end of the internal mammary artery is left intact and the distal end is sutured beyond the site of stenosis. Figure 6-2 shows an internal mammary artery graft

FIGURE 6-2: SAPHENOUS VEIN GRAFT AND INTERNAL MAMMARY ARTERY GRAFT

Note. From *Atlas of Anesthesia: Cardiothoracic Anesthesia* by B. Dorman. Edited by R. Miller (series editor) & J.G. Reves. Copyright 1999, Current Medicine. Used with permission of Images.MD.

on the right. Most CABG surgeries involve a combination of a LIMA graft and saphenous vein grafts. The right internal mammary artery (RIMA) can be used in addition to the left. The decision to use both internal mammary arteries is surgeon and facility specific. The advantage of using both the RIMA and the LIMA is that the patient has the benefit of two very durable arterial grafts. The disadvantage is that the sternal wall is left with a decreased blood supply. This predisposes the patient to an increased risk of sternal wound infection, especially in the patient with diabetes.

In some young patients, revascularization with all-arterial grafts may be considered, with the hope of achieving longer-term patency and avoiding the need for repeat operation. The need for one or more repeat procedures is a concern in younger patients because of increased risk. Lack of an acceptable conduit is also a concern if the procedure must be performed more than once. The radial

artery also can be used as graft material; however, it is prone to spasm because of its thick muscular nature. The risk of spasm can be decreased with the use of nitrates and calcium channel blockers, both intraoperatively and postoperatively. The advantage of the radial artery is its length, which enables it to be used to reach most distal targets. The radial artery is not used unless the patient has adequate patency of the ulnar artery. The radial artery is most often harvested from the patient's nondominant hand.

Clinical Application

Ulnar pulse and distal circulation should be checked postoperatively if the radial artery was harvested for graft material during surgery.

The right gastroepiploic artery supplies blood to the greater curvature of the stomach. When this artery is used as graft material in CABG, a more extensive surgery results because abdominal entry is also required (Ledoux & Luikart, 2010). This artery can be used as a pedicle graft or a free graft.

When patients have no available arterial or venous conduit, cryopreserved saphenous vein grafts or umbilical vein grafts that have been treated with glutaraldehyde can be used. Unfortunately, these grafts have poor long-term patency, so they are used only when no other options are available. Other nonhomologous grafts have been used but also have poor patency. These grafts include bovine internal mammary arteries and synthetic grafts (Eagle et al., 2004).

Advantages

CABG has proven mortality benefits in certain high-risk patient groups, as previously discussed. CABG also has proven long-term success, with graft patency rates at more than 90% at 10 years with the use of arterial conduits (Smith, Allen et al., 2006). CABG allows revascularization to some occlusions that are not accessible using catheter-based techniques.

Contraindications

Patients who have inadequate conduits are not ideal candidates for CABG. Very small coronary arteries distal to the site of stenosis are also a limiting factor in performing CABG. Patients with severe atherosclerosis of the aorta are at very high risk for intraoperative neurological complications and may not be able to undergo traditional CABG requiring cross-clamping of the aorta. Other patient comorbidities may result in an unfavorable risk/benefit ratio for CABG.

Minimally Invasive Techniques

MIDCAB

Minimally invasive CABG (MIDCAB) is performed on a beating heart without cardiopulmonary bypass and without the use of a full median sternotomy to gain access. Access to the heart is usually achieved through a left lateral thoracotomy or through a mini sternotomy. This approach is cosmetically appealing for patients. However, this procedure is technically challenging because visibility is not the same as with a full sternotomy. In addition, if a thoracotomy is used the intercostal nerves can be irritated, producing increased postoperative pain (Niinami, Ogasawara, Suda, & Takeuchi, 2005).

A ministernotomy allows the LAD and right coronary artery (RCA) to be visualized and bypassed using the same incision (Niinami, Ogasawara, Suda, & Takeuchi, 2005). A left thoracotomy approach provides direct visualization of the LAD and access to the LIMA. A right thoracotomy approach is needed to provide visualization of the RCA and access to the RIMA (Hughes & Platt, 2010). Access to both internal mammary arteries is improved with the ministernotomy approach.

To allow for suturing, such medications as beta-blockers or adenosine can be given to slow or temporarily stop the heart. Mechanical stabilizers are also used to hold the coronary artery still while suturing occurs. The advantages of MIDCAB are associated with its avoidance of the full sternotomy and cardiopulmonary bypass circuit. MIDCAB decreases the need for blood transfusions and minimizes the risk of other complications associated with the cardiopulmonary bypass circuit. Patients who have MIDCAB have shorter lengths of hospital stay compared to those who have traditional CABG (Hughes & Platt, 2010) MIDCAB procedures are not frequently done today because the number of lesions that can be bypassed are limited. With the improvements in interventional cardiology procedures, particularly with the addition of drug-eluting stents, patients needing only one or two bypass grafts are often treated with an interventional procedure.

OPCAB

Off-pump CABG (OPCAB) is another less-invasive form of CABG. This surgery is done without cardiopulmonary bypass, but involves a full median sternotomy. A full sternotomy offers better access to bypass the vessels that supply the lateral and posterior walls. Intraoperative techniques are used to lower heart rate, stabilize the coronary arteries, and clear the operative field of blood. As with MIDCAB there are technical challenges for the surgeon when suturing on a moving heart that remains full of blood. In addition, when performing OPCAB on more complex patients, there are intraoperative hemodynamic challenges that can typically be controlled by the perfusionist when the patient is on the cardiopulmonary bypass circuit.

The avoidance of cardiopulmonary bypass with the use of the LIMA and RIMA eliminates the need to clamp the aorta in patients with high-risk aortic atherosclerosis. All patients having CABG have their aortas imaged with transesophageal echocardiography or epiaortic imaging prior to surgery. If an aorta is atherosclerotic it cannot be cross clamped as used in traditional CABG. Even with OPCAB, if a saphenous vein graft is used, the aorta is often clamped at least partially to allow for suturing of the proximal end.

There are several potential advantages to OPCAB that are similar to the advantages of MID-CAB. Many of the advantages are associated with avoidance of the cardiopulmonary bypass circuit, including a reduced need for blood transfusion that results in: 1) less coagulopathy, 2) less hemodilution, and 3) decreased amount of heparin. Other complications that have the potential to be minimized with OPCAB include stroke, atrial fibrillation, and infection (Miller, 2010). The number of OPCAB procedures performed each year has increased since the late 1990s. In the state of New York, 27% of CABG procedures in the year 2000 were done off pump (Racz et al., 2004). Today, some cardiovascular surgical programs do a substantial portion of their procedures as OPCABs. However, the majority of CABG surgeries done in the United States are still traditional CABG procedures (Miller, 2010). OPCAB is a relatively newer technique, and the results of these techniques are expected to improve over time. With increased surgeon experience, the number of OPCAB surgeries is expected to continue to increase, which will result in shorter lengths of stay associated with CABG. Patients receiving OPCAB may be extubated in the operating room and transferred from intensive care to step down care as soon as 12 hours after surgery (Miller, 2010).

Robotics and Other Techniques

Additional techniques for CABG using robotics are also being performed. With robotic surgery, the robot's manipulators receive transmitted instructions from a remote, but interfaced, computer. The surgeon remains at the computer console, where he or she is able to visualize a three-dimensional view. The surgeon uses hand grips at the console and the movements made by the surgeon are duplicated by the robot. Any extraneous movement from the surgeon, such as tremors, is filtered out by system software (Hughes & Platt, 2010). A major advantage of robotic technology is the ability of the robot to manipulate in small spaces where human hands are too large for optimal maneuvering. The cost of this technology as well as the need for extensive surgeon training has limited the widespread use of this technology. Robotic technology can also be used with endoscopic techniques. During endoscopic techniques, small incisions are made in the intercostal spaces. This technology can be used on beating hearts as well as on arrested heart (Hughes & Platt, 2010). Without a full sternotomy, cardiopulmonary bypass cannulation can occur through the femoral artery and vein. Cardioplegic solution can be administered via endovascular techniques (Eagle et al., 2004).

Potential Complications

The use of cardiopulmonary bypass causes a diffuse inflammatory response. This response results in transient multiorgan dysfunction and can also delay recovery after surgery. Various strategies are used to limit the immune response associated with cardiopulmonary bypass:

- Preoperative corticosteroids block complement activation and reduce the levels of proinflammatory cytokines. (Steroids may not be indicated in patients with diabetes.)

- The administration of leukocyte-poor blood and leukocyte depletion via filtration during the perioperative period has been shown to be beneficial in improving myocardial performance during acute or chronic ischemia.

(Eagle et al., 2004)

Patients undergoing CABG today are older and have more comorbidities than patients of the past. However, advances in CABG continue to allow for improved outcomes, even for high-risk patients.

Low Cardiac Output State

The most common cause of mortality after CABG is a low cardiac output state (Eagle et al., 2004). Myocardial damage from a perioperative MI can occur as a complication of CABG and is a common cause of a low cardiac output state. Perioperative MI can occur due to graft spasm or embolization into the graft, or as a complication of cardiopulmonary bypass if myocardial protection is not adequate. Patients with perioperative MI are at increased risk for adverse outcomes. These patients are treated with maximal medical therapy, including antiplatelet agents, beta-blockers, and angiotensin-converting enzyme inhibitors. Low cardiac output after CABG can be caused by reversible conditions after surgery, including acidosis and hypoxemia.

Neurological Complications

The second most common cause of postoperative mortality is postoperative stroke (Eagle et al., 2004). Neurological complications after CABG are classified as type I or type II. Type I deficits include major focal deficits and coma. Type II deficits include various degrees of intellectual deterioration and memory loss. Neurological complications can be caused by intraoperative or postoperative hypoxia, emboli from cardiopulmonary bypass, hemorrhage, or metabolic abnormalities (Eagle et al., 2004). Risk factors for type I and II neurological complications include advanced age and hypertension. Additional risk factors for type I complications include atherosclerosis of the proximal aorta; previous history of neurological disease, UA or diabetes; and intraoperative use of an IABP. Additional risk factors for type II complications include prior CABG, alcohol consumption, dysrhythmias, heart failure, and history of peripheral vascular disease (Eagle et al., 2004).

Type II complications may be related to the brain's own microcirculation, in addition to microemboli during cardiopulmonary bypass. Sophisticated arterial line filters within the cardiopulmonary bypass circuit help protect against microemboli. Type II complications have been associated with periods of hypotension or hypoperfusion and may be reversible. Minimizing type I complications is critical because stroke is the second leading cause of mortality. A type I neurological injury can produce a 21% mortality rate (Eagle et

al., 2004). The use of ultrasound via transesophageal echocardiography or epiaortic imaging to assess the aorta for the presence of atherosclerotic plaque is a technique to help minimize type I complications.

When atherosclerotic plaque is identified in the ascending aorta, the patient is at high risk for an adverse neurovascular outcome. Embolization of atherosclerotic plaque is the most common cause of perioperative stroke (Ledoux & Luikart, 2010). Atherosclerotic emboli can be dislodged from the aortic arch during cannulation for cardiopulmonary bypass or during clamping of the aorta. In very high-risk patients, a no-clamp strategy may be used (Eagle et al., 2004).

Other factors that contribute to postoperative stroke are recent anterior wall MI with left ventricular thrombus and recent stroke. Patients with a recent stroke should not have CABG for at least 4 weeks. If CABG is done within 4 weeks of a stroke, then the patient is at high risk for hemorrhagic complications of stroke. Patients who also have symptomatic or severe carotid stenosis should be treated with carotid endarterectomy prior to CABG. Patients routinely have carotid ultrasound exams prior to surgery to assess for significant carotid stenosis. Carotid endarterectomy is generally not performed in asymptomatic carotid disease unless stenosis is 80% or greater (Eagle et al., 2004).

The risk of neurovascular complications also increases with the time spent on cardiopulmonary bypass. Hyperglycemia can also worsen neurological impairment.

Peripheral neurovascular complications, including brachial plexus injury and ulnar nerve injury, can also occur as complications of surgery.

Atrial Fibrillation

Another complication of CABG is the development of atrial fibrillation postoperatively. Atrial fibrillation occurs in 20% to 40% of postoperative patients and is most commonly seen on the second to third hospital day (Ledoux & Luikart, 2010). If atrial fibrillation persists for more than 24 hours, warfarin can be initiated to prevent clot formation and future stroke. Several patient factors increase the likelihood of developing atrial fibrillation postoperatively:

• chronic obstructive pulmonary disease (COPD) or proximal RCA disease (can cause right ventricular and right atrial enlargement)

• cessation of beta-blockers prior to surgery

• increased cross-clamp time, producing atrial ischemia

• advanced age.
(Eagle et al., 2004)

Increased circulating catecholamines, volume overload, hypoxia, and electrolyte disturbances in the postoperative state can also contribute to the development of atrial fibrillation (Ledoux & Luikart, 2010). Atrial fibrillation extends the length of stay and also greatly increases the risk of postoperative stroke.

The standard therapy for the reduction of postoperative atrial fibrillation is the initiation of beta-blockers preoperatively or very early postoperatively. Patients who were taking beta-blockers preoperatively and have them withdrawn perioperatively are at increased risk for developing atrial fibrillation as a complication of CABG. Amiodarone can be used if beta-blockers are contraindicated.

Wound Infection

Preoperative antibiotic administration is routinely used to help prevent postoperative infection. Cephalosporins are the class of choice. Because an adequate tissue level of antibiotics is required at the time of incision, timing of preoperative antibiotics is important. Preoperative antibiotics should be administered within 30 minutes of incision time (Eagle et al., 2004). Additional antibiotic dosing may be required for longer surgeries. Postoperative intravenous (IV) antibiotics are continued for 1 to 2 days.

Mediastinitis, or deep sternal wound infection, is a serious complication of CABG that results in a mortality rate as high as 25% (Eagle et al., 2004). Sternal wound infections typically manifest several days to 2 weeks after surgery (Ledoux & Luikart, 2010). Skin and nasopharyngeal gram-positive organisms are the leading cause of postoperative deep sternal wound infections (Eagle et al., 2004). Obesity, diabetes, repeat surgery, and excessive use of electrocautery are risk factors. In addition, the use of both internal mammary arteries increases the risk because the sternum receives less blood flow. Superficial wounds are treated with antibiotics and drainage, whereas deep sternal wounds require surgical debridement and closure with a muscle flap (Ledoux & Luikart, 2010).

Several strategies are used during surgery to decrease the risk of mediastinitis and sternal wound infection (See Box 6-1.)

Renal Dysfunction

Renal dysfunction is another potential complication after CABG because cardiopulmonary bypass decreases glomerular filtration rate. The following characteristics place a patient at risk for developing renal dysfunction after bypass: advanced age, heart failure, type I diabetes, preexisting renal dysfunction, and prior CABG (Eagle et al., 2004). Mortality is high for those who develop renal dysfunction perioperatively and is especially high for those who require dialysis. Early recognition of renal insufficiency and assurance of adequate volume administration are key nursing interventions in preventing postoperative renal failure.

Clinical Application

Nephrotoxic medications, including nonsteroidal anti-inflammatory drugs (NSAIDs) and aminoglycoside antibiotics, should be avoided in high-risk patients.

Patients with end-stage renal disease are at very high risk for mortality and morbidity if they undergo CABG. However, their risk for mortality

BOX 6-1: STRATEGIES TO DECREASE STERNAL WOUND INFECTIONS

1. Meticulous aseptic technique
   a) Double gloving of operating room (OR) team.
   b) Reduced OR traffic.
2. Clipping, rather than shaving, hair and avoidance of hair removal.
3. Shorter perfusion times.
4. Avoidance of unnecessary electrocautery.
5. Proper selection and timing of preoperative and perioperative antibiotics.
   a) Preoperative antibiotic timing within 1 hour of incision.
   b) Postoperative antibiotics for 48 hours or less. B-lactam antibiotic is single choice for standard cardiac prophylaxis unless there is a high incidence of methicillin-resistant Staphylococcus aureus (MRSA).
   c) In select high-risk patients a glycopeptide (Vancomycin) may be reasonable as an adjunct.
   d) Vancomycin is not recommended as a sole prophylactic agent. Routine mupirocin is recommended for all patients in staphyloccal colonization.
6. Use of chlorhexidine for patient skin preparation.
7. Use of chlorhexidine mouth rinse preoperatively and postoperatively (American Association of Critical Care Nurses (AACN), 2010).
8. Perioperative glycemic control.

(Eagle et al., 2004; Engelman et al., 2007)

may be even higher if they do not undergo revascularization; therefore, CABG may be considered for some of these patients. Patients with end-stage renal disease have a particularly high risk of developing postoperative infection and sepsis (Eagle et al., 2004).

Pulmonary Complications

Mild pulmonary complications can occur simply as a result of cardiopulmonary bypass. During cardiopulmonary bypass, capillary permeability and pulmonary vascular resistance increase and noncardiac pulmonary edema can occur (Ledoux & Luikart, 2010). Acute respiratory distress syndrome (ARDS) is a serious potential complication. Patients undergoing repeat CABG and those requiring blood transfusions are at higher risk for developing ARDS. Preoperative pulmonary edema should be resolved prior to surgery because pulmonary edema increases with cardiopulmonary bypass.

Most patients experience postoperative atelectasis. Postoperative thoracic and abdominal surgery patients are prone to hypoventilation due to postoperative pain.

Clinical Application

Postoperative pain control is an effective intervention in preventing atelectasis by promoting adequate ventilation.

The most common preoperative pulmonary problem is COPD. Those with moderate to severe COPD, including those with elevated partial pressure of carbon dioxide levels and those who use home oxygen, are at increased risk for postoperative complications. These patients are likely to remain on ventilators longer, which places them at risk of developing nosocomial pneumonia. In addition to their risk of pulmonary complications, these patients also experience an increased risk of ventricular dysrhythmias postoperatively (Eagle et al., 2004).

Clinical Application

Smoking cessation is an important intervention to decrease the risk of pulmonary complications in patients electively undergoing CABG.

All pulmonary infectious processes should also be resolved prior to surgery. Before surgery, it is important for patients to receive incentive spirometry and to perform coughing and deep breathing exercises. This preoperative treatment also provides the instruction for postoperative exercises. If time allows, weight loss should be achieved in obese patients electively undergoing CABG because it can help to decrease the risk of adverse pulmonary effects and other complications.

Clinical Application

It is important to accomplish preoperative respiratory teaching (incentive spirometry and coughing and deep breathing), even in patients without pre-existing lung disease, because postoperative sedation and pain interfere with the patient's ability to learn during the early postoperative period.

Patients who are unable to be extubated in a timely fashion because of pulmonary complications are usually ventilated using low tidal volume. The use of low tidal volume is one lung-protective strategy to limit damage to pulmonary tissue caused by mechanical ventilation. Pneumothorax can also occur as a postoperative complication and can happen at the time of removal of pleural chest tubes.

Postoperative Bleeding

Postoperative bleeding is usually venous in nature and originates from the site of sutures. Bleeding can also occur from pericardial adhesions during a repeat procedure. Blood loss should be less than 300 ml/hr during the first several hours and then should begin to taper. Average total blood loss is approximately 1 L (Ferraris et al., 2005). Patients who experience prolonged cardiopulmonary bypass are at risk for developing coagulapathies postoperatively. Coagulation profiles are drawn postoperatively to determine any deficiencies in clotting factors. Recognized deficiencies are replaced with administration of the appropriate clotting factors. Platelet count should be kept above 100,000/mm³.

Patients who are at high risk for bleeding preoperatively, including those undergoing repeat CABG and those with expected long cardiopulmonary bypass, may receive antifibrinolytic drugs to reduce the risk of bleeding. If postoperative bleeding cannot be adequately controlled, then mediastinal re-exploration may be needed to reduce the risk of cardiac tamponade, a life-threatening postoperative emergency.

Transfusion

Patients having CABG account for 10% of blood transfusions in the United States. However, only 20% of the patients having CABG are the recipients of the vast majority of blood transfusions in this patient population (Eagle et al., 2004). Blood transfusions produce an immunosuppressive effect and increase the risk of nosocomial infection, particularly nosocomial pneumonia. Therefore, the goal is to avoid the need for perioperative transfusion whenever possible. The risk of complications from transfusion increases when the transfused blood is older than 1 month old (Raghavan & Marik, 2005). In patients having CABG, the proinflammatory substances that accumulate during the storage of blood can increase pulmonary complications postoperatively (Raghavan & Marik, 2005).

There is some evidence that many of the detrimental effects of blood transfusions are related to donor white blood cells and how they react with stored red blood cells (RBCs) (Raghavan & Marik, 2005). Depletion of leukocytes can be helpful in blunting this immunosuppressive response. This procedure can occur in the blood bank or at the bedside at the time of transfusion using a filter. Several factors increase the patient's risk of needing a blood transfusion during or after surgery. These risk factors are listed in Box 6-2.

BOX 6-2: RISK FACTORS FOR PERIOPERATIVE BLOOD TRANSFUSION

- Increased age
- Increased time on cardiopulmonary bypass
- Repeat CABG
- Emergent or urgent operation
- Low RBC volume preoperatively
- Preoperative fibrinolytic, anticoagulant, or antiplatelet therapy

(Eagle et al., 2004)

Anticoagulation and Antiplatelet Therapy Prior to Surgery

If a patient is expected to need CABG within 24 hours, then low-molecular-weight heparin (LMWH) is not used as the anticoagulant of choice; unfractionated heparin (UFH) is used instead. LMWH should be stopped 18 to 24 hours before surgery and replaced with UFH, which can be continued until a short time before the incision is made. In addition, a direct thrombin inhibitor, such as bivalrudin, can be continued until immediately before surgery. Warfarin is typically held for 4 days prior to surgery (Ferraris et al., 2007).

Aspirin can be held preoperatively in elective cases, but is not held if the patient has had a recent acute coronary syndrome (ACS) (Antman et al., 2004; Ferraris et al., 2007). The benefits of continuing aspirin therapy in patients with ACSs need to be weighed against the risks of postoperative bleeding. Clopidogrel should be held prior to CABG to reduce the risk of postoperative bleeding. It is recommended to be held for 5 to 7 days before surgery (Eagle et al., 2004; Ferraris et al., 2007). Prasugrel is recommended to be held for at least 7 days prior to surgey (Gold Standard/Elsevier, 2010). The glycoprotein (GP) IIb/IIIa inhibitors tirofiban and eptifibatide need to be discontinued 4 to 6 hours before CABG, and abciximab needs to be stopped 12 to 24 hours before surgery (Ferraris et al., 2007). In patients who proceed to CABG after receiving abciximab, platelet aggregation does not return to normal for 48 hours. These patients receive special precautions during CABG to minimize the risk of bleeding. Such precautions include:

- lower doses of intraoperative heparin
- minimal hemodilution
- platelet transfusion
- possible use of antifibrinolytics, such as e-aminocaproic acid and tranexamic acid

(Bojar, 2005; Eagle et al., 2004)

Patients can donate their own blood during the 30 days prior to surgery to be used as an autologous transfusion if needed during or after surgery. Patients who have adequate hemoglobin levels and do not have unstable or potentially unstable ischemic disease are the best candidates. In other candidates, an option is to use recombinant human erythropoietin (EPO) preoperatively to restore RBC volume before donation of blood for autologous transfusion (Bojar, 2005). In another technique, blood is taken from the patient prior to cardiopulmonary bypass and then reinfused in the patient immediately after bypass. Autotransfusion from mediastinal-shed blood has also been used to decrease the number of blood transfusions. However, some researchers express concern that autotransfusion can stimulate fibrinolysis (Eagle et al., 2004).

Late Postoperative Complications

Weeks to months after CABG, some patients experience an autoimmune response of the pericardial tissue. This response causes inflammation of the pericardium and is termed *postpericardiotomy syndrome*. The pleural space can also be involved. Patients are treated with NSAIDs. Steroids can also be used, if needed.

Cardiac tamponade can also occur late in the postoperative period. It can occur alone or as a complication of postpericardiotomy syndrome. Late tamponade is most typically seen in patients on warfarin (Ledoux & Luikart, 2010).

Special Populations

Patients Who Require Emergency CABG

Any emergent or urgent surgery carries an increased risk of mortality and morbidity. Whenever possible, PCI, an IABP, and medical treatment should be used to stabilize the patient prior to surgery. Failed PCI procedures in patients who are ischemic or who have hemodynamic instability may warrant emergency CABG. Emergency CABG may also be performed at the time of a repair of a mechanical complication of acute MI, such as septal or mechanical rupture. Emergency CABG is not performed in patients with only a small area of myocardium at risk who are hemodynamically stable (Antman et al., 2004).

Patients Who Have Had an Acute MI

Patients who have had acute MIs have higher mortality with CABG for the first several days after the infarction. For patients with large MIs who are stabilized, surgery should be delayed to allow the myocardium to recover. However, some patients with acute MIs are unable to wait to have CABG, including those with left main or triple vessel disease and those with symptomatic valve disease. CABG mortality is elevated for the first 3 to 7 days after an MI (Antman et al., 2004).

Patients Who Have Had a Right Ventricular MI

Patients with large right ventricular MIs are at particularly high risk and may need surgery delayed for up to 4 weeks to allow for recovery of the right ventricle. During surgery, the pericardium is no longer able to contain the acutely injured right ventricle and it dilates. This dilation may even prevent the chest from closing (Eagle et al., 2004).

Older Adult Patients

The greatest increase in CABG is among patients older than 85 years of age. Older adults have an increased risk of mortality and morbidity; however, improvement in functional capacity and quality of life can be achieved in most patients in this age-group (Eagle et al., 2004).

Women

Some studies have found differences in CABG mortality and morbidity rates when comparing women to men, with women having higher complication rates. However, the evidence is conflicting as to whether gender is the determining factor. General consensus is that risk factors and patient comorbidities are more important than gender, and CABG should not be delayed as a treatment option for women (Eagle et al., 2004).

Patients With Diabetes

Patients with diabetes have an increased risk of mortality with CABG compared to patients who do not have diabetes (Woods, Smith, Sohail, Sarah, & Engle, 2004). However, in the Bypass Angioplasty Revascularization Investigation (BARI) Trial, CABG was shown to provide a greater survival benefit to appropriate patients with diabetes than did PCI (Woods et al., 2004). In addition to diabetes, any hyperglycemia during the perioperative period increases risk, especially for sternal wound infections. Hyperglycemia can occur in patients without diabetes due to surgical stress, hypothermia, commonly used postoperative medications, and other complex metabolic changes that occur during CABG (Lorenz, Lorenz, & Codd, 2005). New guidelines from the Society of Thoracic Surgeons recommend target glucose levels less than 180 mg/dL in patients with and without diabetes during the perioperative period. Glycemic control with continuous IV infusion is the best strategy for those patients who have diabetes. If a patient has an anticipated intensive care stay of 3 days or longer, then the target for glucose control is less than 150 mg/dL. In addition to decreasing the risk of sternal wound infection, glycemic control less than 180 mg/dL in patients with diabetes results in a decrease of overall mortality and morbidity and an improvement in long-term survival (Lazar et al., 2009).

Patients with Peripheral Vascular Disease

Patients with peripheral vascular disease commonly have coexisting CHD. Patients with peripheral vascular disease who undergo CABG have an increased short- and long-term risk of mortality.

Patients with Low Ejection Fractions

Patients with low ejection fractions or clinical heart failure also have an increased risk of operative mortality. However, this group of patients, when treated with CABG, also have the greatest survival benefit when compared to treatment with medical therapy. In addition, this population can benefit from symptom relief and improvement in functional capacity (Gibbons et al., 2002).

Patients with Valve Disease

Patients with coexisting moderate to severe aortic stenosis commonly undergo aortic valve replacement at the time of CABG. In addition, patients who have clinically symptomatic mitral valve regurgitation with structural abnormalities undergo mitral valve repair at the time of CABG (Bonow et al., 2008; Eagle et al., 2004). If the mitral valve is structurally normal and regurgitation is not severe, the regurgitation may be caused by reversible ischemia that will be corrected with the revascularization procedure. Combined procedures increase the operative risk of complications and mortality. When a valve procedure is added to CABG, the risk of stroke substantially increases (Bonow et al., 2008; Eagle et al., 2004).

Postoperative Nursing Care

All patients who have undergone open heart surgery are cared for in a similar fashion, regardless of the exact operation performed. They receive care in an intensive care unit for the immediate postoperative period. During this period, patients are on mechanical ventilation for a minimum of 2 to 4 hours (Ledoux & Luikart, 2010) and are monitored via a cardiac monitor. In addition, patients have an arterial line and pulmonary artery catheter in place for invasive monitoring of systemic and intracardiac pressures. The arterial line allows for continuous monitoring of blood pressure, which can be unstable during the early postoperative period. Hypertension or hypotension can occur after surgery. Hypotension frequently occurs in the early postoperative period as the patient warms up. The patient can also experience hypovolemia due to fluid volume alterations associated with cardiopulmonary bypass. The pulmonary artery catheter allows for assessment of preload, afterload, and contractility. Poor cardiac output can occur due to problems with heart rate, preload, afterload, and contractility. Having a pulmonary artery catheter in place provides information regarding which parameter of cardiac output is abnormal. This allows treatment to be directed at the specific cause of the low cardiac output.

Pulmonary artery catheters with the capability of continuous cardiac output and venous oxygen saturation monitoring are commonly used. Venous oxygen saturation levels give an assessment of the amount of oxygen left over after the patient has used a portion of what was delivered. This is called *venous reserve.* The body normally uses approximately 25% of the oxygen that is delivered to the tissues. This leaves an average venous reserve of approximately 75%. When the venous oxygen saturation level (venous reserve) drops, it is because: 1) delivery has dropped, 2) consumption needs have increased, or 3) a combination of a decrease in delivery and increase in consumption. Venous oxygen saturation levels provide a good assessment of the delivery and consumption of oxygen because they measure the patient's venous reserve. Postoperative patients also have temporary epicardial pacing wires in place.

Bradycardiac dysrhythmias (bradydysrhythmias) can occur postoperatively, especially in patients who have received valve repair or replacement. The suture lines from valve surgery are close to the conduction system, and postoperative edema can cause temporary heart block.

Pleural and mediastinal chest tubes connected to water-seal chambers and 20 cm of suction are also used. Stripping of chest tubes postoperatively should be avoided because of the risk of damaging bypass grafts. Mediastinal chest tubes can recover blood during the immediate postoperative period to be used for autotransfusion. Packed RBCs generally are not given unless the hemoglobin level falls below 8 g/dl (Ledoux & Luikart, 2010). Control of hypertension is important during the postoperative period to reduce the risk of bleeding.

Early postoperative aspirin administration, initiated at least within the first 48 hours, is important to prevent saphenous vein graft closure. Aspirin also reduces many other postoperative complications and decreases postoperative mortality (Eagle et al., 2004; Ferraris et al., 2005).

Fast Tracking

Low-risk patients can be selected for fast tracking after CABG. These patients are targeted for early extubation, early ambulation, and early discharge. Special pathways are used to guide care in patients being fast tracked. Patients who are fast tracked are sedated postoperatively with short-acting agents and receive lower doses of opioids to allow for earlier extubation. Patients can be extubated postoperatively when they are awake, respond appropriately, and are able to have pain controlled without using medications that interfere with extubation. Prior to extubation, patients must also have no serious postoperative bleeding and have stable vital signs. Pharmacological strategies to prevent atrial fibrillation are also a key component of fast tracking.

Early ambulation and phase I cardiac rehabilitation exercises are also a part of the fast track program. Patients who undergo traditional CABG and who are fast tracked are generally discharged 3 to 5 days postoperatively. Older patients are commonly more difficult to fast track because of higher numbers of preoperative comorbidities. Patients who receive less invasive forms of surgery generally advance more quickly to extubation, step down care, and discharge.

Postdischarge Care

Administration of postoperative aspirin is continued indefinitely. All patients also receive statin therapy to reduce the progression of vein graft disease. After CABG, patients are placed on a 20- to 25-lb lifting restriction, with no more than 10 lb over the head for 6 to 8 weeks after discharge. Patients generally wait to drive after CABG, even after their restrictions are over, because of chest soreness and fear of injury.

A formal cardiac rehabilitation program referral should be made for all patients prior to discharge. Patients usually begin participation in outpatient cardiac rehabilitation 4 to 8 weeks after surgery. In one long-term study of patients who participated in cardiac rehabilitation after CABG, outcomes at 5 years included increased physical mobility, perception of better health, and perception of better overall life situations. Compared to those who do not participate in cardiac rehabilitation, a larger percentage of those who complete the program are working at 3 years (Eagle et al., 2004).

Assessment of depression and presence of psychosocial support are important nursing interventions in the postdischarge period. Depression occurs in up to 33% of patients after CABG (Eagle et al., 2004). Psychosocial interventions for patients after CABG are similar to those for patients with CHD. These interventions were discussed in detail in Chapter 5.

Clinical Application

Facilitating participation in cardiac rehabilitation is a key nursing intervention in the prevention and treatment of postoperative depression and social isolation.

Many patients and their caregivers experience major psychosocial adjustments after discharge. Adapting to postoperative pain, changes in body image, activity limitations, and financial burdens are a few of the areas for which nurses need to provide support during the discharge transition (Theobald & McMurray, 2004). Telephone follow-up programs are one method of providing postoperative support, especially to assure a smooth home transition in patients who are fast tracked.

Presentation with Angina after Coronary Artery Bypass Grafting

Up to 20% of patients presenting with UA have undergone CABG. These patients are at higher risk for mortality and morbidity than patients who have never received revascularization (Anderson, et al., 2007). Patients who present with ACS or other symptoms suggestive of ischemia after having CABG are generally candidates for cardiac catheterization. It is difficult to distinguish between graft closure and progression of native vessel disease using only noninvasive testing. Most patients who present with ischemia within 30 days of surgery have graft failure due to thrombosis. This acute graft closure can occur in vein grafts and arterial conduits. These patients are usually candidates for PCI to treat the focal stenosis. If multiple vein grafts are stenosed or if the stenotic graft is supplying the LAD, then repeat CABG is often indicated.

Repeat Surgery

Mortality and morbidity risks are higher for patients who undergo repeat CABG. These patients may also have limited available graft options. Long-term results are not as successful with repeat operations as with initial operations.

PERCUTANEOUS CORONARY INTERVENTION

PCI refers to a group of catheter-based technologies used to treat coronary stenosis. PTCA was the first of these catheter-based techniques. Intracoronary stents are now used in the vast majority of PCI procedures. In addition, a variety of other techniques and therapies are used in PCI.

Prior to the use of intracoronary stenting, coronary interventional technique was primarily limited to PTCA. Sometimes referred to as *plain old balloon angioplasty,* PTCA is a catheter-based procedure in which a balloon is inflated at the site of coronary stenosis to increase the vessel lumen diameter. Balloon inflation causes plaque rupture and disruption of the endothelium (see Figure 6-3). PTCA has two primary limitations: acute vessel closure and restenosis. Prior to stents, the acute closure rate during PTCA was approximately 5% and the 6-month restenosis rate was 35% to 45% (Anderson et al., 2007). The risk for acute vessel closure made it necessary for standby of a CABG team in case emergency CABG was needed. Restenosis occurs through different processes, including vessel recoil and remodeling as well as neointimal hyperplasia, which occurs in response to vessel injury. Smooth muscle cells from the media of the vessel migrate through tears to reach the luminal surface. Also, myofibrils from the adventia transform into smooth muscle cells and migrate to the site of injury. This collection of smooth muscle cells can result in restenosis.

Interventional Devices and Adjunct Procedures

Intracoronary Stenting (Bare Metal)

The first U.S. Food and Drug Administration (FDA) approval for an intracoronary stent occurred in 1993 (Deelstra, 2010). Stent design and the associated pharmacology with stent use have improved

FIGURE 6-3: BALLOON INFLATION CAUSING PLAQUE DISRUPTION DURING PTCA

Note. From *Atlas of Heart Diseases: Chronic Ischemic Heart Disease* by E. Powers. Edited by E. Braunwald (series editor) & G.A. Beller. Copyright 1995, by Current Medicine. Used with permission from Images.MD.

significantly since that time. Bare metal and drug-eluting stenting, GP IIb/IIIa and clopidogrel antiplatelet therapy, and newer anticoagulants (such as bivalrudin), have made PCI a safer procedure and have also contributed to substantially improved outcomes. Stenting involves the placement of a metal scaffold-type structure to help prevent elastic recoil and to keep open the lumen of the vessel. Stents can be made from various metals and have different structural designs. Most stents are delivered and expanded with the use of a balloon system (see Figure 6-4). Self-expanding stents are also available. After a stent is deployed and expanded, a high-pressure balloon is typically used to assure that the stent is fully deployed.

Stenting reduces the risk of acute vessel closure, which can lead to ST-segment elevation myocardial infarction (STEMI). Intracoronary stents have also reduced the need for emergency CABG by preventing and treating dissections caused by balloon inflation. Stenting also reduces the percentage of late vessel restenosis. Stents impact restenosis by decreasing the elastic recoil of the vessel and also by decreasing the remodeling that occurs after vessel injury associated with PTCA. Stenting with bare metal stents reduces restenosis rates to approximately 20% to 30% (Deelstra, 2010). Bare metal stents decrease restenosis by impacting vessel remodeling. With the use of intracoronary stenting, results in patients older than 75 years of age are similar to those of younger patients (Smith, Feldman et al., 2006). Intracoronary stenting is usually done in conjunction with balloon angioplasty but it can also be performed without balloon dilatation.

Drug-Eluting Stents

Stents coated with pharmacological agents aimed at decreasing restenosis have been FDA-

FIGURE 6-4: TYPES OF INTRACORONARY STENTS

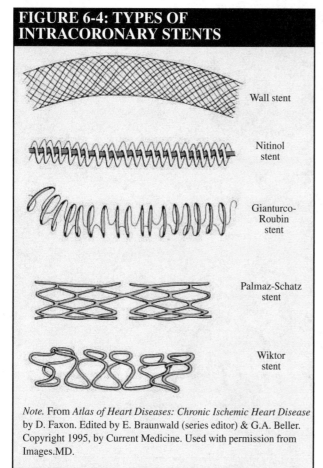

Wall stent

Nitinol stent

Gianturco-Roubin stent

Palmaz-Schatz stent

Wiktor stent

Note. From *Atlas of Heart Diseases: Chronic Ischemic Heart Disease* by D. Faxon. Edited by E. Braunwald (series editor) & G.A. Beller. Copyright 1995, by Current Medicine. Used with permission from Images.MD.

approved since 2003 (Deelstra, 2010). Drug-eluting stents impact restenosis by both preventing vessel remodeling and inhibiting neointimal hyperplasia. The two pharmacological agents initially used with drug-eluting stents were sirolimus and paclitaxel. Only one agent is coated per stent. Both agents are used to specifically prevent in-stent restenosis. Sirolimus is an immunosuppressive agent that is also used to prevent organ rejection during kidney transplantation (MedlinePlus, 2010). This drug reduces cytokine production and inflammation and also inhibits proliferation of smooth cells (Deelstra, 2010). Paclitaxel is an antiproliferative (or antineoplastic) agent that is also used as a chemotherapeutic agent (MedlinePlus, 2008). Newer drug-eluting stents have been approved for use. These drug-eluting stents use the drugs zotorolimus and everolimus.

Drug-eluting stents have shown improved restenosis rates compared to bare metal stents. The initial drug-eluting stents reduced restenosis rates to approximately 10% (Deelstra, 2010). With the use of drug-eluting stents in conjunction with contemporary antiplatelet therapy, restenosis rates with interventional cardiology procedures are often in the single digits. Future drug-eluting stents will include partially biosorbable stents where a bare metal stent will remain after the drug is absorbed, and fully biosorbable stents that will remain in place only long enough to prevent vessel recoil and remodeling. New polymer coatings for stents are also being developed that will have more biocompatible surfaces.

Directional Atherectomy

Directional atherectomy can be used to cut and remove plaque in native vessels or in saphenous vein grafts. A rotating cutter is directed toward the plaque to be removed. Both directional and rotational atherectomy "debulk" coronary arteries containing a large amount of atherosclerotic plaque. Directional atherectomy can be used in calcified lesions. Figure 6-5 displays pictures of devices used for directional coronary atherectomy.

FIGURE 6-5: DIRECTIONAL CORONARY ATHERECTOMY DEVICES

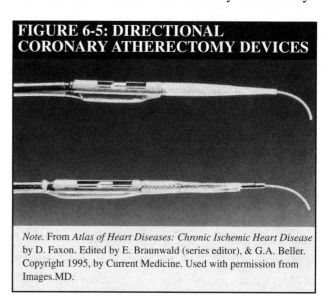

Note. From *Atlas of Heart Diseases: Chronic Ischemic Heart Disease* by D. Faxon. Edited by E. Braunwald (series editor), & G.A. Beller. Copyright 1995, by Current Medicine. Used with permission from Images.MD.

Rotational Atherectomy

Rotational atherectomy involves the use of high-speed rotating blades or burs to remove components of the atherosclerotic plaque. This technique is not used in the presence of acute thrombus. It is used to help prepare for a more successful PTCA and stent procedure when a hard, calcified lesion is present. Rotational atherectomy has permitted intervention in some lesions that previously could only be treated with CABG (Eagle et al., 2004). Creatine kinase (CK)-MB enzymes can be released during this procedure because microparticles are embolized distally. This distal embolization causes platelet activation. The use of GP IIb/IIIa inhibitors can reduce platelet aggregation and limit the release of CK-MB enzymes. Atherectomy procedures have higher rates of complications when performed alone and are typically performed in conjunction with intracoronary stent placement (Smith, Feldman et al., 2006).

Extraction Techniques

Other atherectomy techniques, such as angiojet thrombectomy and transluminal extraction atherectomy, are used for the extraction of visible thrombi within the coronary artery. An angiojet thrombectomy device works by delivering high-velocity saline jets. The jets are also given retrograde to assist in removal of thrombotic material (Deelstra, 2010). When thrombi are removed prior to intervention, the risk of postprocedure complications may be decreased. These techniques are also proposed to remove degenerative graft material and thrombi commonly seen with saphenous vein graft stenosis.

Laser

With laser techniques, tissue is ablated using a combination of photochemical, thermal, and mechanical effects. These techniques are not widely used. Early results demonstrated increased dissection and perforation with ablative techniques (Deelstra, 2010).

Cutting Balloons

Special cutting balloons are now available that can be used to make incisions into the plaque prior to dilatation. This technique allows for greater plaque compression in lesions resistant to balloon dilatation (Deelstra, 2010).

Radiation (Brachytherapy)

Locally delivered ionizing radiation has been used to treat in-stent restenosis. Radiation decreases the intimal hyperplasia associated with in-stent restenosis by interfering with smooth cell proliferation. Both gamma and beta radiation have been used. Patients who have undergone radiation treatment need to be on clopidogrel for an extended period because a reduction in neointimal hyperplasia increases the risk of contact between blood and stent material as well as thrombus formation. Drug-eluting stents have significantly reduced in-stent restenosis and brachytherapy is no longer a routinely used treatment option.

Intravascular Ultrasound

With intravascular ultrasound, a miniature ultrasound transducer on the end of a catheter provides a cross-sectional image of the coronary artery that can be used to evaluate results in high-risk procedures. This technology can guide assessment of lesions that are difficult to visualize with angiography. Intravascular ultrasound can also be used to assess the quality of lesions, including those that are calcific. It can also be used to guide atherectomy procedures and to assure that intracoronary stents are optimally deployed. Optimally deployed stents reduce the risk of in-stent thrombosis.

Coronary Pressure Measurements

Fractional flow reserve measurements are used to assess the maximal coronary blood flow at the area of stenosis. Flow is measured using a pressure wire. The result represents a fraction of what is normally expected with no stenosis. A result of less than 0.75 represents a significant coronary stenosis.

Advantages

Advantages of PCI include low rates of procedure mortality and morbidity. These procedures also take less time to perform and are easier to repeat if needed than is CABG. No general anesthesia, thoracotomy, or cardiopulmonary bypass is required. Patients experience much shorter hospital stays and are able to return to work sooner. Central nervous system complications are also decreased. However, patients must have suitable anatomy to be candidates for PCI. Not all lesions can be reached by a catheter-based technique.

Indications

PCI is performed in a wide range of patients, from stable to unstable and with a varying amount of myocardium at risk. PCI is more effective than medical treatment in relieving angina (Rimmerman, 2010). PCI was historically limited to single vessel proximal CHD; however, with newer techniques, the scope of interventional cardiology has expanded. For patients with two vessel disease, PCI is routinely considered an acceptable alternative to surgery. PCI may even be considered in three vessel disease if left ventricular function is normal and the patient does not have diabetes.

Insufficient evidence is available regarding the mortality benefits of PCI in high-risk patients. Elective PCI is an option for revascularization in patients with normal left ventricular function. However, CABG is recommended for patients with abnormal left ventricular function who have severe symptoms (Gibbons et al., 2002). Some evidence shows that CABG improves survival in patients with diabetes who have three vessel disease (Eagle et al., 2004; Gibbons et al., 2002). However, abciximab, a GP IIb/IIIa inhibitor, has been shown to improve the outcomes of PCI in patients with diabetes (Anderson et al., 2007). Continued advances in PCI may open the door for more PCI procedures in groups of patients who are currently only recommended for CABG.

PCI is not indicated in non-LAD disease, except if ischemia is found on noninvasive testing. PCI is also not performed on lesions with less than 60% stenosis, unless ischemia is found on noninvasive testing. Many patients with chronic angina undergo PCI for control of symptoms, even though there may be no associated survival benefit. As with all medical decisions, physician judgment and, often, patient preferences play an important role in treatment decisions.

Success Rates

Success of PCI procedures is typically defined in four different ways: angiographic success, procedural success, clinical success, and long-term success. These definitions are listed in Table 6-1.

With the use of stents and GP IIb/IIIa inhibitors, angiographic success rates with PCI are as high as 99% (Smith, Feldman et al., 2006). Results of PCI are similar in patients presenting with either stable angina or UA. The limiting factor for long-term success with PCI continues to be restenosis. The majority of restenosis occurs during the 3- to 6-month period after the procedure. It is unusual for restenosis to occur after 12 months (Smith, Feldman et al., 2006). Bare metal stents help eliminate the elastic recoil associated with restenosis, and drug-eluting stents show promise of greatly impacting the neointimal hyperplasia that still limits long-term success. However, the use of drug-eluting stents is new, and long-term outcomes

TABLE 6-1: PCI SUCCESS	
Term	**Definition**
Angiographic success	Substantial enlargement of the vessel lumen at the site of intervention; less than 20% residual stenosis
Procedural success	Angiographic success + Freedom from major hospital complications
Clinical success	Angiographic success + Procedural success + Relief from signs and symptoms of ischemia
Long-term success	Clinical success for longer than 6 months
(Smith, Feldman et al., 2006)	

have not yet been evaluated. Other patient factors that affect long-term success include age, left ventricular function, diabetes, and the presence of diffuse, small, or multivessel disease. Many patients with these factors are referred for CABG.

Complications

Major hospital complications from PCI include death, periprocedural MI, the need for emergency CABG, stroke, renal failure, significant bleeding, and major vascular complications. Significant bleeding is defined as a greater than 3.0 g/dl decrease in hemoglobin level, or bleeding that results in transfusion or extended length of stay (Smith, Feldman et al., 2006). Nurses play an important role in assessing for vascular complications after the procedure. Vascular complications can include:

- occlusion of the artery at the site of access

- vessel dissection (splitting and separation of arterial layers) at the site of entry

- arteriovenous fistula (connection between artery and vein) at the site of entry

- pseudoaneurysm at the site of entry.

A retroperitoneal bleed (resulting from a large hematoma in the retroperitoneum) can be potentially life-threatening. Patients typically experience lumbar pain, hypotension, and a drop in hematocrit. A computed tomography (CT) scan is performed to confirm the diagnosis. The patient is treated with IV fluids and blood transfusion, and surgical repair of the artery may also be needed. Arterial punctures made above the inguinal ligament place the patient at increased risk for retroperitoneal bleed (Shoulders-Odom, 2008).

Patients who are treated with interventional procedures are at increased risk for hemorrhagic and ischemic embolic stroke. Hemorrhagic stroke results from the anticoagulation therapy used during the procedure. A more common complication,

however, is ischemic stroke, which is caused by plaque embolization during the procedure.

The use of contrast agents during PCI increases the risk of renal insufficiency and renal failure after the procedure. Renal dysfunction as a result of contrast is referred to as *contrast-induced nephropathy.* Patients with existing renal insufficiency, older adults, and those with diabetes are at highest risk for renal complications with PCI. It is important that high-risk patients are well hydrated with normal saline solution prior to, during, and after PCI. Careful use of contrast agents (to avoid any overuse during the procedure) is also important in preventing renal complications. Patients with diabetes who are taking metformin need to have the agent held prior to and after the procedure. Contrast-induced nephropathy can produce temporary or permanent renal dysfunction. The definition of post-PCI renal failure includes creatinine greater than 2.0 mg/dl, a greater than 50% increase in baseline creatinine, or the need for dialysis (Smith, Feldman et al., 2006).

Distal microembolization during an intervention can result in postprocedure chest pain and a small rise in cardiac enzymes. Chest pain from embolization of microparticles is usually transient and lessens with time. There is an increased risk of embolization from larger debris during PCI with acute thrombus, saphenous vein graft PCI, and rotational atherectomy (Deelstra, 2010). Stent thrombosis most frequently occurs acutely (within 24 hours) or subacutely (within 30 days) (Shoulders-Odom, 2008). The risk of acute and subacute stent thrombosis has been reduced with improved techniques for stent deployment and aggressive use of antiplatelet therapy. Although these remain very serious complications, they occur in only approximately 1% of patients (Deelstra, 2010). The biggest risk factor for late stent thrombosis is premature discontinuation of dual antiplatelet therapy (Shoulders-Odom, 2008), which is discussed in detail later in this chapter.

Additional complications that can occur during the procedure include spasm and vessel perforation. Spasm is most common during rotational atherectomy and is treated with intracoronary nitroglycerin. Vessel perforation is rare, but can be a very serious complication. When perforation occurs, a balloon is inflated in an attempt to stop blood leakage from the perforated site. Specially coated stents are also used to tack up the vessel wall. If too much blood is lost, tamponade can occur. Pericardiocentesis may be indicated.

Special Circumstances

Emergency PCI

Emergency PCI can usually be performed without additional cardiac assistive devices. If a patient shows signs of hemodynamic instability, has ongoing ischemia, or is in cardiogenic shock, an IABP is inserted to provide cardiac support and improve outcomes. Patients who are in cardiogenic shock and have severely depressed left ventricular function may be placed on full cardiopulmonary support during emergency PCI. Emergency PCI is ideally performed in a setting with onsite surgical backup. If performed in a facility with no onsite surgical backup, there should be the ability to transfer the patient to a cardiac operating room within 1 hour (Smith, Feldman et al., 2006). Emergency PCI as a reperfusion strategy during an acute MI should be done within 90 minutes from contact with Emergency Medical Services (Antman et al., 2004). Primary PCI is superior to fibrinolytic therapy when reperfusion can be achieved within 90 minutes by an experienced operator. If a fibrinolytic is given and is not successful, then PCI is indicated. PCI is termed *rescue* or *salvage* when it is performed after failed fibrinolytic therapy in a patient who is actively ischemic.

Emergency PCI is also beneficial in reducing mortality in patients who develop cardiogenic shock as an early complication of acute MI. PCI is not beneficial when cardiogenic shock is the result of a mechanical complication, such as papillary muscle or septal rupture.

Vein Graft Stenosis after CABG

Patients with acute graft closure (vein graft or arterial conduit) within 30 days of surgery usually have successful PCI to the focal area of stenosis. PCI across suture lines has been accomplished safely within 10 days of surgery (Smith, Feldman et al., 2006).

Vein graft disease can produce very serious and unstable lesions. It can be caused by hyperplasia or atherosclerosis. Vein grafts are at a particularly high risk for developing brittle plaques and thrombotic occlusions. These lesions are very complex.

Patients with late vein graft stenosis (longer than 5 years after surgery) in a graft supplying the LAD and patients with more than one stenotic vein graft generally need repeat CABG (Eagle et al., 2004; Smith, Feldman et al., 2006). Vein graft stenosis that occurs within 5 years of the time of surgery may be able to be effectively treated with PCI. Unfortunately, the use of GP IIb/IIIa inhibitors has failed to substantially improve results of PCI for vein graft stenosis (Smith, Feldman et al., 2006). Ischemia that occurs more than 1 year after CABG can represent new stenosis within the graft or new native vessel disease.

One of the challenges of PCI for vein graft stenosis is the unique brittle nature of the plaques, which can cause embolization of graft material. Extraction devices to remove thrombi prior to intervention have been helpful in preventing distal embolization. In addition, devices have been developed to catch this debris and protect the patient from distal embolization. Distal protection devices include balloons or filters that are deployed distal to the site of intervention to collect debris that dislodges during the procedure. The goal is to prevent small amounts of myocardial damage that can occur due to distal embolization.

Medications Before, During, and After PCI

Oral hypoglycemic agents are usually withheld the morning of the procedure because of the patient's nothing-by-mouth (NPO) status. Metformin should be held for 24 to 38 hours prior to the procedure and should continue to be held for 48 hours after the procedure because of the potential for renal toxicity.

Aspirin should be given prior to PCI. Patients coming in for elective procedures should be instructed to take aspirin at home. If the patient is on clopidogrel at home, it is also continued and taken prior to the procedure. If the patient is receiving LMWH before the procedure, it is typically held the morning of the procedure. If the patient is going to have the procedure done more than 8 hours from the holding of the dose, UFH can be started to maintain adequate anticoagulation before the procedure.

UFH is the anticoagulant of choice during PCI. A GP IIb/IIIa inhibitor is also typically initiated during the procedure and continued for several hours after the procedure. If a GP IIb/IIIa is used during the procedure, then UFH dosages are lowered. UFH is not routinely continued postprocedure in uncomplicated patients and this has helped reduce the number of vascular complications (Shoulders-Odom, 2008). Bivalrudin is an alternative anticoagulant that can be used during interventional procedures. When bilvarudin is used as the anticoagulant, a GP IIb/IIIa inhibitor is not needed in low-risk patients.

Additional antiplatelet therapy is initiated before or during the procedure and continued afterward. Typically, 300 mg or higher of clopidogrel (or 60 mg of prasugrel) are given as a loading dose, before, during, or immediately after the procedure. Patients with non-STEMI who are high risk and receiving an invasive strategy should have both clopidogrel (or prasugrel) and a GP IIb/IIIa inhibitor initiated prior to procedure, preferably as

soon as possible (Anderson et al., 2007; Kushner et al., 2009). Clopidogrel (75 mg) or prasugrel (10 mg) daily is continued for a recommended 12 months in patients with bare metal stents. The absolute minimum time of 1 month in patients with bare metal stents can be used in patients at high risk for bleeding. The minimum duration of therapy for daily clopidogrel or prasugrel is 12 months for all drug-eluting stents. Many patients with drug eluting stents will remain on clopidogrel or prasugrel indefinitely. In addition to taking clopidogrel or prasugrel after stenting procedures, patients will go home on aspirin doses of 162 to 325 mg daily for a period of time, before having the dose lowered to a maintenance level of 75 to 162 mg daily (King et al., 2007).

The administration of aspirin and clopidogrel after stenting procedures is referred to as dual antiplatelet therapy. Dual antiplatelet therapy must be continued until the stent is completely endothialized and no longer thrombogenic. Drug-eluting stents take longer to endothialize than bare metal stents because the eluting drug is inhibiting tissue growth. Premature discontinuation of dual antiplatelet therapy can result in the serious complication of late in-stent thrombosis, which most often results in MI. It is recommended that the interventional cardiologist discuss the patient's ability to comply with dual antiplatelet therapy for the recommended time frame before implanting a drug-eluting stent. If there any concerns, a bare metal stent can be used instead (King et al., 2007).

Clinical Application

Many patients have financial barriers to medication compliance that is of particular concern with clopidogrel requirements after stenting procedures. In addition, many patients see multiple physicians and may be scheduled for procedures during which the physician would prefer the patient stop clopidogrel. Therefore, it is important to specifically ask patients about their ability to afford clopidogrel therapy and to refer patients as appropriate to manufac-

turer assistance programs and other available resources. In addition, patients must know that only their interventional cardiologist can give permission for them to discontinue their clopidogrel. Any request by another physician must be cleared by the cardiologist.

Before the procedure, it is important to assess for allergy to iodine-based contrast agents. If a patient has never been exposed to an iodine-based contrast agent, assess for an allergy to shellfish because many contain organic iodine. If a patient has an iodine allergy, he or she will be premedicated with steroids and antihistamines to avoid an anaphylactic reaction.

Intraprocedure Care

Patients normally receive conscious sedation during PCI. Arterial access is achieved with sheath insertion, most typically via the femoral artery. If the femoral artery cannot be accessed, then the radial or brachial artery can be used. Radial access is being used by some physicians more frequently to minimize the postprocedure vascular complications. Common procedure technique involves the threading of a guidewire across the lesion, followed by the advancement of the interventional device over the guidewire. Heparin is typically the anticoagulant used during the procedure to avoid thrombotic complications associated with the insertion of foreign devices. Bedside activated clotting times are monitored during the procedure to assure the appropriate level of anticoagulation. Ischemia from balloon inflation may cause or increase dysrhythmias during the procedure. To protect renal function, isosmolar agents are recommended in patients with chronic kidney disease, and in those with any renal dysfunction, doses of renally cleared drugs should be adjusted (King et al., 2007).

Postprocedure Nursing Care

A major focus of postprocedure nursing care is the prevention of complications related to the vascular access site. The arterial sheath is generally removed 4 to 6 hours after the procedure, or as soon as clotting times allow, unless a vascular closure device is used. Upon return to the nursing unit, bedside activated clotting times are drawn until they return to acceptable levels and the arterial sheath can be safely removed. Earlier sheath removal is associated with fewer bleeding and vascular complications (Shoulders-Odom, 2008). After the arterial access sheath is removed, hemostasis is a priority. Hemostasis can be achieved with manual pressure, the use of a C-clamp, or the use of a commercial compression device. Pressure is applied for a minimum of 20 minutes to achieve hemostasis. Research has not shown a significant difference in complication rates between the various methods of compression to achieve hemostasis (Shoulders-Odom, 2008). An increasing number of interventional cardiologists are using the radial artery as an access site to minimize the bleeding complications often associated with groin access. Use of the radial artery allows for increased patient comfort and mobility as well as easier access for holding pressure during sheath removal.

If a vascular closure device is used, the arterial sheath is removed in the interventional laboratory. The most common vascular closure devices in use are VasoSeal or AngioSeal, Duett, and Perclose (or the newer generation StarClose) (Deelstra, 2005). The most common vascular closure devices and their mechanisms of action are described in Table 6-2. The benefits of vascular closure devices include improved patient comfort and earlier ambulation. Associated risks of these devices include infection, bleeding from the site, and leg ischemia, which can potentially result in the need for vascular surgery (Deelstra, 2010). Vasovagal response is a potential complication of arterial sheath removal. Hypotension, bradycardia, diaphoresis, nausea, and vomiting can also occur. This response is triggered by pain and anxiety associated with the sheath removal process. If the patient is hypovolemic, the response is exagger-

TABLE 6-2: COMMON VASCULAR CLOSURE DEVICES AND MECHANISMS OF ACTION	
Closure Device	**Mechanism of Action**
VasoSeal	• Collagen delivered to surface of femoral artery (extravascular) • Platelets attracted to collagen and seal is formed • Collagen reabsorbs in 6 weeks
Angio-Seal	• Seals the puncture site between two absorbable structures: 1) suture anchor below, 2) collagen plug above • Structures dissolve within 90 days
Perclose	• Arteriotomy is sutured for immediate hemostasis
StarClose	• Staples are used to create a purse-string closure
Duett	• Liquid mixture of thrombin and collagen is delivered to puncture site
(Shoulders-Odom, 2008)	

ated. Treatment involves fluids, atropine and, whenever possible, the elimination of pain and anxiety.

After arterial sheath removal, the access site should be frequently assessed for external bleeding or development of a hematoma. A hematoma occurs when there is a collection of blood in the soft tissue.

Clinical Application

Patients should be instructed to immediately report any feeling of warmth or moisture, which may indicate bleeding, and any new burning at the insertion site, which commonly accompanies the development of a hematoma.

Pressure is applied to treat bleeding or hematoma formation that occurs after arterial sheath removal. Most hematomas are self-limiting and resolve without further treatment. Hematomas can result in femoral nerve compression (Shoulders-Odom, 2008). Any large hematoma should be assessed for a pulsatile mass or the presence of a bruit. These assessment findings can indicate the presence of a pseudoaneurysm. A pseudoaneurysm occurs when hemostasis does not produce an adequate amount of thrombus formation at the puncture site. This lack of thrombus leaves a communicating track between the artery and surrounding tissue. Ultrasound can confirm the presence of a pseudoaneurysm. Large pseudoaneurysms will require treatment with either ultra-

sound guided compression or ultrasound guided thrombin injection. Surgical intervention may be required if these treatments are not successful.

In addition, nurses must frequently assess for other potential neurovascular complications. Nursing assessment includes frequent pulse, pain, and sensation checks to the area distal to the insertion site. After sheath removal, these assessments are typically done every 15 minutes for the first hour and then with decreasing frequency if the patient remains free from complications.

The clinical trial Standards of Angioplasty Nursing Techniques to Diminish Bleeding Around the Groin (SANDBAG) found the following nursing interventions effective in preventing postprocedure groin bleeding:

- nurse-to-patient ratio of 1:1.5 or less during the sheath removal process

- prompt removal of the sheath within 4 to 6 hours of the procedure

- patient comfort measures, including pain medication and head of bed elevation to 30 degrees

- avoidance of a sandbag, which has been shown not to decrease bleeding but to increase discomfort

- patient ambulation 8 hours after sheath removal. (Deelstra, 2010)

Adequate hydration preprocedure and postprocedure is an important component to preventing renal complications related to contrast administration. NPO status prior to the procedure increases the importance of IV hydration. Hydration with 0.9% normal saline solution is considered the gold standard in preventing contrast-induced nephropathy. Other strategies that are sometimes used to prevent contrast-induced nephropathy include hydration with a sodium bicarbonate drip (154 mEq of sodium bicarbonate/L) and pretreatment with n-acetylcysteine. These treatments have been the subject of some research, but are not yet included in evidence-based practice guidelines. Evidence-based practice guidelines support the use of isosmolar contrast agents in patients with chronic kidney disease (Kushner et al., 2009).

Assessment of blood urea nitrogen and creatinine levels is important in the postprocedure evaluation. Whenever possible, nephrotoxic drugs should be held for 48 hours prior to and after PCI. Examples of common nephrotoxic drugs include metformin, NSAIDs, and some antibiotics. Metformin is important because patients with diabetes have an increased risk of developing postprocedure nephropathy.

Patients should also be monitored for recurrent ischemia after PCI. The ST-segment should be monitored in the leads evaluating the vessel receiving intervention. Any chest pain postprocedure should be evaluated with a 12-lead ECG. There are several causes of chest pain after an interventional procedure, including:

- sensation from presence of stent, which is benign
- transient spasm of vessel
- occlusion of side branch
- distal embolization of microemboli
- acute vessel closure or acute thrombosis.

(Shoulders-Odom, 2008)

Chest pain as a result of acute vessel closure or acute thrombosis warrants a return visit to the interventional laboratory.

Many patients are cared for in specialized postinterventional units. Patients without complications who undergo elective procedures are discharged within 24 hours. Patients with PCI during an acute MI have extended stays that vary, based on the amount of myocardial damage.

Postdischarge Instructions

Elective PCI patients are generally discharged the day after the procedure, limiting time during the inpatient hospital stay for patient education regarding risk factor reduction. Patients should be encouraged to participate in outpatient cardiac rehabilitation programs so they can receive the same education and support for risk factor modification as those who have had surgery. Place special emphasis on the importance of risk reduction to manage disease progression in these patients.

Clinical Application

PCI has a shorter recovery period than CABG and does not provide the long-term reminder of a midsternal scar. For this reason, after PCI, patients may minimize the importance of their CHD and their future risks. It is important that they fully understand that PCI does not treat the underlying disease process and that aggressive risk reduction is critical in managing the underlying disease.

TRANSMYOCARDIAL LASER REVASCULARIZATION

Transmyocardial laser revascularization (TMLR) is limited to patients who have angina that is refractory to maximal medical treatment and who are not candidates for other forms of revascularization. Patients who are candidates for this surgery, but not other forms of revascularization, usually have very diffuse small vessel disease. During this procedure, a series of transmural endomyocardial channels are created with lasers to improve myocardial blood supply. These channels are created on the epicardial surface and go through to the endocardium. The typical number of channels ranges from 20 to 40, with the size of the channels approximately 1-mm wide. The physiology behind the treatment is more complex than simply creating channels for oxygenated blood to flow from the endocardium up through the myocardium to the epicardium. Two theories are proposed regarding the mechanism of action: 1) the laser treatment stimulates angiogenesis and causes improvement in regional blood flow to the ischemic area of myocardium, and 2) the laser treatment creates denervation of the myocardium and an improvement of symptoms (Bridges et al., 2004).

TMLR has been effective in improving anginal symptoms, functional capacity, and quality of life. This procedure is typically done in the cardiac surgery suite as a standalone surgery, or it can be done with CABG, when not all ischemic areas can be reached by grafting. Percutaneous options are currently being investigated.

CONCLUSION

Advancements continue to improve the safety and outcomes associated with CABG and PCI revascularization options. These advancements improve treatment options and outcomes for patients with CHD.

Interventional cardiologists and thoracic surgeons are also coming together in some situations to complement each other and perform hybrid revascularization procedures. An example of a hybrid revascularization procedure is a LIMA to the LAD via a robotic procedure and additional interventional techniques to the RCA and circumflex arteries. The major challenge to hybrid procedures is timing. Antiplatelet therapy (including clopidogrel), which is a standard part of post-PCI treatment, is also routinely held for several days prior to elective CABG procedures.

With the increasing older adult population, the number of revascularization procedures continues to increase. The impact of nursing on the care of these patients before, during, and after these procedures is important. Revascularization does not alter the underlying disease process; therefore, patient education and risk factor reduction remain key nursing elements in all settings.

EXAM QUESTIONS

CHAPTER 6
Questions 47-53

Note: Choose the one option that BEST answers each question.

47. The patient who would be a good candidate for CABG is

    a. a patient with 90% left main occlusion.

    b. a patient with less than 50% LAD occlusion and less than 50% circumflex occlusion.

    c. a patient with an RCA lesion with normal left ventricular function.

    d. a patient with very diffuse and very small vessel disease.

48. The term OPCAB refers to

    a. the use of thoracotomy instead of sternotomy.

    b. patients who are fast tracked to be discharged in less than 5 days.

    c. CABG surgery without the use of cardiopulmonary bypass.

    d. combination open heart surgery and percutaneous procedure.

49. Which patient in the following list is at high risk for an adverse neurovascular complication after CABG?

    a. A previously healthy 50-year-old woman undergoing cardiopulmonary bypass

    b. A patient with an atherosclerotic aorta undergoing cardiopulmonary bypass

    c. A patient undergoing OPCAB

    d. A 67-year-old man having a MIDCAB to the LAD with no known history of hypertension

50. A component of a fast-track pathway after CABG would include

    a. extubation by the third postoperative day.

    b. anticipated discharge between postoperative days 7 and 8.

    c. liberal use of opioid medications to increase patient comfort during the ventilator weaning process.

    d. pharmacological strategies to prevent postoperative atrial fibrillation.

51. Recent advances in PCI that have improved safety and long-term outcomes include

    a. beta-blocker and calcium channel blocker administration to relax coronary arteries and improve blood flow immediately after the procedure.

    b. permanent implantable radiation to prevent stents from developing initial restenosis.

    c. the use of an IABP prior to all procedures.

    d. intracoronary stents, clopidogrel, GP IIb/IIIa inhibitors, and direct thrombin inhibitors.

continued on next page

52. Key nursing interventions immediately after
    PCI include

    a. assessing for vascular complications and
       assuring adequate hydration.

    b. monitoring blood sugar level every hour for
       4 hours.

    c. limiting fluids and holding all medications
       for 6 hours after the procedure.

    d. performing range-of-motion on the
       affected extremity to avoid vascular
       complications.

53. Key patient education and discharge planning
    principles after revascularization include

    a. assuring patients that there will be no
       activity restrictions after discharge.

    b. assuring patients that they no longer have
       CHD.

    c. informing patients that aggressive risk
       factor modification is necessary to manage
       their underlying CHD.

    d. informing patients that it is normal to
       continue to have angina after
       revascularization.

CHAPTER 7

HEART FAILURE

CHAPTER OBJECTIVE

After completing this chapter, the learner will be able to describe current strategies for the management of heart failure.

LEARNING OBJECTIVES

After completing this chapter, the learner will be able to

1. define the clinical syndrome of heart failure and the hallmark manifestations of the syndrome.

2. explain the most common cause of heart failure.

3. describe the difference in pathophysiology between systolic and diastolic dysfunction.

4. describe two neurohormonal responses to heart failure that produce negative end results over time.

5. describe the one positive neurohormonal response in heart failure.

6. define the two classifications of medications used to slow progression of left ventricular remodeling and heart failure disease progression.

7. describe two nonpharmacologic treatments for heart failure.

8. describe key nursing considerations regarding patient education in patients with heart failure.

INTRODUCTION

Understanding heart failure and its management is very important in cardiovascular nursing. Approximately 5 million people in the U.S. live with heart failure today, and 550,000 new cases are diagnosed annually. Moreover, 300,000 patients die each year of heart-failure related causes. After being diagnosed with heart failure, approximately 50% of patients die within 5 years (Hunt et al., 2009). Heart failure as a primary diagnosis accounts for approximately one million hospital admissions annually. There are another two million admissions annually when heart failure is a secondary diagnosis. One third of hospitalized patients are readmitted within 90 days because of further decompensation (Hobbs & Boyle, 2009). In addition, another 20 million people with asymptomatic cardiac impairment are likely to develop heart failure symptoms within a 5-year period (Soine, 2010).

The increasing number of people with heart failure is attributed to several factors, including the aging population, improved short-term survival of patients after a myocardial infarction (MI) (placing this group in the high-risk category for development of heart failure in the future), and an increased awareness of heart failure and established guidelines, resulting in increased diagnosis and management of the syndrome (Hunt et al., 2009).

Definition

Heart failure is a complex clinical syndrome that can result from any cardiac disorder that impairs the ability of the ventricle to either fill properly or eject optimally. This syndrome results in a pathologic state in which the heart is unable to pump enough oxygenated blood to meet the metabolic needs of the body (Hunt et al., 2009).

Patients with heart failure present with one or both of the hallmark manifestations:

1. dyspnea and fatigue, which may impact exercise tolerance

2. extracellular fluid (ECF) retention, which can cause peripheral edema and pulmonary congestion.

(Hunt et al., 2009)

Patients may have only one of the two manifestations of heart failure at any given time. For this reason, the term "heart failure" is more accurate than "congestive heart failure." With either dyspnea and fatigue or ECF retention, the patient's functional capacity and quality of life are affected.

CLINICAL PRESENTATION

Most patients with heart failure present with decreased exercise tolerance due to dyspnea or fatigue. Because these presenting symptoms are nonspecific, many patients are not readily diagnosed with heart failure. These symptoms are sometimes attributed to deconditioning associated with the aging process. Many patients with heart failure also have coexisting conditions (such as pulmonary disease) that contribute to exercise intolerance. These coexisting conditions make differential diagnosis challenging.

Symptom assessment is more difficult in older patients. Many older adults do not experience exertional dyspnea because they have developed more sedentary lifestyles to accommodate their decreased functional capacity.

Clinical Application

When assessing for exertional dyspnea, remember to do so within the context of the patient's activity level. The nurse must ask the patient about dyspnea with exertion and must also assess the degree to which the patient has been exerting himself or herself. A patient who sits in a chair for the majority of the day may not present with the same complaint of dyspnea on exertion as a patient attempting to complete activities of daily living (ADLs).

Patients may also present with ECF overload, manifested as peripheral edema or abdominal swelling. Anorexia commonly accompanies abdominal swelling. Additional findings during a physical exam that indicate fluid overload are the presence of a third heart sound (S_3) and jugular venous distention. Patients with pulmonary congestion present with dyspnea on exertion, orthopnea, and paroxysmal nocturnal dyspnea. Pulmonary congestion usually occurs when the ventricle rapidly fails. Many patients with left ventricular end-stage heart failure have no signs of pulmonary congestion. Regardless of initial presentation, progressive changes in symptoms over time are common to most patients with heart failure.

Clinical Application

When assessing for a third heart sound, listen at the 5th intercostal space, left midclavicular line with the bell of the stethoscope. Normal S_1 and S_2 sound like "lub dub." When the 3rd heart sound is added it will sound like "lub dub da" or "I Believe" or "Kentucky."

ETIOLOGY

A variety of cardiac disorders can cause heart failure, but the most common cause is left ventricular dysfunction (Hunt et al., 2009). The most common cause of left ventricular dysfunction is ischemic coronary heart disease (CHD), followed by hypertension. The American Heart Association (AHA) reports that up to 75% of patients with heart failure have hypertension (Hunt et al., 2009). Because CHD and hypertension increase the risk of heart failure, strategies to reduce risk and control disease progression in these disorders are also key in reducing heart failure risk.

Other causes of left ventricular dysfunction include:

- valvular disease
- thyroid disease
- viral infection
- alcohol abuse
- idiopathic (no known cause).

When a patient presents with heart failure syndrome and left ventricular dysfunction is suspected or identified, the following questions can help determine the cause:

- Does the patient have a history of ischemic CHD or associated risk factors, including diabetes, hypertension, hyperlipidemia, or peripheral vascular disease?
- Does the patient have a history or evidence of valvular heart disease?
- Has the patient been exposed to chest irradiation or had any exposure to cardiotoxic agents?
- Does the patient's lifestyle involve any illicit drug or excessive alcohol use?
- Does the patient have a family history of idiopathic cardiomyopathy or unexplained, sudden cardiac death?
- Is there any suspicion for noncardiac causes, such as:
  - hyperthyroidism
  - infectious process
  - collagen vascular disorder
  - pheochromocytoma?

(Hunt et al., 2009)

INITIAL EVALUATION OF PATIENTS WITH HEART FAILURE

Recommendations from the American College of Cardiology (ACC) and AHA Guidelines for the Management of Heart Failure include:

1. thorough history and physical examination to identify cardiac and noncardiac conditions that contribute to the development and acceleration of heart failure

2. initial and ongoing assessment of functional capacity, based on the patient's ability to perform routine ADLs

3. initial and ongoing assessment of fluid volume status

4. initial electrocardiogram (ECG) and chest radiogram

5. initial two-dimensional echocardiogram with Doppler to assess the function of the left ventricle

6. initial lab work evaluation, including complete blood count, electrolytes, blood urea nitrogen, creatinine, blood glucose, thyroid-stimulating hormone, liver function studies, and urinalysis.

Because of the high association between ischemic CHD and heart failure, most patients with chest pain of unknown etiology presenting with the clinical syndrome of heart failure also undergo cardiac catheterization (Hunt et al., 2009).

PATHOPHYSIOLOGY

The AHA/ACC staging system classifies heart failure as a progressive disorder. In this model of progression, left ventricular dysfunction begins with an initial insult to the myocardium. Even without further identifiable insults, left ventricular dysfunction continues to progress.

Left ventricular dysfunction can range from predominantly diastolic dysfunction to predominantly systolic dysfunction. Patients with heart failure can also have a combination of systolic and diastolic dysfunction. Patients with combined systolic and diastolic dysfunction have a worse prognosis than those with isolated systolic or diastolic dysfunction (Hobbs & Boyle, 2009).

Systolic Dysfunction

In predominant systolic dysfunction, ejection is a problem. With substantial dilation of the ventricle, reduced wall motion occurs and the heart is unable to contract effectively. The patient's ejection fraction (percent of blood the ventricle ejects per beat relative to the total amount of blood in the ventricle) decreases. A normal ejection fraction is greater than or equal to 55%. An ejection fraction less than 50% percent generally defines systolic dysfunction (Soine, 2010). Systolic dysfunction is found in two thirds of patients with heart failure (Hunt et al., 2009). This type of heart failure is now referred to as *heart failure with reduced ejection* rather than systolic heart failure (Soine, 2010). The reason for this new terminology is that patients with systolic dysfunction seldom have normal diastolic function. The terminology of systolic heart failure implies that diastolic function is normal, and this is not typically the case.

Patients with systolic dysfunction also have low cardiac output. As a result, left ventricular end-diastolic volume (preload) increases and can lead to pulmonary congestion. Dilated cardiomyopathy (ischemic or idiopathic) is a common cause of systolic dysfunction. However, cardiomyopathy should not be used interchangeably with systolic heart failure. Cardiomyopathy is a structural disorder associated with the development of heart failure, but heart failure is a clinical syndrome characterized by the presentation of certain symptoms. Cardiomyopathy is discussed in detail in the next chapter.

Diastolic Dysfunction

The remaining one third of patients with the clinical syndrome of heart failure have predominant diastolic dysfunction. In predominant diastolic dysfunction, the ventricle is not dilated and ejection fraction remains within normal limits. In diastolic dysfunction, however, the ventricle has impaired relaxation and does not fill properly. This type of heart failure is now called *heart failure with normal or preserved ejection fraction* (Soine, 2010). Again, the rationale for the new terminology is that patients with predominant diastolic dysfunction seldom have completely normal systolic function, even though the ejection fraction is still preserved.

Diastolic dysfunction is commonly associated with chronic systemic hypertension and left ventricular hypertrophy. The aging process affects the elastic properties of the heart. In particular, older women are at high risk for diastolic dysfunction. Ischemic heart disease and restrictive or hypertrophic cardiomyopathy can also cause diastolic dysfunction. In these conditions, the ventricle can become stiff or noncompliant. A noncompliant ventricle is unable to completely relax during diastole, impairing filling (see Figure 7-1). In some cases the ejection fraction is elevated to levels of 70% to 75%. This elevation in ejection fraction

FIGURE 7-1: LEFT VENTRICULAR DIASTOLIC DYSFUNCTION

Normal

Diastolic dysfunction

Ejection fraction is normal or decreased

Note. From *Essential atlas of Heart Diseases: Heart Failure.* Edited by Eugene Braunwald (series editor) & W.S. Colucci. Copyright 2004, by Current Medicine. Used with permission from Images.MD.

occurs because there is no contractile deficit in diastolic dysfunction. In diastolic dysfunction the total volume in the ventricle at the end of diastole may actually be less because of the stiffness and noncompliance of the left ventricle. Therefore, ejection of 70% of volume does not result in a greater cardiac output.

In diastolic dysfunction, end-diastolic pressures are elevated; however, volumes remain low to normal. To increase diastolic filling, the pressure in the left atria increases. When increased left atrial pressure rises above the pressure in the pulmonary capillaries, pulmonary edema can result. Patients with diastolic dysfunction commonly become symptomatic with exertion when heart rate is increased. When heart rate is increased, ventricular filling time is reduced. Increased levels of circulating catecholamines also increase heart rate and worsen diastolic dysfunction.

Three conditions are required for diagnosis of diastolic dysfunction: 1) signs and symptoms of heart failure, 2) normal or slightly increased ejection fraction, and 3) increased diastolic filling pressure and abnormal relaxation of the left ventricle (Hunt et al., 2009). For practical purposes, the diagnosis of diastolic heart failure is made in patients presenting with the clinical syndrome of heart failure with no evidence of systolic dysfunction.

Table 7-1 summarizes the comparison between systolic and diastolic heart failure. Figure 7-2 compares the concentric hypertrophy of diastolic heart failure with the eccentric hypertrophy of systolic heart failure. Remember that patients can have coexisting systolic and diastolic dysfunction.

Echocardiography

Two-dimensional echocardiography with Doppler flow studies is the most frequently used diagnostic test in evaluating patients with the clinical syndrome of heart failure. A noninvasive, cost-effective diagnostic tool, the echocardiogram can identify systolic and diastolic dysfunction, including a measurement of ejection fraction. When systolic dysfunction is identified, the echocardiogram can assist in determining the etiology. Regional wall-motion abnormalities indicate ischemic CHD as the cause, whereas global dysfunction indicates a non-ischemic origin. An echocardiogram can also identify other causes of heart failure, such as valvular or pericardial disease. Although an echocardiogram can provide essential information regarding the possible cause of heart failure, it cannot identify the exact cause.

Left and Right Ventricular Failure

The left and right ventricles are part of a closed circulatory system. Right ventricular failure usually results from prolonged left ventricular failure. Isolated right ventricular failure can occur with right ventricular MI, pulmonary hypertension, or chronic severe tricuspid regurgitation. Signs of right ventricular heart failure include weight gain, jugular venous distention, peripheral edema, abdominal swelling, and hepatomegaly.

Neurohormonal Responses to a Failing Heart

Neurohormonal responses are the body's response to decreased cardiac output and poor

TABLE 7-1: SUMMARY COMPARISON OF SYSTOLIC AND DIASTOLIC DYSFUNCTION			
Systolic dysfunction	Two thirds of patients with heart failure	Decreased left ventricular contractility and ejection fraction	Most common cause is CHD resulting in myocardial infarction or chronic ischemia
Diastolic dysfunction	One third of patients with heart failure	Impaired left ventricular relaxation and abnormal filling	Usually related to chronic hypertension or ischemic heart disease

FIGURE 7-2: COMPARISON OF CONCENTRIC HYPERTROPHY OF DIASTOLIC DYSFUNCTION AND ECCENTRIC HYPERTROPHY OF SYSTOLIC DYSFUNCTION

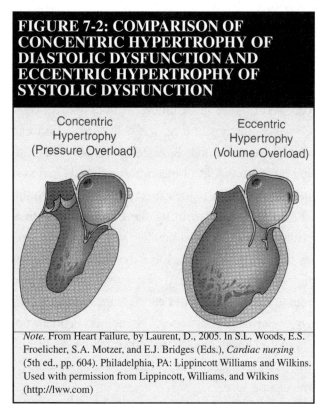

Concentric Hypertrophy (Pressure Overload)

Eccentric Hypertrophy (Volume Overload)

Note. From Heart Failure, by Laurent, D., 2005. In S.L. Woods, E.S. Froelicher, S.A. Motzer, and E.J. Bridges (Eds.), *Cardiac nursing* (5th ed., pp. 604). Philadelphia, PA: Lippincott Williams and Wilkins. Used with permission from Lippincott, Williams, and Wilkins (http://lww.com)

organ perfusion. Initially, these responses are helpful in improving cardiac output and organ perfusion. Over time, however, these responses actually lead to clinical deterioration. Several neurohormonal responses have been identified in the progression of left ventricular dysfunction. Among the most important and well-understood of these responses are sympathetic nervous system (SNS) stimulation and activation of the renin-angiotensin-aldosterone system (RAAS).

Other neurohormonal responses to heart failure include increased circulating levels of endothelin, vasopressin (also known as antidiuretic hormone), and cytokines (Hunt et al., 2009). The same compensatory mechanisms that initially help preserve cardiac output and blood pressure actually cause progressive deterioration of myocardial function in the long term.

Neurohormonal Responses in Heart Failure

Sympathetic Nervous System Stimulation

One of the first responses to a failing left ventricle is activation of the SNS. As the left ventricle

begins to fail, cardiac output and blood pressure decrease. This fall in blood pressure activates the baroreceptors and vasomotor regulatory centers in the medulla. The result is an increased level of circulating catecholamines, which stimulate alpha- and beta-adrenergic receptors to increase heart rate, increase peripheral vasoconstriction (increase afterload), and increase contractility. Over time in chronic heart failure, beta-receptors become less able to respond to circulating catecholamines. This decreased response to circulating catecholamines is called *beta-receptor down regulation* and is an attempt to protect the failing heart from chronic overstimulation of the SNS (Soine, 2010). Beta-receptor down regulation contributes to the exercise intolerance associated with heart failure. Chronic stimulation of the SNS also accelerates the ventricular remodeling process.

Increased heart rate, afterload, and contractility help maintain cardiac output and blood pressure, but also have the negative effect of increasing myocardial oxygen demand. Over time, this increased stimulation of the SNS can worsen ischemia and cause cardiac dysrhythmias and sudden cardiac death. Circulating catecholamines, along with angiotensin II, have an influence on increasing cellular calcium, which contributes to the development of cardiac dysrhythmias in heart failure (Opie, 2004). Additionally, over activation of the SNS causes direct adverse effects on the structure and function of the heart. These cardiotoxic properties are responsible for the beta-receptor down regulation seen with chronic heart failure (Soine, 2010).

Renin-angiotensin-aldosterone System

Activation of the RAAS is another compensatory neurohormonal response to a failing heart. The RAAS is activated as the kidneys respond to decreased renal perfusion. It is also activated by an increase in SNS stimulation. When the RAAS is activated, circulating levels of renin, angiotensin II, and aldosterone increase. Angiotensin II is a potent vasoconstrictor, thus systemic vascular resistance and afterload increase. Aldosterone is a mineralocorticoid responsible for sodium and water retention. When sodium is retained by the body, so is water; therefore, preload increases. Enhanced preload increases end-diastolic volume in the ventricles, which further dilates the ventricles and enhances the ventricular remodeling process. If the left ventricle becomes overstretched, contractility is depressed.

Vasopressin and Endothelin

In chronic heart failure, angiotensin II and osmotic stimuli produce an increase in vasopressin release, causing a reabsorption of water and additional vasoconstriction. Levels of endothelin (an endogenous hormonal vasoconstrictor) are elevated in heart failure in response to angiotensin II, vasopressin, and circulating catecholamines (Soine, 2010). Figure 7-3 summarizes the neurohormonal responses of the SNS and RAAS.

Clinical Application

Current treatment for heart failure involves inhibition of neurohormonal systems with beta-blockers and angiotensin-converting enzyme (ACE) inhibitors. Patients typically do not understand the neurohormonal blockade associated with these medications or the importance they play in stopping disease progression. If patients think that these medications are only used to treat hypertension and that their blood pressures are normal, they may be less compliant because they do not fully understand the impact of therapy.

Inflammatory Response

Cytokine levels are also elevated in heart failure, producing local and systemic inflammatory responses. Local inflammatory responses occur early in the course of the disease; systemic responses occur later in the course. Cytokines, neurohormones, mechanical stress, and certain physiological conditions can promote cell growth (hypertrophy) and cell death (apoptosis) (Soine,

FIGURE 7-3: VICIOUS CYCLE OF NEUROHORMONAL RESPONSES IN HEART FAILURE

Note. From *Atlas of Heart Diseases: Heart Failure* by M. Givertz & W. Colucci. Edited by E. Braunwald (series editor) and W.S. Colucci. Copyright 2004, by Current Medicine. Used with permission from Images.MD.

FIGURE 7-4: NEUROHORMONAL RESPONSES OF THE RAAS AND SNS IN HEART FAILURE

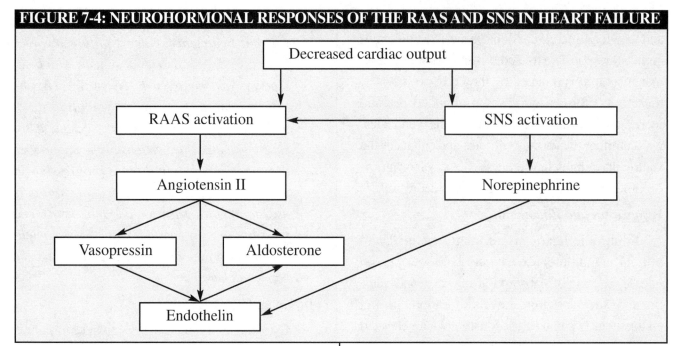

2010). Hypertrophy and apoptosis are seen in the ventricular remodeling process. Figure 7-4 shows the vicious cycle of heart failure caused by uninterrupted neurohormonal responses.

Positive Neurohormonal Response

The release of the hormones atrial natriuretic peptide and brain natriuretic peptide (BNP) from cardiac myocytes is the one beneficial neurohormonal response in heart failure. These hormones have the positive effect of systemic and pulmonary vasodilation and also enhance sodium and water excretion.

Other neurohormonal responses work to counteract the vasoconstrictive effects of the SNS and RAAS stimulation. However, the vasoconstrictive effects of neurohormonal activation commonly overpower these counterefforts.

Table 7-2 summarizes the results of neurohormonal responses to heart failure.

Left-ventricular Remodeling

Left-ventricular remodeling is another response to the initial left ventricular injury. Remodeling is a process of pathological growth, whereby the ventricles hypertrophy and then dilate. Ventricular remodeling occurs due to myocyte hypertrophy in

response to either pressure or volume overload in the ventricles. When pressure overload occurs, the myocytes thicken and concentric hypertrophy results. When volume overload occurs, the myocytes elongate and eccentric hypertrophy results (Opie, 2004). Concentric and eccentric hypertrophy are shown in Figure 7-2.

The process of ventricular remodeling is very complex at the cellular level. Concentric hypertrophy causes left-ventricular wall thickening and leads to an increased risk of subendocardial ischemia. Eccentric hypertrophy and eventual dilation can cause regurgitation of the mitral valve and elevated left atrial pressures. These effects accelerate the remodeling process.

Another component of ventricular remodeling includes necrosis and apoptosis of cardiac myocytes. Necrosis (accidental cell death) occurs in response to deprivation of oxygen. Apoptosis (programmed cell death) is stimulated by several factors, including angiotensin II, cytokines, and cellular injury from hypoxia (Soine, 2010). Myocyte loss in either form can facilitate slippage of myocytes. In response to slippage, a reparative fibrosis occurs that makes the ventricle stiffer.

TABLE 7-2: SUMMARY OF RESULTS OF NEUROHORMONAL STIMULATION IN HEART FAILURE

SNS	• Stimulation of RAAS and endothelin • Vasoconstriction (increased afterload), increased heart rate, increased contractility • Aggravation of ischemia • Potentiation of dysrhythmias • Acceleration of ventricular remodeling • Direct toxicity to cardiac myocytes
RAAS	• Arterial vasoconstriction from angiotensin II • Stimulation of vasopressin and endothelin • Sodium and water retention from increased aldosterone • Endothelial dysfunction from increased aldosterone • Organ fibrosis from increased aldosterone
Vasopressin	• Reabsorption of water • Vasoconstriction
Endothelin	• Vasoconstriction • Fluid retention • Increased contractility • Hypertrophy
Cytokines	• Pro-inflammatory response • Contribution to apoptosis (programmed cell death) • Contribution to cardiac cachexia (systemic inflammatory response)
Natriuretic peptides*	• Systemic and pulmonary vasodilatation • Increased sodium and water excretion • Suppression of other neurohormones
Nitric oxide*, bradykinin*	• Arterial smooth muscle relaxation and vasodilation, some prostaglandins*
* Neurohormonal response with positive benefit in heart failure	

This process of ventricular remodeling is complicated by other physiological responses beyond the scope of this chapter. Remodeling is also enhanced by the prolonged activation of the SNS, RAAS, and other neurohormonal responses, including endothelin production (Opie, 2004). In addition to norepinephrine, other substances produced in the activation of neurohormonal responses may have direct cardiotoxic effects.

ONGOING ASSESSMENT IN HEART FAILURE MANAGEMENT

Functional Capacity

The New York Heart Association (NYHA) classification is the most commonly used system to assess functional capacity (see Table 7-3).

Patients classified as NYHA class IV have 20% overall annual mortality (Hunt et al., 2009). The NYHA classification system has limitations

TABLE 7-3: NEW YORK HEART ASSOCIATION FUNCTIONAL CLASSIFICATIONS			
Class I	**Class II**	**Class III**	**Class IV**
Cardiac disease with no resulting limitation on physical activity	Cardiac disease with slight limitation on physical activity	Cardiac disease with marked limitation on physical activity	Cardiac disease resulting in inability to carry out any physical activity without discomfort
Ordinary activity free from fatique, palpitations, dyspnea, and anginal pain	Comfortable at rest but ordinary activity results in fatigue, palpitations, dyspnea, or anginal pain	Comfortable at rest but less-than-ordinary activity results in fatigue, palpitations, dyspnea, or anginal pain	Possible symptoms of cardiac insufficiency at rest
(Hunt et al., 2001)			

because of the subjectivity involved in the assessment process. In addition, NYHA functional capacity class assessment does not always progress in a systematic way. Patients can move between classes throughout the progression of the disease. NYHA classifications do not correspond with the ACC/AHA stages of heart failure progression. Other tools that are used to assess functional capacity include the 6-minute walk test, maximal exercise testing, and peak oxygen consumption (Hobbs & Boyle, 2009; Hunt et al., 2009).

Clinical Application

Because patients commonly decrease their activity levels to adjust to declining functional capacity, it is important to ask specific questions regarding the level of activity the patient is able to tolerate. For example, ask, "Is there any leisure activity you are no longer able to do that you wish you still could do?" An additional question to assess activity levels is, "Tell me what you do on a typical day."

Fluid Volume Status

Several ongoing physical parameters are assessed to determine ECF volume status, including

- weight

- amount of jugular venous distention

- edema of legs, abdomen, sacral area, or scrotum

- presence of organ congestion: hepatomegaly or rales.

The most reliable sign of ECF overload is jugular venous distention (Hunt et al., 2009). Most patients with peripheral edema also have ECF overload; however, peripheral edema also has non-cardiac causes, making the finding of peripheral edema less specific to heart failure. Most patients with compensated chronic heart failure do not have audible rales or crackles in their lung fields on physical examination. Rales or crackles are generally a sign of rapid onset of heart failure. Therefore, the absence of pulmonary rales should not be considered an adequate measure of optimal fluid volume status. Short-term assessment of ECF volume status is best measured by a change in daily weight.

Clinical Application

Patients should be instructed to weigh themselves daily first thing in the morning, after urinating, and prior to eating. They should be instructed to use the same scale and wear the same amount of clothing. A weight gain of more than 2 lb in 24 hours or more than 3 lb in a week should be reported to the physician. Keep in mind that 1 lb of weight = 1 pt of fluid. (This particular application is related to patient education and patient self-care. Patient's weigh themselves in pounds at home so that is why patients are instructed in pounds).

Many physicians have patients adjust their diuretic doses at home based on daily weights. With the assessment of daily weights and appropriate intervention, ECF volume can be managed on an outpatient basis and many hospital admissions can be avoided.

Laboratory Values

Routine measurement of electrolytes and renal function is important in the patient with heart failure, as many of these levels become altered because of the disease process and/or treatment. Monitoring potassium levels is particularly important in heart failure patients because diuretics can cause hypokalemia. Many heart failure patients are also on digoxin, and hypokalemia increases the risk of digoxin toxicity. In contrast, other medications used in the treatment of heart failure, such as ACE inhibitors, angiotensin II receptor blockers (ARBs), and aldosterone antagonists, can predispose patients to hyperkalemia. Patients taking loop diuretics who experience the expected side effect of hypokalemia and who also take one or more medications that can predispose patients to hyperkalemia are unlikely to be ordered potassium supplements. Thyroid levels should be assessed because hyperthyroidism and hypothyroidism can contribute to heart failure (Hunt et al., 2009).

TREATMENT GOALS FOR PATIENTS AT RISK FOR AND WITH HEART FAILURE

The majority of major clinical trials have evaluated treatment strategies for systolic dysfunction. Few large-scale clinical trials have evaluated the treatment of isolated diastolic dysfunction. Clinical practice guidelines exist for treatment of systolic dysfunction; these guidelines are addressed in this section. However, many patients with diastolic dysfunction are on many of the same medications. Treatment goals for diastolic dysfunction aim to control hypertension, heart rate, and blood volume.

The 2005 ACC/AHA Heart Failure Guidelines organized treatment strategies based on the "Stage" of heart failure (Hunt et al., 2009). These stages are demonstrated in Table 7-4. Unlike the NYHA classification system that is based on symptoms, the staging system is based on the progression of the disease process, including risk, anatomical changes, and symptoms. The NYHA classification system is based on the patient's activity levels and related symptoms at the time of evaluation. The patient may move up and down the scale based on his or her current situation. When evaluating the staging system, the first two stages (A and B) are actually void of any evidence of heart failure. However, these two stages provide the key to long-term prevention, as therapies in these stages are focused on preventing the development of left ventricular remodeling and, ultimately, heart failure. Stages C and D focus on therapies for patients with signs and symptoms of heart failure. Treating patients appropriately in stages A and B would hopefully eliminate the movement of patients to stages C and D.

Clinical Application

Medications are provided to patients for either a mortality benefit or symptom relief. When administering medications to a patient, it is important to evaluate why the patient is receiving that particular medication. This also helps the nurse provide better education for the patient. For example, in Stage B, beta-blockers and ACE inhibitors are indicated for patients with low ejection fractions, when no symptoms of heart failure exist. In this stage, the medications are used for their long-term mortality benefit.

TABLE 7-4: ACC/AHA STAGES OF HEART FAILURE

	Stage A	Stage B	Stage C	Stage D
Presentation	At high risk for HF but without structural heart disease or symptoms of HF. HTN CAD DM Obesity Metabolic syndrome Family history CM	Structural heart disease but without signs or symptoms of HF. Previous MI LV remodeling including LVH and low EF. Asymptomatic vascular disease	Structural heart disease with prior or current symptoms of HF. Know structural disease and SOB, fatigue, reduced exercise tolerance.	Refractory HF requiring specialized interventions. Marked symptoms of HF at rest despite maximal medical therapy.
Treatment Strategies	Treat HTN Treat DM Smoking cessation Treat lipids Regular exercise DC alcohol/drug use ACE-inhibitors in in select patients.	All measures as stage A. ACE-I in select patients. Beta blockers in in select patients. Implantable defibrillators.	All measures under stages A and B. Sodium restriction Daily weight Diuretics Medications in select patients. Digitalis Aldosterone antagonists Hydralazine/nitrates CRT Implantable defibrillators.	All measures under stages A, B, and C. Mechanical assist Transplantation Palliative care Hospice

(Hunt et al., 2005)

Risk Control in Patients with Structural Heart Disease

When a patient has evidence of structural heart disease, aggressive measures should be put in place to reduce risk. Strict control of blood pressure, both systolic and diastolic, should be maintained in patients with hypertension. Blood pressure targets lower than 130/80 mm Hg should be established for patients with diabetes and renal disease. When combination drug therapy is required to manage hypertension, those medications effective in treating both heart failure and hypertension become the preferred medications. These include diuretics, ACE inhibitors or ARBs, and beta-blockers. Diabetes increases the risk of heart failure and also worsens outcomes for those with heart failure. ACE inhibitors have been shown to limit end-organ damage in patients with diabetes, even if hypertension is not present (USDHHS, 2004). ARBs have also been shown to prevent heart failure in high-risk patients, including those with vascular disease, hypertension, and diabetes (Hunt et al., 2009).

Any patient with CHD should have aggressive control of risk factors to decrease the risk of future coronary events and to reduce the risk of heart failure development. Treatment of hyperlipidemia in patients with previous MI has been shown to reduce the risk of heart failure (Braunwald et al., 2002). After an MI, all patients should be started on beta-blockers, and most patients are also started on ACE inhibitors or ARBs. These medications help reduce left ventricular remodeling after MI. Aggressive efforts to reperfuse patients during acute MI are important in preserving myocardial function in the short-term and preventing heart failure in the long-term.

Patients with contributing lifestyle habits, such as smoking, illicit drug use, or excessive alcohol consumption, should be counseled regarding the impact of these habits on the development of heart failure. Coexisting noncardiac disorders, such as thyroid disease, should be treated because untreated tachycardia associated with hyperthyroidism can cause cardiomyopathy, while hypothyroidism contributes to decreased myocardial contractility.

Treatment in Patients with Asymptomatic Chronic Left Ventricular Systolic Dysfunction

Patients with asymptomatic chronic left ventricular systolic dysfunction should be managed with ACE inhibitors or ARBs and beta-blockers, because these two classifications of medications have been proven to slow the progression of left ventricular dysfunction. There is no data to support the use of digoxin in these patients because digoxin has minimal impact on disease progression (Hunt et al., 2009). Diuretics are not indicated because these patients show no signs or symptoms of fluid overload.

Treatment in Patients with Symptomatic Left Ventricular Dysfunction

Patients with symptomatic left ventricular dysfunction are generally considered as having active heart failure. These patients are managed with ACE inhibitors or ARBs and beta-blockers to slow disease progression. In addition, they are placed on diuretics and moderate sodium restrictions to control ECF volume status. Daily weight can be used to guide diuretic therapy. Diuretic therapy can also improve symptoms, increase cardiac function, and improve exercise tolerance (Hunt et al., 2009). However, diuretics do not improve survival and may cause renal and metabolic side effects (Hobbs & Boyle, 2009). Patients may also be prescribed digoxin to improve symptoms and exercise toler-

ance. Physical activity should be encouraged in all heart failure patients, except those in an acute decompensated state. Physical activity is encouraged to prevent deconditioning, which contributes to exercise intolerance.

PHARMACOLOGICAL TREATMENT FOR HEART FAILURE

Angiotensin-Converting Enzyme Inhibitors and Angiotensin II Receptor Blockers

ACE inhibitors interfere with the conversion of angiotensin I to angiotensin II in the RAAS system. In addition, they enhance the action of kinins. Both actions are responsible for their positive impact in heart failure. These medications interfere with the ventricular remodeling process, slow disease progression, and reduce the risk of death (Calclasure, Kozlowski, & Highfill, 2001; Hobbs & Boyle, 2009; Hunt et al., 2009; Soine, 2010). ACE inhibitors also improve symptoms and contribute to a sense of well-being. Benefits are seen in all stages of heart failure, although it may take several weeks to months for the effects to be seen.

ACE inhibitors remain the first choice for interruption of the RAAS in chronic heart failure and should be given to all patients with current or prior symptoms of heart failure who have a reduced ejection fraction (Jessup et al., 2009). ARBs (an alternative to ACE inhibitors) directly block angiotensin II. ARBs are indicated in patients who cannot tolerate ACE inhibitors because of cough or angioedema. Candesartan was the first ARB to be approved by the U.S. Food and Drug Administration (FDA) for the treatment of heart failure (Hunt et al., 2009).

Beta-Blockers

Beta-blockers are indicated in heart failure to block the neurohormonal responses of chronic

SNS stimulation. Multiple studies have proven a mortality benefit in patients treated with beta-blockers. Beta-blockers have several beneficial effects, including favorably affecting ventricular remodeling and apoptosis. Beta-blockers can decrease dysrhythmias and ischemia by decreasing heart rate and contractility, thereby decreasing myocardial oxygen consumption. Beta-blockers are indicated in heart failure stages B, C, and D.

Beta-blockers are initiated in low doses and slowly titrated upward. Beta-blockers are not initiated when the patient is in fluid overload or a decompensated state. Patients who show signs of decompensation after a maintenance dose of beta-blocker therapy has been administered generally do not have beta-blocker therapy discontinued.

Clinical Application

When chronic oral therapy with ACE inhibitors and beta blockers has been established, these agents should generally be continued if the patient needs to be hospitalized for an acute exacerbation. *An exception would be in a patient who is hemodynamically unstable during his or her acute exacerbation* (Jessup et al., 2009).

Aldosterone Antagonists

An aldosterone antagonist, such as spironolactone or eplerenone, can be beneficial in patients with heart failure who experience symptoms at rest. In a large-scale, long-term trial, low-dose spironolactone reduced the risk of death in patients already taking ACE inhibitors. The greatest benefit was seen in those patients who were also taking beta-blockers and digoxin (Hunt et al., 2009). Hyperkalemia is a potential side effect, especially when patients are already on ACE inhibitors. The addition of aldosterone antagonists is recommended in stage C in those patients continuing to experience NYHA classification III or IV heart failure while on an ACE inhibitor, beta-blocker, and diuretic.

Medications used in treatment for heart failure are summarized in Table 7-5. Specific medications by class are listed in Table 7-6.

TABLE 7-5: SUMMARY OF HEART FAILURE MEDICATIONS BY CLASS

ACE inhibitors and ARBs	• Interrupt the neurohormonal responses of the RAAS and favorably impact disease progression • Reduce mortality and morbidity
Beta-blockers	• Interrupt the neurohormonal responses of the SNS and favorably impact disease progression • Reduce hospitalizations ** Not initiated in acute decompensated state*
Diuretics	• Decrease ECF load and improve symptoms in an overload state • Maintain ECF volume status and sodium balance • Have no impact on mortality *Loop diuretics with the addition of a thiazide diuretic if needed*
Digoxin	• Improves symptoms, exercise tolerance, and quality of life • Used in patients who are symptomatic on the above three medications • No mortality impact *Dosage is usually 0.125 mg; toxicity can occur with normal serum levels*
Aldosterone antagonists	• Reserved for patients with moderate to severe heart failure *Cannot be used if creatinine level is greater than 2.5 mg/dl because* of the *risk of hyperkalemia*

TABLE 7-6: EXAMPLES OF MEDICATIONS BY CLASS

ACE inhibitors	ARBs	Beta-blockers	Loop diuretics	Aldosterone antagonists
Captopril	Candesartan	Carvedilol	Furosemide	Spironolactone (nonselective)
Enalapril		Metoprolol	Torsemide	Eplerenone (selective)
Lisinopril		Bisoprolol	Bumetanide	
Ramipril				

Hydralazine and Isosorbide Dinitrate

A combination of hydralizine and isosorbide dinitrate should be added to the treatment regimen for African Americans with moderate to severe symptoms of heart failure on optimal treatment with beta-blockers, ACE-inhibitors, and diuretics (Jessup et al., 2009). In clinical trials utilizing combinations of hydralazine and isosorbide dinitrate in addition to or in place of standard therapy with ACE inhibitors, there was no conclusive evidence of benefit. However, retrospectively, a significant benefit was noted in the African American population. This benefit was significant enough for the ACC/AHA to add this as a class I recommendation to the updated heart failure guidelines in April 2009.

Diuretics

Diuretics are added to the treatment regimen for heart failure stage C when the patient presents with symptoms of fluid overload. Loop diuretics work at the loop of Henle to increase sodium and water excretion. After fluid overload has been resolved, diuretics are usually continued to maintain fluid volume status. Few heart failure patients are able to maintain optimal ECF balance without the use of a diuretic.

Diuretics improve symptoms more rapidly than any other drug and can also increase cardiac function and improve exercise tolerance. Optimal use of diuretics is also key to the effectiveness of ACE inhibitor and beta-blocker therapies. ACE inhibitor therapy is less effective and patients are less likely to tolerate beta-blocker therapy if the diuretic dose is too low and ECF overload is present. The risk of hypotension and

renal insufficiency are increased with ACE inhibitor use if the diuretic dose is too high.

Digoxin

Digoxin is a weak inotropic agent, but its benefits in heart failure come from its other effects, including reducing sympathetic outflow and suppressing renin secretion. Digoxin can improve symptoms and decrease the rate of hospitalization but has not been proven to reduce mortality (Hobbs & Boyle, 2009). A dose of 0.125 mg per day (lower than once thought necessary to be effective) is recommended in most patients (Hunt et al., 2009). Digoxin is recommended in stage C for patients with heart failure who remain symptomatic despite treatment with ACE inhibitors, beta-blockers, and diuretics.

Contraindicated Medications

Although ACE inhibitors, ARBs, beta-blockers, diuretics, and digoxin are used in the treatment of heart failure, certain medications should be avoided in patients with heart failure. Most antiarrhythmics are poorly tolerated in patients with heart failure because of their proarrhythmic and cardiodepressant effects. Amiodarone is the only antiarrhythmic that does not adversely affect survival in patients with heart failure (Hunt et al., 2009).

Calcium channel blockers, with the exception of amlodipine, adversely affect survival in patients with systolic dysfunction. Amlodipine has a neutral effect in heart failure and can be used if needed to treat coexisting angina or hypertension. Patients with heart failure should be instructed to avoid the use of nonsteroidal anti-inflammatory drugs (NSAIDs), which can cause sodium retention and peripheral vasoconstriction. These medications diminish the efficacy of diuretics and ACE inhibitors, while enhancing the likelihood of toxic renal effects.

NONPHARMACOLOGICAL TREATMENT STRATEGIES FOR HEART FAILURE

Exercise Training

Controlled trials have shown that exercise training improves symptoms, quality of life, and exercise capacity in patients with heart failure. This beneficial effect is additive to the effects of optimal medical therapy (Hunt et al., 2009). Exercise training in patients with heart failure is best accomplished in a formally structured program, such as cardiac rehabilitation. Studies show that many of the hemodynamic abnormalities associated with chronic heart failure improve with exercise training. The physiological benefits of exercise training for patients with chronic heart failure occur in skeletal muscle as opposed to in the heart itself (Myers, 2010).

Cardiac Resynchronization Therapy

Cardiac resynchronization therapy (CRT) is indicated in patients with moderate to severe heart failure and those with wide QRS complexes who are symptomatic despite optimal medical therapy. In resynchronization therapy, a biventricular pacemaker is placed with leads in both the right and left ventricles. A lead is also implanted in the right atrium to allow for atrial pacing. Resynchronization is common in heart failure because approximately one third of the patients with a low ejection fraction and NYHA class III or IV heart failure have bundle branch block that causes the right and left ventricles to depolarize at different times (Jessup et al., 2009). When this occurs, the walls of the right and left ventricles do not contract simultaneously. This dyssynchrony decreases myocardial function and

cardiac output. There is also an associated increase in mortality in patients with cardiac dyssynchrony (Jessup et al., 2009). Resynchronization therapy with a biventricular pacemaker allows the right and left ventricles to contract simultaneously, thereby improving cardiac performance. Studies show clinical improvement in exercise tolerance, quality of life, and mortality after resynchronization therapy in patients with moderate to severe heart failure (Jacobson & Gerity, 2010; Jessup et al., 2009). Evaluation of CRT continues in the research arena. As more data is collected, more information is known regarding who will receive the greatest benefit from this treatment and when. CRT is exciting technology that is having a great impact when used in the right patient at the right time. More information on CRT is discussed in Chapter 12.

Clinical Application

It is important to remember that CRT is a therapeutic treatment used in heart failure. These devices are not placed because of heart rate issues. With this in mind, when ventricular pacing occurs, therapy is delivered. If there is no ventricular pacing, then there is no synchrony between the right and left bundle. It is important to differentiate this patient population from the patient population with pacemakers implanted to maintain normal heart rates.

SPECIAL ISSUES IN HEART FAILURE

Sudden Death

Patients with heart failure are at high risk for sudden cardiac death. They can also die of progressive pump failure and congestion or end-organ failure from systemic hypoperfusion. Although more than 50% of patients with heart failure have episodes of nonsustained ventricular tachycardia, it is not necessarily the simple progression to sustained ventricular tachycardia that increases the risk of sudden death (Hunt et al., 2009). Sudden death in patients with heart failure is commonly associated with an acute ischemic event or bradydysrhythmias. For this reason, interventions in heart failure are aimed at preventing sudden death, rather than treating asymptomatic ventricular dysrhythmias.

Treatments used to decrease the risk of sudden cardiac death in heart failure include:

- beta-blockers

- amiodarone

- implantable cardioverter-defibrillators (ICDs).

Most antiarrhythmic drugs are poorly tolerated in patients with heart failure. However, amiodarone (although a class III antiarrhythmic) also has vasodilatory properties and is generally well tolerated by such patients. Because of the toxicity associated with amiodarone, it is not routinely used in treatment for heart failure. However, it is used in patients with a history of sudden cardiac death, ventricular fibrillation, or sustained unstable ventricular tachycardia (Hunt et al., 2009). ICDs are indicated in the following patients with heart failure: survivors of cardiac arrest and those with sustained ventricular tachycardia, inducible ventricular tachycardia during an electrophysiology study, or ejection fraction less than 35% 40 days after an MI (Jessup et al., 2009). ICDs are discussed in further detail in Chapter 12.

Acute Decompensated Heart Failure

Patients with acute decompensated heart failure commonly present with the following clinical signs: tachycardia, tachypnea, pallor, diaphoresis, inspiratory crackles or rales, jugular venous distention, peripheral edema, hepatomegaly, ascites, extra heart sounds (S_3 and often S_4), and a possible mitral regurgitation murmur. Additionally, patients may also experience an increase in the symptoms of dyspnea and fatigue. An evaluation for common disease processes that may precipitate an episode of acute heart failure should be carried out in the patient pre-

senting with an exacerbation of or new onset heart failure. Some of those precipitating factors include:

- acute MI or ischemia

- severe hypertension

- atrial and ventricular dysrhythmias

- infections

- pulmonary emboli

- renal failure

- medical or dietary noncompliance.

(Jessup et al., 2009)

Brain Natriuretic Peptide Levels

Brain natriuretic peptide (BNP) levels are used as a diagnostic indicator in patients presenting with signs of decompensation. Plasma concentrations of BNP are elevated in patients with decompensated heart failure with fluid overload. This diagnostic tool is also helpful when a patient's primary complaint is shortness of breath, yet the etiology is unclear. A BNP level less than 100 pg/ml has a high negative predictive value; therefore, it can be used to eliminate heart failure as the cause of dyspnea. BNP levels greater than 500 pg/ml at the time of discharge are highly associated with readmission within 30 days. BNP levels can remain chronically elevated in end-stage heart failure (Hunt et al., 2009). BNP levels may be elevated for reasons other than heart failure, such as pulmonary hypertension and pulmonary emboli. BNP levels should be used in conjuction with other available clinical informtion for heart failure and not as a stand alone definitive diagnostic test (Jessup et al., 2009).

Diuretics

Diuretics are the first-line strategy for the treatment of acute decompensated heart failure with volume overload. If currently on diuretic therapy, an intravenous (IV) dose equal to the oral dose is recommended. Because early intervention may be associated with improved outcomes in patients hospitalized with heart failure, the ACC/AHA recommends diuretic therapy begin at the earliest presentation – emergency department or outpatient clinic (Jessup et al., 2009). Jugular venous distension is one of the most useful tools in evaluating the effects of diuretic therapy. Additionally, a decrease in pulmonary congestion, peripheral edema, and body weight all demonstrate the effectiveness of diuretic therapy (Hunt et al., 2009).

Ultrafiltration

Ultrafiltration is a mechanical method of removing excess fluid through a semipermiable membrane according to a pressure gradient. The process of ultrafiltration occurs with a machine much like a dialysis machine. However, unlike dialysis, the goal is fluid removal only and not particles such as electrolytes. The fluid removal process with ultrafiltration is slow and occurs over many hours and sometimes days. When a patient is nonresponsive to diuretics or if the degree of renal dysfunction is severe, ultrafiltration may be needed to solve the problem of fluid overload (Jessup et al., 2009).

Inotropic Therapy

Patients in acute decompensated heart failure may require IV administration of a positive inotrope. Dobutamine, a sympathomimetic, and milrinone, a phosphodiesterase inhibitor, are the commonly used IV inotropes. Milrinone has vasodilator properties, in addition to inotropic properties.

Vasodilator Therapy

Patients in acute decompensated heart failure may also need vasodilator therapy to help reduce preload or afterload. Nesiritide, a synthetic BNP, is one vasodilator used in treatment for acute decompensated heart failure. Nesiritide is a venous and arterial vasodilator, so it reduces both preload and afterload. Other vasodilators used in acute decompensated heart failure include nitroglycerin and nitroprusside. IV nitroglycerin is usually given in low doses as a venous vasodilator, and nitroprusside is used predominantly as an arterial vasodilator. These medications should only be used in patients with an adequate blood pressure.

Patient Monitoring and Care

Patients admitted with acute decompensated heart failure require careful observation until stabilized. Evaluation of the effects of treatment should include:

- careful measurement of intake and output
- vital sign evaluation
- daily weight measurement (same time each day)
- daily supine and standing blood pressure
- frequent assessment of perfusion and congestion status.

(Jessup et al., 2009)

End-Stage Heart Failure

Patients with end-stage refractory heart failure have special management issues. These patients need very careful control of their ECF volume status because many of their symptoms are related to sodium imbalances causes by ECF overload. ACE inhibitors and beta-blockers are effective in patients with end-stage refractory heart failure; however, these patients may not tolerate these medications well and, therefore, lower doses may need to be used. Patients should not receive these medications if the systolic blood pressure is less than 80 mm Hg or if they show signs of hypoperfusion. Patients should not be initiated on beta-blockers if they have symptomatic ECF retention or require IV inotropic support.

End-stage heart failure patients may decompensate frequently and may need to be admitted for IV inotropic or vasodilator therapy. After the patient is stabilized and oral medications are resumed, the patient must be observed for a period to assure the oral regimen is sufficient to avoid further decompensation. Patients unable to be weaned from IV inotropic support may be candidates for at-home, continuous, inotropic support. This measure is a final option, used only for palliative relief in end-stage disease. Intermittent inotropic therapy at one time was an option for end-stage heart failure treatment. This therapy is no longer recommended in the management of end-stage heart failure because it has been shown to increase mortality (Hunt et al., 2009).

Transplantation

Cardiac transplantation is the only established surgical treatment for refractory heart failure. Unfortunately, this treatment option is available only to a small group of patients each year. Most patients with end-stage heart failure do not meet criteria for cardiac transplantation. Transplantation is indicated only for patients with severe functional impairment who require continuous IV inotropic support. These candidates need to be otherwise healthy. The survival rate at 1 year has improved over time and is currently greater than 87% (Ledoux & Luikart, 2010). After transplantation, patients remain on lifelong immunosuppression therapy, placing them at risk for additional complications.

Left Ventricular Assist Devices

Left ventricular assist devices can be used to provide hemodynamic support to failing hearts for patients waiting for cardiac transplantation and those who are not candidates for transplantation. Some left ventricular assist devices can be surgically implanted. Complications with left ventricular assist devices are common and can be life threatening. For this reason, the use of these devices is limited.

Prognosis and Referral to Palliative Care and Hospice

Physicians should discuss end-of-life care issues with patients with end-stage heart failure while they are still able to participate in the decision-making process. A palliative care referral can be made at any time after the diagnosis of a chronic medical condition for which there is no cure. The primary goal of palliative care is quality of life. A referral to palliative care does not prohibit the patient from continuing active treatment, but rather offers adjunctive resources and support to help with decision making and address psychosocial aspects of care.

Hospice care is another option for end-stage disease management that is often underutilized. A prediction of death within 6 months is traditionally a criterion for admission to hospice services. Because sudden cardiac death is one of the major causes of death in heart failure patients, the time of death is difficult to predict. Many patients with end-stage heart failure have periods of good quality of life during the final 6 months. Hospice admission policies need to be flexible enough to allow end-stage heart failure patients to participate in these palliative programs when appropriate. Healthcare providers who specialize in treating patients with heart failure also need to be more attentive to end-of-life care in this population and initiate more patient dialogue and appropriate hospice referrals.

PATIENT EDUCATION

Heart failure is the final pathway for many cardiac disorders. Heart failure care is complex and involves continuity across the continuum. Research shows that careful monitoring and follow up make a difference. Nurses play an important role in the monitoring and follow-up care of patients with heart failure. Nurses also contribute substantially to patient and family education. Teaching the patient and family self-management strategies is key in the effective management of heart failure. Addressing healthcare literacy is key in this patient population to effectively teach self-management strategies. Through discharge education, postdischarge telephone follow up, and nurse-led heart failure clinics, nurses are making a difference in the management of heart failure. One study demonstrated that one hour of education delivered by a nurse educator at the time of hospital discharge resulted in improved clinical outcomes, increased self-care, and reduced cost of care (Hunt et al., 2009). Patients are an integral part of the management of heart failure. Self-care, which incorporates self-management and maintenance, can have an impact on the management of this disease process (Moser & Reigel, 2008).

Discharge instructions should include six specific areas of care:

1. Recognition and response to signs and symptoms of worsening heart failure

2. Daily weight monitoring

3. Discharge medications (with an emphasis on adherence, persistence, and follow up for dose adjustments up to recommended doses)

4. Diet/sodium restriction

5. Activity level

6. Follow-up appointments
(Jessup et al., 2009)

These six areas of focus for discharge instructions are consistent with the quality indicators measured for the Centers for Medicare & Medicaid Services (CMS) and The Joint Commission.

Clinical Application

Healthcare illiteracy can exist in the presence of literacy. Even patients who are able to read may not be able to adequately understand the complexities of instructions used in healthcare. Several strategies can help improve health literacy:

*   *Create a trusting relationship.*

*   *Slow down when providing instructions.*

*   *Use commonly understood words, rather than medical terminology.*

*   *Focus on practical information about self-care, rather than details about pathophysiology.*

*   *Ask patients to teach back what they have learned.*

(Potter & Martin, 2005)

Additional resource information on this very important topic of health literacy can be found in the healthcare literacy fact sheets available for download at the Center for Health Care Strategies, Inc. Web site.

Recognition of Signs and Symptoms

Patients need to understand how to recognize the signs and symptoms of worsening heart failure. Recognizing changes in activity tolerance is key. As activity intolerance is decreasing, heart failure symptoms may be increasing. Some patients and families find it helpful to keep an activity diary as an objective record of their activities and tolerance.

Daily Weights

Daily weights can be the most sensitive indicators for accurately assessing ECF status. A scale with large numbers for visibility is important for older adult patients. Some patients require family assistance with weighing themselves because they cannot independently step onto and off of a scale. Scales with grab bars are beneficial but, because of their cost, may not be an option for all patients.

Clinical Application

Asking about the presence of a working scale at home is a key nursing intervention.

Clinical Application

Patients should be aware that the measurement of daily weights is not for the evaluation of adipose tissue, but the evaluation of fluid retention.

Nurses should instruct patients to keep a chart of daily weight and to take the chart with them to their physician office visits. Patients should also be instructed to report any gain of 3 lb in 2 days or greater than 3 lb in 1 week (Moser & Reigel, 2008). Some hospitals have programs that allow patients to call in and report their weights each day to a nurse or a computer system. Patients with weight gain and patients who do not call in are identified to receive further follow-up.

Clinical Application

It is important for patients to report their weight gain even if they do not have any other symptoms.

Medication Adherence

Medication adherence is critical to the effective management of heart failure. Patients are more compliant when they fully understand the benefits of therapy. It is important to make sure that the patient understands the benefits of therapy, including those medications that may not improve symptoms, but improve long-term mortality. Patients with heart failure are on multiple medications, which can cause a variety of compliance issues. A careful assessment of any financial concerns regarding prescribed medications is also important. Nurses should discuss any financial concerns with physicians so that every effort can be made to prescribe the most cost-effective, yet appropriate, medication regimen. Social services should be consulted to assure that patients receive all available healthcare support services. Home healthcare can be invaluable in assessing the home environment and evaluating medication compliance and understanding in that setting.

Physical limitations affecting adherence include poor vision and poor dexterity. Nurses should assess the patient's ability to read the small print on labels and open vials, and divide pills, if necessary. Nurses should also instruct patients to report any perceived side effects to their physician before stopping any medications. Because of the effects of NSAIDs on diuretic and ACE inhibitor therapy, nurses should instruct patients to avoid the use of these medications.

Patients should always carry with them a complete list of medications and their doses, especially to every physician office visit. Nurses can facilitate this practice by providing a comprehensive, legible list of medications with a current date printed on a wallet card. Nurses should review all admission and discharge medications to ensure that the necessary medications are ordered and that different physicians did not inadvertently order two medications in the same drug classification.

Diet/Sodium Restriction

Patients with heart failure also need information regarding adherence to a moderate, sodium-restricted diet. In the presence of a sodium restriction, diuretic therapy is more effective (Moser & Reigel, 2008). In many cases, patients do not realize the hidden sodium content in processed foods. Because many foods contain high amounts of sodium, patients and their caregivers must learn how to read food labels. Patients with heart failure should limit their sodium intake to 2 to 3 g per day, unless ordered otherwise. Fresh foods are the best choice for low sodium content. Frozen foods typically contain less sodium than do canned foods.

Clinical Application

Many patients understand not to use the salt shaker, but do not understand how to read a food label. Instruct patients to look for the "sodium" content in foods when reading labels. Also instruct patients to look for portion size to determine the amount of sodium in each serving. Keeping a diary of daily sodium intake may be helpful for some patients in tracking their sodium consumption.

Physical Activity and Socialization

Physical activity should be promoted in all patients with heart failure to prevent deconditioning. Most patients benefit from exercise training in a formal cardiac rehabilitation program. Participation in this type of program also provides interaction with other people and the opportunity for a healthcare provider to assess the patient at regular intervals.

Patients with heart failure are at risk for isolation and depression if they have limited activity tolerance. Many hospitals and communities have support groups for patients and families living with heart failure. Nurses should carefully assess support systems and opportunities for socialization in patients who are homebound.

Follow Up

Close physician or advanced practice nurse follow-up care is critical to the successful management of heart failure. Patients need to understand the importance of keeping all scheduled appointments, even when they are feeling well. Many medications are titrated to optimal doses on an outpatient basis. Nurses need to assess for any barriers to keeping office appointments, such as lack of transportation or conflicting work schedules of family members. Key components of patient education for patients with heart failure are summarized in Box 7-1.

Additional resources for patient education can be found at the Heart Failure Society of America Web site (www.hfsa.org).

Clinical Application

There are many reasons for non-adherence in the patient with heart failure. It is essential that the nurse listens carefully to the patient and asks specific questions to fully appreciate the patient's understanding of discharge instructions. Asking the simple question, "Do you have any questions?" does not ascertain the patient's understanding of the instructions. A more appropriate question might be framed in a manner that demonstrates understanding, such as, "What are you going to do when your weight increases 3 pounds over 2 days?"

Additionally, it is important to assess for patient resources. For example, daily weights cannot be performed if a patient does not have a scale.

BOX 7-1: PATIENT EDUCATION CHECKLIST

- Recognition of signs and symptoms
  - Activity intolerance: activity diary
  - ECF retention: daily weight
    » Assess for home scale
- Medication compliance
  - Review benefits of therapy
  - Provide wallet card with current medication list
    » Assess for and eliminate barriers to accurate and consistent administration
- Diet/Sodium limitation
  - Label reading
  - Avoiding processed and canned foods
- Physical activity plan
  - Cardiac rehabilitation
- Support system and socialization opportunities
- Follow-up with primary cardiac care providers

CONCLUSION

Heart failure is a chronic condition in which nurses play an important role in patient management. Nurses have a tremendous opportunity to collaborate with interdisciplinary team members to maximize patient outcomes. Research regarding the management of heart failure is ongoing, and practice guidelines are works in progress. The role of nurses in the management of heart failure will continue to expand. All nurses should understand the importance of heart failure prevention strategies in patients who are at risk for CHD and those who have CHD but do not yet have heart failure.

Additionally, there is a current focus on efforts to decrease hospital readmission rates in this vulnerable patient, by focusing on the transition between hospital and home. The Hospital to Home improvement initiative, sponsored by the Institute for Healthcare Improvement and the ACC, is one such initiative in which nurses can actively contribute to improving quality outcomes in this patient population. More information regarding this initiative and the opportunity to improve care in this patient population can be found on the Hospital to Home Web site (http://www.h2hquality.org).

EXAM QUESTIONS

CHAPTER 7
Questions 54-63

Note: Choose the one option that BEST answers each question.

54. The hallmark symptoms of heart failure are

    a. rapid heart rate with syncope.

    b. chest pain with positive myocardial enzymes.

    c. dangerously low heart rate requiring a pacemaker.

    d. dyspnea and fatigue or fluid retention.

55. Heart failure is most commonly a result of

    a. digoxin toxicity.

    b. ischemic CHD.

    c. an untreated viral infection.

    d. renal failure.

56. Systolic left ventricular dysfunction is best defined as

    a. impaired ability of the left ventricle to contract and effectively eject blood.

    b. impaired ability of the left ventricle to relax and fill.

    c. heart failure with an elevated systolic blood pressure.

    d. heart failure in which the heart stops beating during systole.

57. Neurohormonal responses in heart failure, which over time lead to clinical deterioration, include

    a. activation of the liver to release glycogen stores.

    b. increased production of cholesterol to make more needed hormones.

    c. activation of the SNS and RAAS.

    d. increased production of hemoglobin to increase oxygen capacity.

58. The one positive neurohormonal response in chronic heart failure, which results in vasodilation, is increased release of

    a. norepinephrine.

    b. cytokines.

    c. BNP.

    d. vasopressin.

59. Medications commonly used in the treatment of heart failure to interrupt neurohormonal responses, reduce ventricular remodeling, and decrease mortality include

    a. ACE inhibitors and beta-blockers.

    b. ACE inhibitors and calcium channel blockers.

    c. calcium channel blockers and nitrates.

    d. beta-blockers and nitrates.

60. Which of the following statements is true concerning the use of diuretics in heart failure?

    a. Diuretics have common life-threatening side effects and are only used in severe decompensation.

    b. Diuretics are used in patients with past and present signs of fluid overload.

    c. Diuretics are used because they reduce mortality.

    d. Diuretics should only be used in patients who cannot tolerate ACE inhibitors.

61. Cardiac resynchronization therapy (CRT) is used in heart failure to

    a. restore sinus rhythm in patients with atrial fibrillation.

    b. defibrillate patients out of life-threatening dysrhythmias.

    c. restore synchrony between right and left ventricle depolarization by pacing both ventricles at the same time.

    d. restore synchrony between the heart and lungs by dilating the pulmonary artery.

62. A true statement regarding end-stage heart failure is

    a. all patients diagnosed with end-stage heart failure die within 6 months from the time of diagnosis.

    b. most patients with end-stage heart failure are candidates for and receive cardiac transplantation.

    c. most patients come to the hospital daily for infusion of an IV inotrope.

    d. many patients can have periods of good quality of life, even after they are diagnosed as having end-stage disease.

63. Key patient education nursing interventions in heart failure include instruction on

    a. recognizing signs and symptoms of hypoglycemia.

    b. the importance of daily weights and reporting weight gain.

    c. eating foods high in sodium.

    d. maintaining bed rest to avoid episodes of exacerbation.

CHAPTER 8

CARDIOMYOPATHY

CHAPTER OBJECTIVE

After completing this chapter, the learner will be able to recognize the three main types of cardiomyopathy and their physiological differences.

LEARNING OBJECTIVES

After completing this chapter, the learner will be able to

1. define cardiomyopathy.

2. identify the three primary types of cardiomyopathy.

3. differentiate the pathophysiology associated with each type of cardiomyopathy.

4. identify tools utilized for the diagnosis of cardiomyopathy.

5. recognize the primary treatment goals for cardiomyopathy.

6. describe the difference between hypertrophic obstructive cardiomyopathy and hypertrophic nonobstructive cardiomyopathy.

7. recall one medication to avoid with hypertrophic obstructive cardiomyopathy that is useful in the treatment of other types of cardiomyopathy.

INTRODUCTION

The term "cardiomyopathy" refers to abnormal myocardial performance caused by diseases of the myocardium. In a scientific statement released by the American Heart Association (AHA), Maron et al. (2006) defined cardiomyopathy as follows:

> Cardiomyopathies are a heterogeneous group of diseases of the myocardium associated with mechanical and/or electrical dysfunction that usually (but not invariably) exhibit in appropriate ventricular hypertrophy or dilation and are due to a variety of causes that frequently are genetic (p. 1809).

The classification of these disorders can become confusing and the term cardiomyopathy can refer to a wide variety of disorders. These disorders may be classified as primary or secondary cardiomyopathies. Primary cardiomyopathies are disorders affecting the heart muscle alone and are the least common forms of cardiomyopathy. Secondary cardiomyopathies are more common and myocardial involvement is due to a larger systemic disorder. There are three main categories or types of cardiomyopathy: 1) dilated cardiomyopathy (DCM); 2) restrictive cardiomyopathy (RCM); and 3) hypertrophic cardiomyopathy (HCM) (Porth, 2005). In 1996, the World Health Organization (WHO) added two additional categories: arrhythmogenic right ventricular cardiomyopathy and peripartum cardiomyopathy (Porth, 2005). The classification of each type is based on clinical, structural, functional, and hemodynamic criteria (Schoen & Mitchell, 2010). The end result of all types of cardiomyopathy is dysfunction of the myocardium. As knowledge about cardiomyopathy grows, causes are identified for what was once considered idiopathic cardiomyopathy. For the purpose of this text, the discussion in this chapter will focus on the three main types of cardiomyopathy. In addition to this discussion, the chapter will introduce in less detail two of the newer types of cardiomyopathy: 1) arrhythmogenic right ventricular cardiomyopathy (ARVC) and 2) Takotsubo cardiomyopathy. As information is becoming available for these newer disease processes, they are being recognized in the clinical setting on a more regular basis.

DILATED CARDIOMYOPATHY

Definition

An enlarged, dilated cardiac chamber is the hallmark characteristic of DCM. This dilation can affect one or all four cardiac chambers. As the chamber enlarges, its ability to contract becomes impaired, resulting in systolic dysfunction (see Figure 8-1).

Prevalence

DCM is the most common form of cardiomyopathy and represents the largest group of heart failure cases (Bott-Silverman, 2009). Although the exact number of people with DCM is difficult to determine, the population is large. The AHA and the American College of Cardiology (ACC) stage heart failure into four categories (see Table 8-1). Most people who fall into stages B, C, or D have one type of cardiomyopathy. It has been estimated that idiopathic DCM occurs in 0.4 per 1,000 of the general population (Bott-Silverman, 2009). African Americans have an increased risk of developing

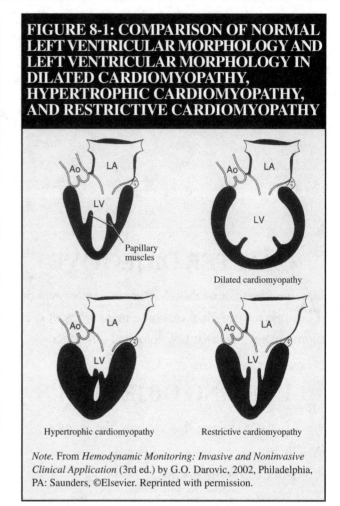

FIGURE 8-1: COMPARISON OF NORMAL LEFT VENTRICULAR MORPHOLOGY AND LEFT VENTRICULAR MORPHOLOGY IN DILATED CARDIOMYOPATHY, HYPERTROPHIC CARDIOMYOPATHY, AND RESTRICTIVE CARDIOMYOPATHY

Dilated cardiomyopathy

Hypertrophic cardiomyopathy

Restrictive cardiomyopathy

Note. From *Hemodynamic Monitoring: Invasive and Noninvasive Clinical Application* (3rd ed.) by G.O. Darovic, 2002, Philadelphia, PA: Saunders, ©Elsevier. Reprinted with permission.

DCM due to increased presence of risk factors, such as hypertension. African Americans with DCM also have a higher mortality rate than Caucasian Americans (Bozkurt & Mann, 2007).

Causes

There are a wide variety of causes of DCM. The most common identifiable cause of DCM is ischemic cardiomyopathy that results from damage to the myocardium from mycocardial infarction (MI). Ischemic DCM is responsible for approximately 60% of the patients with symptoms of heart failure (Bott-Silverman, 2009). DCM also has a variety of nonischemic causes (see Box 8-1). Among some of the more common causes are valvular heart disease and alcohol or drug toxicity. Regardless of the cause of damage to the myocytes, myocardial fibrosis occurs. The end result is dilation of the cardiac chambers, causing impaired mechanical function of the heart.

TABLE 8-1: AMERICAN HEART ASSOCIATION/AMERICAN COLLEGE OF CARDIOLOGY STAGING OF HEART DISEASE

Stage	Description
A	Patients at risk for heart failure with no structural heart disease
B	Patients with structural heart disease without symptoms of heart failure
C	Patients with past or present heart failure symptoms
D	Patients with advanced disease

(Hunt et al., 2009)

BOX 8-1: CAUSES OF DILATED CARDIOMYOPATHY

- Idiopathic
- Ischemic heart disease
- Genetic disorders
- Hypertension
- Viral or bacterial infection
- Valvular heart disease
- Chemotherapy
- Peripartum syndrome related to toxemia
- Cardiotoxic effects of drugs or alcohol

Unfortunately, as the myocardium dilates and myocardial dysfunction occurs, the physiologic response to decreased cardiac function results in further myocardial damage and dysfunction. This process is referred to as *ventricular remodeling,* and therapeutic treatment is aimed at preventing, slowing, and reversing the process.

Pathophysiology

The primary dysfunction in DCM involves ventricular dilation and a decreased ability of the ventricle to contract. For example, MI causes myocardial necrosis or cell death at the site of the infarct, and scar tissue replaces healthy myocytes. Myocardial contractility in the area of the scar tissue no longer occurs. This decrease in contractility in one area increases stress on other areas of the myocardium. Over time, the ventricle begins to dilate. As the ventricular chamber enlarges, the myocardial fibers stretch to the point that they become overstretched and can no longer forcefully contract. This loss of contractile function is referred

to as *systolic dysfunction.* As contractile function is lost, the ventricle is unable to eject its contents and ejection fraction decreases, as does stroke volume and cardiac output. As a result of this decreased ejection of ventricular contents, volume in the ventricle at the end of systole increases. When the left atrium empties into the left ventricle during diastole, the increased residual volume in the ventricle prevents the atrium from emptying completely. The increased volume in the left atrium subsequently increases the pressure in the left atrium. The left atrium dilates to compensate for the increased volume and subsequent pressure. This atrial dilation can provide adequate compensation for some time. Ultimately, however, this compensation fails and the increased volume and pressure in the atrium are reflected back into the pulmonary system. Pulmonary failure occurs and symptoms of left-sided heart failure develop. As left ventricular function deteriorates, the right ventricle ultimately fails as well, resulting in right-sided heart failure.

Many compensatory mechanisms occur as the ventricular chamber dilates. Normally, as the ventricular wall dilates, it becomes thinner. In some instances, the ventricular wall may actually increase in thickness to help maintain cardiac contraction, as seen with aortic regurgitation. Although they maintain a normal structure, the mitral and tricuspid valves develop a "functional" regurgitation as dilation of the ventricle increases. When the ventricle dilates, the valve opening also dilates, resulting in an inability of the leaflets to come together completely and impairing the ability of the valve to function normally. Papillary muscle dysfunction may also occur due to the dilation of the ventricular walls.

The neurohormonal system becomes activated in response to the decrease in forward ejection of blood. As ejection fraction decreases, the body responds to the decrease in cardiac output. The renin-angiotensin-aldosterone system (RAAS) activates, causing vasoconstriction of the arteries and retention of fluids and sodium. This vasoconstriction increases afterload and causes an already poorly contracting ventricle to pump harder as it attempts to overcome arterial vasoconstriction and eject its contents. Fluid retention places an increased burden on the already overloaded system, and heart failure develops. A full discussion of the response of the neurohormonal system was covered in the discussion of heart failure in Chapter 7.

Heart rate normally increases when cardiac output decreases. In the early stages of DCM, this response is adequate to maintain perfusion. However, as the disease process progresses, this response is no longer enough to compensate for the

contractile defect. (See Figure 8-2 for a diagram of the basic physiologic changes in DCM.)

Clinical Presentation

Symptoms of DCM are directly related to the severity of the disease process and generally develop over time. Most commonly, patients present with symptoms related to low cardiac output, including weakness, fatigue, and decreased activity tolerance (Schoen & Mitchell, 2010). Because symptoms develop slowly, patients make adjustments in activity levels to compensate for the changes, commonly without being aware that they are doing so. Shortness of breath, dyspnea on exertion, and orthopnea occur as pulmonary edema develops. Because failure of the left ventricle generally occurs before failure of the right ventricle, left-sided heart failure symptoms appear before right-sided symptoms (see Table 8-2). Symptoms of right-sided failure are usually a late development. Some conditions, such as right ventricular infarctions and pulmonary hypertension, can cause direct damage to the right ventricle. In these cases,

FIGURE 8-2: BASIC PHYSIOLOGIC PROGRESSION OF DILATED CARDIOMYOPATHY

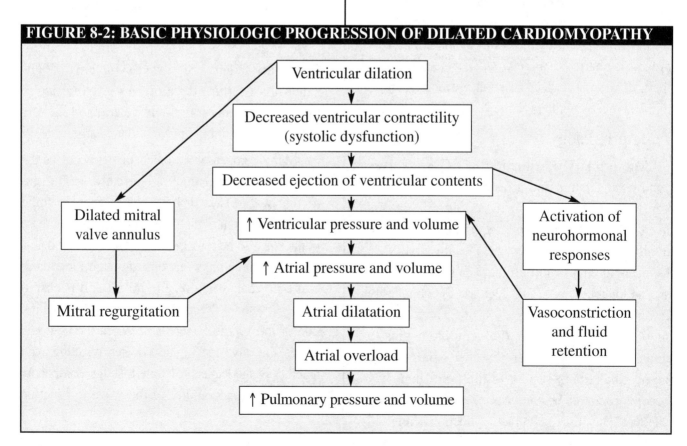

TABLE 8-2: HEART FAILURE SYMPTOMS: RIGHT-SIDED VERSUS LEFT-SIDED

Right-Sided Heart Failure	Left-Sided Heart Failure
Dependent edema	Dyspnea
Distended jugular veins	Paroxysmal nocturnal dyspnea
Enlarged, tender liver	Orthopnea
Ascites	Crackles in lungs

right ventricular failure may occur without any damage to the left ventricle.

Clinical Application

It is important to question patients about their normal level of activity to determine exercise intolerance. Those having symptoms with minimal activity are more seriously ill than those who can participate in activities on a regular basis.

Physical Examination

Findings during the physical examination vary depending on the severity of the disease (see Table 8-3). The severity of DCM depends on the degree of systolic dysfunction. Patients are usually alert until the end stages of the disease process. As perfusion decreases over time, cerebral perfusion eventually will be affected and changes in mental status will occur. The skin may be cool and pale, and cyanosis may be present late in the disease process. When palpating a pulse, the examiner may note an irregularity in the strength. Pulsus alternans (an alternation between weak and strong beats) can occur. Resting tachycardias are not unusual as the heart rate rises in an attempt to compensate for decreased stroke volume. Sustained heart rates greater than 140 beats per minute usually result in rapid decompensation. Heart rate may also be irregularly irregular if the patient is in atrial fibrillation, which is not uncommon. Blood pressure is generally low, with a narrowed pulse pressure. As pulse pressure narrows, systolic and diastolic blood pressure readings move closer to each other. Patients may also experience orthostatic hypotension.

TABLE 8-3: PHYSICAL EXAMINATION FINDINGS IN DILATED CARDIOMYOPATHY

Neurological	• Alert and oriented
Skin	• Cool and dry • Cyanotic (late)
Pulse	• Pulsus alternans
Heart rate	• Elevated
Blood pressure	• Normal to low • Narrowed pulse pressure
Heart examination	• Apical impulse displaced • Additional heart sounds (S_3 or S_4) • Mitral or tricuspid regurgitation murmur
Lung sounds	• Crackles
Jugular vein	• Distended
Liver	• Enlarged • Hepatojugular reflux
Edema	• Peripheral • Ascites

Examination of the heart reveals a displaced apical impulse. At the apex of the heart, a pulse can normally be palpated with each beat. The apical impulse is normally palpable at the fourth or fifth intercostal space, at the left midclavicular line. As the ventricle dilates and changes shape and size, the location of the apex of the heart shifts to the left and down. The apical impulse also decreases in force as the force of contraction decreases with disease progression. During auscultation, a normal first heart sound (S_1, or "lub") and second heart sound (S_2, or "dub") are present. Additionally, a third heart sound (S_3) may be audible immediately after the S_2. The S_3 is best discovered with the bell of the stethoscope when the patient is lying on his or her left side. This sound is loudest at the fifth intercostal space to the left of the sternum if the patient has right-sided heart failure and at the fifth intercostal space at the midclavicular line if the patient has left-sided heart failure (Buss & Thompson, 2010). The S_3 is an indication of an increase in extracellular fluid (ECF) volume and should resolve if the overload is corrected. In addition to the extra heart sound, mitral and tricuspid regurgitation murmurs may be audible. As stated earlier, dilation of the ventricle increases the size of the valve annulus, resulting in mitral and tricuspid regurgitation. These are systolic murmurs, best heard with the diaphragm of the stethoscope, and occur between the S_1 and S_2. Mitral regurgitation murmur is a blowing murmur that is best heard at the apex of the heart. Tricuspid murmur is a blowing or scratchy murmur best heard at the fourth or fifth intercostal space, left of the sternal border (Buss & Thompson, 2010).

Lung sounds are clear early in the disease process. However, as the disease progresses and heart failure occurs, crackles develop, indicating pulmonary edema. Dullness to percussion or diminished breath sounds could indicate pleural effusion, which can also occur with heart failure. Resting dyspnea is a sign of severe impairment.

Other examination findings consistent with right-sided heart failure include jugular venous distension, hepatojugular reflux, liver engorgement, edema, and ascites. All of these findings are directly related to the amount of failure present. Jugular veins are distended when the patient lies with the head elevated at a 45-degree angle. The liver is enlarged and often times tender. Hepatojugular reflux is present when pressure is applied to the liver and the jugular veins become distended. Peripheral edema is generally present, and ascites may also occur.

Clinical Application

Confusion and disorientation should be carefully evaluated because patients with DCM commonly develop atrial fibrillation and are at high risk for the development of emboli.

Clinical Application

Asking patients to tightly squeeze your hand while listening to their hearts enhances murmurs and the additional heart sound in DCM.

Clinical Application

Peripheral edema alone is not confirmation of heart failure because not all peripheral edema is the result of a dysfunctional myocardium.

Diagnosis

Chest X-ray Film

An enlarged cardiac silhouette is visible on chest X-ray film. Pulmonary congestion and pleural effusion may also be visible, if present.

Echocardiogram

The echocardiogram is very useful in the diagnosis of DCM. Echocardiography can provide information about the size of the heart's chambers as well as wall thickness. In DCM, all four chambers may be enlarged; however, the left ventricle is the largest of all the chambers and may also be the only chamber enlarged. Myocardial wall thickening is usually not present because the chamber walls are normal and often thin.

The echocardiogram is also useful in assessing ventricular function. Assessment of ventricular wall motion and ejection fraction provides valuable information about the ability of the dilated heart to contract. Normal ejection fraction is 55% to 65% (Bond, 2010). DCM is characterized by progressive cardiac dilation and systolic dysfunction (Schoen & Mitchell, 2010). In addition to an ejection fraction less than 40%, there is co-existing hypertrophy with an increased size of the left ventricle at the end of diastole (Bott-Silverman, 2009; Schoen & Mitchell, 2010). Echocardiography can also indicate the presence of thrombi in the ventricular cavity.

Cardiac Catheterization (arteriogram)

Cardiac catheterization is beneficial only if it is necessary to determine whether the patient has coronary heart disease (CHD). Although catheterization provides information about wall motion and ejection, noninvasive cardiac echocardiography is a better choice.

Electrocardiogram

An electrocardiogram (ECG) will most commonly show sinus tachycardia and dysrhythmias, such as atrial fibrillation and ventricular ectopy. Left bundle branch block may be noted, as the dilated ventricle causes changes in the conduction pattern through the bundle branches. Large QRS complexes (characteristic of ventricular hypertrophy) may be present as well.

Clinical Application

Hypertrophic changes on the ECG may cause ST-segment and T wave changes that mimic myocardial ischemia. Careful patient assessment and ECG analysis is needed to differentiate between ischemia and the changes associated with hypertrophy.

Medical Therapy

Medical therapy for DCM is essentially the same as therapy for heart failure. The chapter on heart failure (Chapter 7) covers the treatment options in full detail.

Medical therapy is aimed at the reduction of mortality and symptom relief. Interrupting the harmful neurohormonal response is key to the treatment of DCM. With this in mind, medication can provide the following effects, which will decrease the neurohormonal response:

1. reduction of preload
2. reduction of afterload
3. improvement in contractility.

Preload Reduction

When fluid overload is present, preload reduction is needed. Reduction of preload is accomplished with diuretics. Decreased ECF volume allows the ventricle to become less dilated. The smaller ventricle decreases some of the regurgitation that occurs because of overstretched valve rings. As increased ECF volume is decreased, the stretch on the heart decreases, as does myocardial oxygen demand.

Venous vasodilators, such as nitrates, also decrease preload by dilating the veins, allowing more blood to remain in the vascular system and sending less to the heart. Angiotensin-converting enzyme (ACE) inhibitors help reduce volume by blocking the RAAS effects that have been activated.

Aldosterone antagonists, such as spironolactone and eplerenone, may be added to help with the diuretic effect, if the patient continues to have symptoms at rest. More importantly, newer studies show that the addition of this class of medication can reduce mortality, especially in patients with ejection fractions less than 35% (Hunt et al., 2009).

Afterload Reduction

Reduction of afterload is accomplished with arterial vasodilators. Arterial dilation reduces the work of the ventricle as it attempts to eject its contents. Arterial vasoconstriction is a normal response to decreased cardiac output. This response makes the process of ejecting blood from the ventricle more difficult and puts a greater strain on an already struggling heart. Hydralazine (Apresoline) and ACE inhibitors are the medications of choice for decreasing afterload. In fact, any patient with an ejection fraction less than 40%, with or without symptoms, should be started on an ACE inhibitor because these drugs have been shown to decrease long-term mortality (Jessup et al., 2009).

Clinical Application

Arterial vasodilators decrease blood pressure. Patients on arterial vasodilators should be instructed to report any symptoms of low blood pressure, such as dizziness when standing up.

Contractility

Increased contractility is achieved first by decreasing afterload. Usually, as afterload decreases, contractility increases. Digoxin is the oral medication of choice to assist with contractility. Digoxin does not improve mortality rates but it does improve exercise capacity, improve quality of life, and decrease hospitalizations. This medication is most effective in patients who have low ejection fractions.

Other Considerations in Medical Therapy

Beta-blockers

Standard treatment for patients with left ventricular dysfunction includes the administration of beta-blockers. Although beta-blockers should not be initiated during an episode of acute heart failure, they should be started when the failure is under control. Carvedilol (Coreg), metoprolol (Lopressor), and bisoprolol (Zebeta) have been found in multiple studies to decrease mortality and morbidity in heart failure (Soine, 2010). Beta-blockers are used for their mortality benefit in the treatment of patients with low ejection fractions.

Antidysrhythmic therapy

Patients with DCM may experience ventricular dysrhythmias that require treatment. Medication choices should be made carefully because some medications can cause further depression of the myocardium. Currently, amiodarone is the medication of choice because of its vasodilator properties (Gold Standard/Elsevier, 2010; Hunt et al., 2009). Attempts should be made to convert patients from atrial fibrillation by either mechanical or pharmacological options. If conversion cannot be achieved, then rate control is essential. Digoxin and beta-blockers can be helpful in rate control.

Anticoagulation therapy

The utilization of anticoagulation therapy is controversial. Patients with DCM are at increased risk for embolization due to insufficient contraction of the large ventricular chambers. Additionally, these patients are also at high risk for the development of atrial fibrillation. Anticoagulation is recommended for patients with evidence of a left ventricular thrombus, a previous embolic event, or atrial fibrillation (Hunt et al., 2009).

Dietary restrictions

A salt restriction of 2 to 4 g per day, depending on the severity of the disease process, may be necessary. Excessive salt leads to ECF retention. Simply eliminating table salt can decrease salt intake by 1 to 2 g per day. Fluid restrictions are only necessary in the late stages of the disease process, when medical therapy is no longer effective in controlling volume.

Clinical Application

Patients with DCM are commonly prescribed multiple medications. It is essential to ensure that the patient understands the importance of each medication and the value of compliance with the medication regimen.

Clinical Application

Teach patients to read food labels and how to determine the amount of sodium in the food they are eating. Patients may not understand that sodium is salt and should be educated to look for the word sodium on the food label to determine the amount of salt in the food.

Exercise

A sedentary lifestyle in this population leads to cardiac deconditioning. Exercise should be encouraged. Cardiac rehabilitation programs can be very beneficial in helping develop appropriate exercise programs and cardiac conditioning.

Surgical Therapy

Cardiac Resynchronization Therapy

One of the newest therapies available for patients with DCM is cardiac resynchronization therapy (CRT). This therapy is reserved for patients with New York Heart Association (NYHA) heart failure class III or IV. These patients must also be on maximum medical therapy, without benefit, and have ejection fractions less than 35% (Jessup, 2004). The final key criterion is evidence that the right and left ventricles are not contracting at the same time. This dyssynchrony is evident by a bundle branch block pattern (wide QRS complexes) on an ECG. As ventricular dilation becomes greater, the ventricles no longer contract at the same time. Pacemaker wires are placed in the normal location of the right atrium for atrial pacing and in the right ventricle for right ventricular pacing. A third wire is placed via a coronary vein on the left ventricle free wall. With this placement the right and left ventricles are stimulated simultaneously, resulting in synchronous contraction of the right and left ventricle. This resynchronization of the right and left ventricles has shown improvement in cardiac output, exercise tolerance, and quality of life as well as long term outcomes. (See Chapter 12 for further discussion regarding CRT.)

Implantable Cardioverter-defibrillators

Patients at high risk for sudden death from ventricular dysrhythmias may need implantable cardioverter-defibrillators (ICDs). As the ventricle becomes larger and ejection fraction decreases, the risk of sudden death increases. According to the ACC/AHA, approximately 50% to 75% of those patients with a reduced ejection fraction and symptomatic heart failure have had episodes of nonsustained ventricular dysrhythmias (Hunt et al., 2009). In patients with low ejection fractions, ICDs are commonly implanted as part of the procedure for CRT. (See Chapter 12 for a more detailed discussion of ICDs.)

Other Surgical Procedures

Cardiac transplantation is a surgical option that is available to a limited number of patients nationally. The ACC/AHA reports that only about 2500 people with heart failure benefit from cardiac transplantation annually (Hunt et al., 2009). Other surgical attempts in the treatment of dilated cardiomyopathy are limited. Some surgical procedures that demonstrated benefit early on, but did not provide improvement in long-term outcomes, were cardiomyoplasty and left ventriculectomy, also known as the *Batista procedure.* The Batista procedure involves cutting out part of the left ventricle and sewing the remaining walls together to decrease the size of the ventricle. Cardiac myoplasty involves wrapping a muscle from the patient's back around the heart. A pacemaker wire is placed in the muscle and the muscle is stimulated to contract in conjunction with the heart, assisting contraction. Left ventricular assist devices may be implanted to support the patient until a heart for cardiac transplantation is available.

Outcomes

DCM is the final disease process for many other disorders and diseases that affect the myocardium. Death is usually due to progressive heart failure but can also be caused by sudden cardiac death, pulmonary emboli, or embolic stroke. The lower the ejection fraction, the poorer the prognosis. Patient follow up and compliance with treatment regimen seems to impact outcomes. Chapter 7 outlines the nurse's role in educating patients with heart failure. Patient understanding impacts compliance and, therefore, outcomes in this disease process.

RESTRICTIVE CARDIOMYOPATHY

Definition

RCM is characterized by restrictive filling of one or both of the ventricles, with normal or near normal systolic function (Bott-Silverman, 2009). This restriction to filling results in a decreased ability of the chamber walls to expand during cardiac filling, causing a decrease in the volume in the ventricle at the end of diastolic filling time (see Figure 8-1).

Prevalence

RCM is the least common form of cardiomyopathy and accounts for approximately 5% of all primary heart muscle diseases (Goswami, 2008). Men and women are equally affected. This process can be seen in children as well as adults; however, it appears to be better tolerated by adults.

Causes

As with other cardiomyopathies, RCM has both primary and secondary causes (see Box 8-2). Each cause results in different processes that restrict the myocardium. Some patients present with hemodynamics representative of RCM, but no cause can be determined. Amyloidosis is responsible for 90% of RCM cases in North America (Darovic, 2002). In this disease process, protein fibrils (amyloid) deposit in the tissues of the body and impair organ function. These protein fibrils are deposited throughout the myocardium, resulting in a firm, rubbery heart with thick, but not dilated, ventricular walls. Not all patients with amyloidosis develop cardiac involvement; however, amyloid heart disease has a very poor prognosis.

BOX 8-2: CAUSES OF RESTRICTIVE CARDIOMYOPATHY

Primary Causes
- Endomyocardial fibrosis
- Löffler's endocarditis
- Idiopathic RCM

Secondary Causes
- Infiltrative disorders
  - Amyloidosis
  - Sarcoidosis
  - Radiation carditis
- Storage diseases
  - Hemochromatosis
  - Glycogen storage disorders
  - Fabry's disease

(Bott-Silverman, 2009)

Although not prevalent in North America, endomyocardial fibrosis is relatively common in children and young adults in Africa and the Tropics. Fibrosis of the ventricular endocardium and subendocardium that extends to the mitral and tricuspid valves greatly decreases ventricular chamber function. Patients who have undergone radiation treatments may develop radiation-induced myocar-

dial fibrosis. This fibrosis is not evident until several years after treatment.

Pathophysiology

Normally, as ventricular diastole begins, the atrioventricular valves open and the contents of the atria passively empty into the ventricles. At the end of ventricular diastole, the atria contract and add an additional volume of blood to the ventricles. During ventricular filling, the ventricular walls expand, stretching the cardiac muscle fibers and allowing for adequate filling.

In patients with RCM, the ability of the ventricular walls to expand is limited because of the disease process occurring in the myocardium. This limitation in chamber expansion decreases the heart's ability to adequately fill the ventricle during diastole. This decrease in diastolic filling results in a decrease in the volume of blood the ventricle is then able to eject during systole, and stroke volume is decreased. Generally, the ability of the myocardium to contract is not affected. If the disease process is infiltrative, contractile function can become impaired as the disease progresses. In addition to decreased stroke volume, a concurrent decrease in the forward flow of blood occurs because the ventricle is unable to accept all of the contents from the atrium. Therefore, an increase in intravascular volume occurs and blood backs up into the lungs (left-sided failure) and the body (right-sided failure), resulting in heart failure.

Clinical Presentation

Patients with RCM experience an inability to complete normal daily activities because of fatigue and weakness. These symptoms are due to decreased stroke volume and an inability to compensate for increased metabolic demands. Normally, any increase in activity causes heart rate to increase. This increase in heart rate should provide an increase in circulating blood volume to support the increase in demand. For patients with RCM, an increase in heart rate decreases cardiac output because it decreases the amount of time the ventricle has to fill during diastole. Patients with ECF already have a decreased ability to fill the ventricle during diastole because of the restriction of the myocardial wall. Shorter diastolic times compound the problem and less volume is available in the ventricle for ejection, resulting in a decrease in stroke volume and, subsequently, cardiac output. Decreased cardiac output results in symptoms of fatigue and weakness.

Clinical Application

Anything that would normally cause the heart rate to increase, including activity, decreased blood pressure, fever, shivering, and low blood volume, results in a further decrease in stroke volume in patients with RCM.

Hypotension and syncope may be present in patients with amyloidosis. Other symptoms are caused by the heart failure that occurs. The patient experiences biventricular failure because the disease process is not limited to one ventricle. Right-sided failure may be more prominent early because the impaired function of the right ventricle helps decrease the load on the left side of the heart, decreasing the left-sided failure.

The patient may experience palpitations caused by atrial fibrillation, which is common with RCM. Disturbances in cardiac conduction are not uncommon in infiltrative disorders.

Physical Examination

On physical examination, signs of heart failure (including jugular venous distention, edema, and ascites) are present with associated signs of low cardiac output, including cool extremities, hypotension, and possibly lethargy, depending on the progression of the disease. Hypotension is not uncommon in amyloidosis. Peripheral pulses are decreased and become weaker as the disease progresses and stroke volume continues to decrease.

Auscultation of the heart reveals normal S_1 and S_2 and the presence of an S_3 that is caused by decreased compliance of the ventricle. Systolic murmurs of mitral or tricuspid insufficiency may be audible because the valve opening dilates in conjunction with atrial dilation from volume overload. Amyloidosis may also infiltrate the papillary muscles, resulting in regurgitation of the mitral or tricuspid valve.

Diagnosis

Aortic stenosis, cardiac tamponade, HCM, and hypertensive heart disease should all be ruled out when considering a diagnosis of RCM (Goswami, 2008) because all of these disorders result in diastolic dysfunction. The most important process that must be differentiated is constrictive pericarditis, because it can mimic RCM. The clinician must differentiate these two processes so appropriate intervention can be started (see Table 8-4).

Chest X-ray Film

The size of the ventricles on chest X-ray film appears normal, although the atria may be dilated. If the patient is presenting with heart failure, pulmonary congestion may be present. In constrictive pericarditis a calcified pericardium may be seen on a lateral chest X-ray film.

Echocardiogram

In RCM, cardiac echocardiography shows enlarged atria. The ventricles are normal in size without thickened walls unless an infiltrative disease process is present that causes increased wall mass. Normal contractility is also noted. The ventricular cavity size appears normal or reduced. In patients with amyloidosis, abnormal myocardial textures (such as a speckled appearance of the myocardium) may be noted (Carroll & Crawford, 2009). The echocardiogram also shows any mitral and tricuspid regurgitation caused by atrial enlargement.

TABLE 8-4: CLINICAL FEATURES OF CONSTRICTIVE PERICARDITIS AND RESTRICTIVE CARDIOMYOPATHY

Clinical Features	Constrictive Pericarditis	Restrictive Cardiomyopathy
History	Prior history of pericarditis or condition that causes pericardial disease	History of systemic disease (such as amyloidosis or hemochromatosis)
General exam		Peripheral stigmata of systemic disease
Heart sounds (non-murmurs)	Pericardial knock, high frequency sound	Presence of loud diastolic filling sound, third heart sound, low frequency sound
Murmurs	No murmurs	Murmurs of mitral and tricuspid insufficiency
Chest X-ray	Pericardial calcification	No change from prior normal X-ray film

(Goswami, 2008)

Clinical Application

The echocardiogram is most helpful in differentiating constrictive pericarditis from RCM.

Cardiac Catheterization (angiogram)

A complete cardiac catheterization may not be necessary unless CHD is suspected. Invasive hemodynamic measurements provide valuable information about the hemodynamics associated with the disease process. As restriction occurs, filling pressure of each ventricle increases and stroke volume decreases. Again, differentiating between constrictive pericarditis and RCM is important, and the measurements of pressures on the right and left sides of the heart assist in the differential diagnosis. In RCM, the right- and left-sided ventricular filling pressures are increased; however, left-sided filling pressures are generally higher than those of the right side by 5 mm Hg or greater. In constrictive pericarditis, filling pressures are generally equal.

Endomyocardial Biopsy

An endomyocardial biopsy obtained from the septal wall of the right ventricle is useful for the diagnosis of unexplained RCM for a variety of disease processes (Cooper et al., 2007). Multiple specimens must be obtained from multiple sites because many of these disease processes spread in a patchy, scattered pattern. A biopsy can positively identify infiltrative disorders and provide a defini-

tive diagnosis of RCM (see Figure 8-3). In some instances, a biopsy of abdominal fat may be used to diagnose amyloidosis and a cardiac biopsy can be avoided. Hemochromatosis can be diagnosed through a series of lab tests.

Electrocardiogram

Generally, QRS voltage is low and the ECG shows some nonspecific ST-segment and T wave changes. Large P waves are indicative of atrial enlargement. This change, however, is a late sign of atrial enlargement. Cardiac conduction abnormalities occur as the disease infiltrates the conduction system. Atrial fibrillation is common in patients with RCM. Ventricular dysrhythmias are common in patients with cardiac amyloidosis.

Medical Treatment

Medical treatment is supportive and aimed at the reduction of symptoms, with a focus on:

- reduction of diastolic dysfunction
- treatment of dysrhythmias
- treatment of thromboembolic complications
- treatment of the underlying disease process.

Reduction of Diastolic Dysfunction

Although no medications directly affect restriction, treatment is aimed at reducing the effects of the restriction, including increased ECF volume and decreased stroke volume. Diuretics are the

FIGURE 8-3: RIGHT INTERNAL JUGULAR APPROACH TO MYOCARDIAL BIOPSY

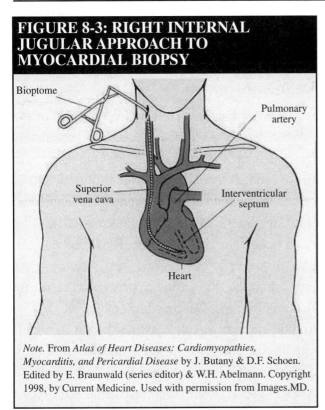

Note. From *Atlas of Heart Diseases: Cardiomyopathies, Myocarditis, and Pericardial Disease* by J. Butany & D.F. Schoen. Edited by E. Braunwald (series editor) & W.H. Abelmann. Copyright 1998, by Current Medicine. Used with permission from Images.MD.

medication of choice to reduce increased ECF volume. Careful assessment of volume status is essential in the treatment of RCM. Reduction of ECF volume is necessary to prevent symptoms of heart failure; however, overreduction of volume further decreases the already decreased filling of the ventricle. Patients with severe RCM have a very narrow range of acceptable volume.

Clinical Application

Patients with RCM should be closely monitored for signs of decreased cardiac output that may result from overdiuresis. Signs and symptoms include hypotension (especially orthostatic hypotension); lethargy; increased heart rate; and increased blood urea nitrogen levels.

Arterial vasodilators, such as ACE inhibitors, may be useful in decreasing afterload and allow for a more effective contraction by the ventricle. However, ACE inhibitors also contribute to diuresis, so volume status must be considered when utilizing ACE inhibitors with diuretics. Any vasodilator that affects the veins decreases the volume entering the heart (preload). This decrease in volume decreases

the amount of volume available for ventricular filling. In many cases, treatment should be initiated with very low doses, with the patient being carefully monitored. ACE inhibitors are poorly tolerated in patients with amyloidosis (Goswami, 2008).

Treatment of Dysrhythmias

Atrial fibrillation is the most common dysrhythmic complication in RCM (Carroll & Crawford, 2009). Loss of atrial contraction can contribute to a decrease in ventricular filling; therefore, a normal sinus rhythm is preferable to atrial fibrillation. A variety of antiarrhythmic medications proven to treat atrial fibrillation may be used. Digoxin may be used cautiously for ventricular rate control, with close monitoring for laboratory or clinical signs of toxicity (Carroll & Crawford, 2009). Beta-blockers and calcium channel blockers may be used to assist with rate control as high heart rates are poorly tolerated in this population. As RCM worsens, conduction system abnormalities develop. Heart blocks (including complete heart blocks) may develop, resulting in the need for a permanent atrioventricular pacemaker. Ventricular dysrhythmias may also develop. Treatment of these dysrhythmias is based on the patient's hemodynamic response and whether the dysrhythmias are sustained or life threatening. These dysrhythmias should be treated in a usual manner, with no specific treatment differences for RCM.

Treatment of Thromboembolic Complications

Patients with endocardial fibrosis are at highest risk for thromoembolism. However, many patients with RCM are at risk for thrombus formation (Carroll & Crawford, 2009). In patients with atrial fibrillation, thrombi can form in the enlarged atrium at the location of the atrial appendage. Thrombi are also a concern in patients with low cardiac output states and mitral or tricuspid valve regurgitation. In these patients, anticoagulation with warfarin should be considered.

Treatment of Underlying Disease Process

Treatment of the underlying disease process varies. Although amyloidosis has no cure, steroids and chemotherapy may be helpful in slowing the progression of the disease. Cardiac transplantation has limited benefits in amyloidosis because the amyloid infiltrates the transplanted organ. Chelation therapy or phlebotomy can be used to treat hemochromatosis, depending on the cause of the iron overload (Carroll & Crawford, 2009).

Clinical Application

Inotropic assistance (medications that increase contractility) is not usually beneficial in RCM because ventricular contraction is not impaired.

Surgical Treatment

Cardiac transplantation is beneficial in idiopathic and familial RCM (Goswami, 2008). Transplant of both the heart and liver is indicated in hemochromatosis. Its usefulness in infiltrative disorders, such as amyloidosis and sarcoidosis, is questionable because these disorders affect the new organ after transplant is completed. In fibrotic endocarditis, excision of the fibrotic endocardium may provide symptomatic relief. Replacement of regurgitant valves may also provide symptomatic relief; however, both of these procedures have a fairly high mortality rate.

Outcomes

Prognosis is poor in patients with RCM, with a 50% mortality rate at 10 years for those with idiopathic RCM (Carroll & Crawford, 2009). Amyloidosis carries the highest mortality, with the 2-year mortality rate being greater than 80%, and survival at 4 years approaching zero percent (Carroll & Crawford, 2009; Darovic, 2002).

HYPERTROPHIC CARDIOMYOPATHY

Definition

HCM is characterized by hypertrophy of the myocardium (see Figure 8-1). Associated with this increase in muscle mass is a decrease in ventricular filling and a decrease in cardiac output. Other causes of ventricular hypertrophy, including long-standing hypertension and aortic stenosis, must be ruled out before a diagnosis of HCM can be made. This disease process has had many names in the past, including idiopathic hypertrophic subaortic stenosis. The WHO's recommendation of "hypertrophic cardiomyopathy" as the correct terminology for this disease process has been widely accepted. HCM is a general term that covers all cases; however, a subgroup of patients with HCM develop HCM with obstruction. When obstruction develops, the process is referred to as *hypertrophic obstructive cardiomyopathy* (HOCM).

Prevalence

HCM is found in one in every 500 adults, or 0.2% of the United States population, and affects women and men equally (Maron et al., 2003). It is the most common reason for sudden cardiac death in young adults.

Causes

Most cases of HCM are inherited. This autosomal dominant trait is caused by gene mutations (Maron et al., 2003). Research findings suggest there is a mutation of sarcomeric protein genes, resulting in a disarray of myocytes (Howie, 2008).

Pathophysiology

In HCM, a generalized disarray of the cardiac myofibrils occurs, along with hypertrophy of the myocytes (see Figure 8-4). Cardiac cells take on a variety of shapes and myocardial scarring and fibrosis occur. These changes result in myocardial walls that become very thin and stiff. The left ventricle is usually affected, with little affect on the right ventricle. The changes may be symmetrical; however, asymmetrical septal hypertrophy is the most common finding (see Figure 8-5). In asymmetrical septal hypertrophy, the ventricular septum experiences the greatest increase in wall thickness, oftentimes up to twice its normal size. Involvement of the septum may be limited to the upper one third, the lower two thirds, or the entire length of the septum (see Figure 8-6).

FIGURE 8-4: NORMAL MUSCLE STRUCTURE VERSUS MUSCLE STRUCTURE IN HCM

Normal Muscle Structure   **Myocardial Disarray**

Note. From Hypertrophic Cardiomyopathy Association. Reprinted with permission. http://www.4hcm.org

FIGURE 8-5: HCM WITH ASYMMETRICAL SEPTAL HYPERTROPHY

Note the increase in the septal wall is greater than the lateral wall of the left ventricle.

Note. From Mayo Foundation for Medical Education and Research. Copyrighted and used with permission of Mayo Foundation for Medical Education and Research, all rights reserved. Retrieved August 13, 2010, from http://www.mayoclinic.org/hypertrophic-cardiomyopathy/examples.html

FIGURE 8-6: HCM WITH ASYMMETRICAL SEPTAL HYPERTROPHY INVOLVING THE UPPER PORTION OF THE SEPTAL WALL

Note. From Mayo Foundation for Medical Education and Research. Copyrighted and used with permission of Mayo Foundation for Medical Education and Research, all rights reserved. Retrieved August 13, 2010, from http://www.mayoclinic.org/hypertrophic-cardiomyopathy/obstruction.html

Ventricular chamber size decreases as the enlarging ventricular walls close in on the ventricular chamber. The thick, stiff walls resist filling. The most prominent hemodynamic effect is decreased ventricular filling. This decreased ability to fill during diastole is referred to as diastolic dysfunction. As ventricular diastole begins, the mitral valve opens and the contents of the left atrium passively empty into the left ventricle. Normally, 70% to 75% of left ventricular filling occurs during this passive stage. In the presence of HCM, early passive filling is slowed due to the stiff, small left ventricle. The second part of diastole is atrial contraction, when the atrium contracts (atrial kick) and delivers an additional volume (25% to 30% of total volume) to the ventricle. A normal ventricle can hold approximately 150 ml of volume and normally ejects 55% to 65% of that volume with each beat. A stiff, noncompliant ventricle can neither hold 150 ml of volume nor accept the amount of volume (70% to 75% of total) normally provided during passive filling because of the high pressure in the left ventricle. Therefore, atrial kick becomes essential in delivering the volume needed to fill the ventricle.

Clinical Application

ECF volume balance in patients with HCM is critical. Because the ventricular chamber is no longer able to expand during filling, the ventricle must fill fully in order to produce adequate stroke volume.

Clinical Application

The development of atrial fibrillation results in a loss of atrial kick. Without atrial kick, ventricular filling (preload) decreases, with an associated decrease in stroke volume.

To compensate for the decreased volume in the ventricle, systolic function becomes hyperdynamic. The ejection fraction that is normally 55% to 65% rises and a greater portion of the ventricular contents are ejected. Ejecting 70% to 80% of a smaller volume helps maintain normal stroke volume.

HOCM occurs when the upper one third of the intraventricular septum becomes hypertrophied. The enlarged septum then obstructs the left ventricular outflow tract (see Figure 8-7). The left ventricular outflow tract is the path the blood in the left ventricle must follow when ejected from the ventricle. Obstruction occurs because of a combination of events. The septal wall enlarges into the left ventricular cavity, including the outflow tract area. Additionally, the anterior leaflet of the mitral valve is drawn toward the septum, as forceful left ventricular contraction produces high-velocity blood flow. The rapid current of blood pulls the anterior leaflet toward the outflow tract as it passes the leaflet, resulting in early closure of the aortic valve and a greatly decreased ejection fraction (see Figure 8-7). Referred to as *systolic anterior motion* (SAM), this obstruction by the anterior leaflet can be life threatening. It is estimated that 30% to 50% of patients with HCM have obstruction (Nishimura & Holmes, 2004).

Mitral valve regurgitation develops as HCM progresses. As papillary muscles become hypertrophied, valve leaflets may also become thick and the annulus calcified. As the left atrium dilates to compensate for the increased pressure and volume in the atrium, the mitral valve ring enlarges as well. These processes contribute to a valve that does not close properly, leading to regurgitation.

Atrial dilation occurs as the atrium attempts to compensate for the increased volume and pressure that results from decreased left ventricular filling. As hypertrophy of the left ventricle increases, forward flow decreases, resulting in decreased cardiac output. Additionally, ECF overload occurs with a backup of the additional volume in the lungs.

Clinical Presentation

Many patients with HCM remain asymptomatic for years. In many cases, HCM is first identified during routine screening of relatives of a known HCM patient. An episode of sudden death is fre-

FIGURE 8-7: HYPERTROPHIC CARDIOMYOPATHY DURING RELAXATION AND CONTRACTION

HCM During Relaxation

HCM During Active Contraction

Note the protrusion of the septum into the outflow tract at rest. As the ventricle contracts (shown in the picture on the right), the anterior leaflet of the mitral valve pulls into the outflow tract and nearly touches the septal wall, causing a nearly complete occlusion of outflow.

Note. From Mayo Foundation for Medical Education and Research. Copyrighted and used with permission of Mayo Foundation for Medical Education and Research, all rights reserved. Retrieved August 13, 2010, from http://www.mayoclinic.org/hypertrophic-cardiomyopathy/obstruction.html

quently the first clinical presentation of HCM in children and young adults. Symptoms usually develop as the disease progresses; however, the severity of the disease process does not always relate to the severity of symptoms. Symptoms may be closer related to the severity of the diastolic dysfunction or mitral regurgitation. The most common symptoms are dyspnea, chest pain, syncope or presyncope, and sudden death.

Dyspnea

Ninety percent of patients presenting with symptoms cite dyspnea as the most prevalent problem (Zevitz, 2006). As the size of the left ventricular chamber becomes smaller, the pressure in the left ventricle increases because the left ventricle is unable to accept the full volume from the left atrium. Left atrial pressure consequently increases, and the left atrial chamber dilates in an attempt to compensate for the increased volume in the atrium. The increase in pressure is ultimately referred back to the pulmonary system. As pulmonary pressures increase, the patient is predisposed to bouts of pulmonary congestion, resulting in dyspnea. Dyspnea is commonly related to activity. Any increase in activity normally increases heart rate to provide an increase in circulating blood volume to support the increase in demand. As with RCM, the normal cardiac response of an increase in heart rate is detrimental to patients with HCM. Increased heart rate decreases the amount of time the ventricle has to fill during diastole, and patients with HCM already have a decreased ability to fill because of restriction of the myocardial wall. An increase in heart rate further decreases diastolic filling time. The hyperdynamic walls of the heart continue to eject a larger-than-normal percentage of the volume in the ventricle, which is helpful to a point. As filling decreases, so does the total volume available for ejection. More important in patients with HCM is the increase in the backup of volume. Increased heart rate allows less and less volume to move forward through the left ventricle. The volume coming from the right side of the heart ends up in the pulmonary system because the left atrium is already full, and pulmonary edema develops.

Chest Pain

Chest pain caused by an imbalance in myocardial oxygen supply and demand is a common symptom of HCM. The increased left ventricular wall mass and hypercontractile state of the ventricle causes an increase in left ventricular myocardial oxygen demand. Several factors contribute to a decrease in myocardial oxygen supply. First, the decrease in cardiac output caused by decreased left ventricular filling does not deliver the oxygenated blood needed. Second, the increased myocardial mass requires more oxygenated blood due to its size. Finally, the coronary arteries are small and have difficulty dilating because of the increased myocardial mass; therefore, they are less able to deliver the needed oxygenated blood. While the patient is at rest, blood supply may be adequate to meet the body's needs. However, with increased stress or exercise, the increased myocardial oxygen demand of the thickened ventricular wall can no longer be met, resulting in angina. Angina can be caused by CHD in addition to increased wall mass, but CHD usually does not occur in HCM.

Syncope

Normally, during exercise, arterial blood vessels dilate to increase blood flow to the system and blood pressure decreases. The normal compensatory mechanism of the heart is to increase cardiac output to compensate for the decreased pressure. The body increases heart rate to increase cardiac output. This system keeps blood pressure in a normal range and allows a patient to tolerate the exercise. As noted earlier, in patients with HCM, increased heart rate does not increase cardiac output because diastolic filling time is decreased, actually decreasing cardiac output. Patients with HCM experience decreased blood pressure during exercise, resulting in dizziness, light-headedness, and blackout spells. Exercise may also cause ventricular or atrial dysrhythmias, resulting in syncopal episodes.

Sudden Death

Sometimes, the first indication of HCM is a sudden cardiac death event. The degree of hypertrophy generally relates to the incidence of dysrhythmias. Ventricular fibrillation is the rhythm that causes 80% of the sudden cardiac deaths in HCM (Zevitz, 2006). A ventricular wall thickness of 30 mm or greater is associated with an increased risk of sudden death dysrhythmias (Maron et al., 2003), whereas a wall thickness less than 15 mm is associated with no risk of sudden death dysrhythmias. Life-threatening dysrhythmias tend to occur in patients younger than 40 years of age. Undiagnosed HCM is one of the most common causes of sudden death in young adults. These life-threatening dysrhythmias generally occur when the young adult engages in strenuous activity.

Other Symptoms

Patients may also present with complaints of fatigue and activity intolerance, which are caused by decreased cardiac output. Palpitations are also a common concern. Oftentimes, palpitations are due to hyperdynamic contraction of the heart. Because of the forcible heartbeat, the patient can actually feel each contraction of the ventricle. An irregular heart rate may also be noted because atrial fibrillation can occur as a result of atrial dilation. Atrial fibrillation results in a loss of atrial kick, which provides active filling during ventricular diastole.

This loss results in a large decrease in cardiac output because the hypertrophic ventricle counts on atrial kick for ventricular filling. Therefore, atrial fibrillation is poorly tolerated and the patient exhibits signs of low cardiac output and decreased perfusion.

Physical Examination

A bisferiens carotid pulse is characteristic of patients with HOCM. The initial upstroke of the carotid pulse is brisk because there is initially no difficulty ejecting blood through the outflow tract. As systole progresses, left ventricular outflow tract obstruction may occur. This obstruction results in a collapse of the pulse and then a secondary rise.

Clinical Application

Because HCM may be confused with aortic stenosis, it is important to note that, in aortic stenosis, the carotid pulse has a delayed upstroke and amplitude.

During cardiac examination, the point of maximal impulse (located at the apex) is forceful and brisk because of the force of contraction. Upon auscultation of the heart, an additional sound is heard (S_4) just before the S_1. An S_4 is best heard with the bell of the stethoscope placed at the 5th intercostal space at the left midclavicular line, with the patient in the left lateral position. This S_4 is not audible in patients with atrial fibrillation.

Patients with HOCM have a classic crescendo-decrescendo systolic murmur. This murmur is best heard at the apex of the heart, at the fifth intercostal space to the left of the sternum or at the fifth intercostal space to the left of the midclavicular line. This murmur can be heard equally well with the bell or diaphragm of the stethoscope and is described as harsh or rough (Buss & Thompson, 2010). Proper identification of the murmur assists in differentiating aortic stenosis from HOCM. The HOCM murmur becomes louder during Valsalva's maneuver, whereas the aortic stenosis murmur becomes quieter. Decreased venous return during Valsalva's maneuver decreases ventricular size and

increases the obstruction, therefore increasing the sound of the murmur. Any factor that decreases venous return to the heart increases the murmur in HOCM (see Box 8-3).

BOX 8-3: FACTORS THAT DECREASE VENOUS RETURN TO THE HEART

- Valsalva's maneuver
- Position change from squatting to standing
- Tachycardia
- Venodilating drugs (such as nitroglycerin)
- Decreased ECF volume from blood loss or diuretics

Mitral regurgitation is not uncommon in HCM. This blowing murmur is heard throughout systole (holosystolic) and is best heard at the fifth intercostal space to the left of the midclavicular line. This murmur does not change in the way a left ventricular outflow obstruction murmur does. This murmur may also radiate to the axillae, whereas left ventricular outflow obstruction murmurs do not.

Crackles may be present in the lung bases if the patient is experiencing heart failure. Right-sided heart failure is a late sign because left-sided failure generally occurs first. Other possible findings on examination include tachypnea and tachycardia. Apical irregularities may be noted if the patient is in atrial fibrillation or experiencing ventricular ectopy.

Diagnosis

Chest X-ray Film

In most cases, chest X-rays are not helpful because HCM usually does not increase ventricular size. The heart generally appears normal in size. The left atrium may be slightly larger than normal and increases in size as the disease progresses. Signs of pulmonary congestion may be present.

Echocardiogram

Echocardiography is the tool of choice for diagnosing HCM. The diagnosis of HCM is easily established utilizing echocardiography. A wide variety of information can be obtained during echocardiography that leads to a diagnosis of HCM (see Table 8-5).

Cardiac Catheterization

For diagnosis of HCM, echocardiography has become the diagnostic tool of choice. Cardiac catheterization provides no additional information for the diagnosis. Most patients with HCM do not have CHD. They may have small vessels due to the increased muscle mass. A mismatch occurs as the small vessels are unable to supply the enlarged myocardium with the needed oxygen. This mismatch, although a supply and demand issue, is not CHD. Cardiac catheterization is useful in patients at high risk for CHD. If cardiac catheterization is necessary, the ventricular cavity and left ventricular outflow tract gradients can be assessed.

Electrocardiogram

On a 12-lead ECG, changes consistent with left ventricular hypertrophy are usually present. These changes include large QRS complexes with abnormal T waves. The absence of ECG changes does not rule out HCM. Deep symmetrical inversion of T waves in leads V_1 to V_6 usually accompanies the large QRS complexes in patients with HCM. In patients experiencing chest pain, these T-wave inversions need to be carefully evaluated by a physician experienced in 12-lead ECG interpretation because these changes may indicate myocardial ischemia. The ECG may also show bundle branch blocks, including left anterior hemiblock, right bundle branch block, and left bundle branch block. Cardiac dysrhythmias, such as atrial fibrillation, may also be discovered using an ECG.

Medical Treatment

Treatment for HCM is aimed at relieving symptoms, preventing complications, and reducing the risk of sudden death. No clinical evidence supports treating patients who are asymptomatic. The data for this population are small because many patients are unaware of the disease process until symptoms appear.

Beta-blockers

The medication type of choice in the initial treatment of HCM with or without obstruction is a beta-blocker (Zevitz, 2006), which provides symptomatic improvement and can increase exercise tolerance. The greatest benefit is seen with patients who are only experiencing symptoms with exertion or exercise. The normal beta response to sympathetic stimulation is an increase in contractility, heart rate, and conduction of impulses from the atrium to the ventricle. Beta-blockers block these normal responses. As previously stated, the primary problem associated with HCM is filling of the ventricle during diastole. The ventricles in

TABLE 8-5: ECHOCARDIOGRAM FINDINGS IN HYPERTROPHIC CARDIOMYOPATHY	
Echocardiogram Parameters Evaluated	**Echocardiogram Findings in HCM/HOCM**
Wall thickness	Increased
Symmetry of septal wall thickness	Septal wall greater than other walls of left ventricle
Left ventricular size	Usually normal
Hyperdynamic left ventricular function	Ejection fraction > 70%
Left atrial size	Usually dilated
Mitral valve leaflets	Systolic anterior motion of anterior mitral leaflet (in obstructive cases)
	Thickened, elongated anterior leaflet
	Mitral regurgitation
Left ventricular outflow tract	Obstruction to flow may be present

patients with HCM are actually hyperdynamic so there is no issue with contractility. Beta-blockers slow heart rate. By decreasing heart rate, the diastolic filling time of the ventricle lengthens, providing more time for the atrium to fill the ventricle. Beta-blockers decrease the resting heart rate and also limit the ability of the heart rate to increase in response to stimulation such as exercise. In addition to preventing an increase in contractility, beta-blockers actually allow for ventricular relaxation. This relaxation again allows for better diastolic filling, especially passive filling. The decrease in contractility and heart rate with increased filling also benefits the patient by decreasing myocardial oxygen demand. A decrease in myocardial oxygen demand should also decrease any myocardial ischemia that is occurring from the increase in muscle mass and decrease in coronary artery size.

Clinical Application

Beta-blockers can cause fatigue, impotence, and sleep disturbances, especially with initial dosing. These symptoms, especially the fatigue, generally ease over time as the patient's body adjusts to the medication. Patients should be made aware of these effects and should be encouraged to continue taking the medication as the body adjusts to the changes.

Calcium Channel Blockers

Another type of medication used in both obstructive and nonobstructive HCM is a calcium channel blocker. The non-dihydropyridine calcium channel blockers have been shown to decrease symptoms, particularly chest pain (Opie & Gersh, 2009). Calcium channel blockers also assist in decreasing contractility. Verapamil is the calcium channel blocker of choice because it decreases ventricular contractility and improves myocardial relaxation, resulting in increased ventricular filling. Verapamil may be used when beta-blockers have not provided the expected benefit or in patients with asthma (Maron et al., 2003).

Clinical Application

Nifedipine and other dihydropyridine calcium channel blockers should be avoided in patients with HCM because of the potent vasodilatory actions that may have detrimental effects.

There is evidence that supports the use of disopyramide (Norpace) in the treatment of patients with symptomatic HOCM, especially those with symptoms of obstruction at rest (Maron et al., 2003). In additon to being a class I antiarrhythmic, disopyramide is a negative inotrope, which decreases ventricular contractility and is used primarily for its negative inotropic benefit. By decreasing contractility, the effect of the outflow obstruction and the mitral regurgitation should diminish. Disopyramide should be used in conjunction with a beta-blocker because it may cause an increase in ventricular rate in atrial fibrillation. Disopyramide also has the ability to prolong the QT interval and cause an increase in ventricular dysrhythmias. The utilization of disopyramide should be limited to patients with severe obstructive disease.

Generally, beta-blockers are the first medication of choice. If beta-blockers do not provide symptom relief, calcium channel blockers are substituted. There is currently no evidence that supports utilizing beta-blockers with calcium channel blockers (Maron et al., 2003).

Antidysrhythmic Therapy

Atrial fibrillation is the most common dysrhythmia associated with HCM. Atrial fibrillation is poorly tolerated in two thirds of the patients with HCM or HOCM (Maron et al., 2003). Every attempt should be made to convert atrial fibrillation back to normal sinus rhythm. The loss of atrial contraction and potentially high ventricular heart rates contribute to decreased ventricular filling and, quite often, rapid hemodynamic deterioration. Either pharmacologic conversion or mechanical cardioversion is acceptable. Beta-blockers help control ventricular rate. Amiodarone is also useful in both obstructive and nonobstructive disease with ventricular or atrial dysrhythmias. Digoxin should be avoided in patients with HOCM because it increases contractility, thereby increasing the obstruction. Anticoagulation protocol should be followed, as with anyone who may have atrial fibrillation.

Other Medications

Diuretics should be used cautiously in patients with HCM because volume status is very important. With the hypertrophy that has developed, preload is already decreased because of the ventricle's inability to expand during filling. Any further loss of filling can result in a decrease in cardiac output.

ACE inhibitors and nitroglycerin preparations should be avoided in patients with HOCM because of their ability to vasodilate and their ability to decrease preload. Both of these effects can increase the outflow obstruction and greatly decrease cardiac output.

Clinical Application

Any medication that increases contractility should be strictly avoided in patients with HOCM. An increase in contractility increases any outflow obstruction and greatly decreases cardiac output. This effect can be life threatening. Examples of drugs that increase contractility include digoxin, dobutamine, dopamine, epinephrine, and norepinephrine.

Nonobstructive Disease Progression

Some patients never develop obstructive disease. These patients can be more difficult to treat, and therapy may be less effective in providing symptom relief. Beta-blockers and calcium channel blockers are beneficial in decreasing heart rate and improving diastolic function. However, over time, the hypertrophic heart evolves into a dilated myocardium and the clinical picture becomes similar to DCM with the development of systolic dysfunction. As patients develop symptoms of heart failure, diuretics, ACE inhibitors, and digoxin may be helpful.

Ultimately, cardiac transplantation may be considered as the heart deteriorates.

Endocarditis Prophylaxis

Infective endocarditis prophylaxis was previously recommended by the ACC in patients with evidence of outflow obstruction, both resting and with exercise, before dental work or surgical procedures (Maron et al., 2003). In 2007, the AHA published new guidelines for the prevention of endocarditis. With this publication, the recommendation for endocarditis prophylaxis in the above mentioned population is no longer in place (Wilson et al., 2007). There is no evidence that supports the use of prophylaxis in nonobstructive disease.

Pregnancy

Because many patients with HCM are young, the issue of pregnancy must be addressed. According to the ACC and the European Society of Cardiology (ESC) Clinical Expert Consensus Document on Hypertrophic Cardiomyopathy (Maron et al., 2003), there is currently no evidence that pregnancy should be avoided in patients with HCM. The mortality risk may be slightly higher; however, that risk is generally associated with women who are already at high risk for other reasons. Normal vaginal deliveries may occur without difficulties.

Surgical Treatment

Cardiac Pacemakers

Dual-chamber cardiac pacing (pacing both the atrium and ventricle) has been utilized to assist in symptom relief. Although dual-chamber pacing is not a primary treatment, some patients report improvement in symptoms with cardiac pacing. There has been a particular benefit noted for patients older than 65 years of age (Maron et al., 2003). Dual-chamber pacing allows for more aggressive treatment with medications that can decrease heart rate.

Ventricular Septal Myectomy

Patients with marked outflow obstruction may be considered for surgical removal of a portion of the hypertrophied septum that is contributing to the outflow obstruction. This surgical procedure is reserved only for those patients on maximum medical therapy who continue to experience severely limiting symptoms and are classified as NYHA functional class III or IV (Maron et al., 2003).

During the procedure, a small amount of the septum is removed from just below the base of the aortic valve, resulting in an enlarged outflow tract (see Figure 8-8). This procedure immediately decreases outflow tract obstruction and SAM of the anterior leaflet of the mitral valve. Mitral valve replacement or repair may also occur during the procedure, depending on the situation. Myectomy without valve replacement is becoming a low-risk procedure, with a relatively low operative mortality rate among all age-groups (Maron et al., 2003). Symptoms immediately improve and some litera-

ture suggests that improvements are sustained for as long as 30 years. Most patients improve from NYHA class III or IV to class II or III. Survival rates are greater than 83% at 10 years (Salberg, 2004). Patients may develop left bundle branch block as a result of the procedure, but pacemakers are rarely necessary.

Percutaneous Alcohol Septal Ablation

A second nonsurgical alternative to septal myectomy is percutaneous alcohol septal ablation (PASA). This procedure is relatively new, but has become an acceptable treatment option. Candidates for PASA are patients with obstruction who are symptomatic and NYHA class III or IV on maximum medical therapy (Maron et al., 2003). However, if mitral valve involvement is advanced and requires repair or replacement, then surgery is the preferable option. PASA is a noninvasive procedure without the risks associated with a major surgery. This procedure may be appropriate for older adult patients who are not good operative candidates.

PASA is performed in the cardiac catheterization laboratory. A catheter is placed in the left anterior descending coronary artery. The catheter is then advanced into one of the septal perforator branches that provide blood flow to the septum. When the appropriate septal perforator is located, ethyl alcohol is injected (see Figure 8-9). The alcohol infiltrates the surrounding myocardial tissue as a toxic agent and a controlled MI occurs. The enlarged septal tissue eventually shrinks and the outflow obstruction is relieved. This reduction in tissue size does not occur immediately and may actually continue to occur for up to 1 year after the procedure. In young patients, the benefits of the surgical procedure outweigh the postprocedure dysrhythmia risk of PASA. A larger percentage of patients require permanent pacing after PASA than after myectomy.

FIGURE 8-8: SURGICAL MYECTOMY

During Surgery

FIGURE 8-9: ALCOHOL SEPTAL ABLATION

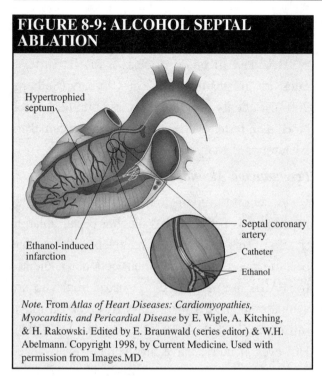

Note. From *Atlas of Heart Diseases: Cardiomyopathies, Myocarditis, and Pericardial Disease* by E. Wigle, A. Kitching, & H. Rakowski. Edited by E. Braunwald (series editor) & W.H. Abelmann. Copyright 1998, by Current Medicine. Used with permission from Images.MD.

Sudden Cardiac Death

On the whole, life expectancy in patients with HCM is normal; however, sudden cardiac death is the most serious complication. In most cases, sudden cardiac death is the event that leads to a diagnosis of HCM. Sudden cardiac death occurs most frequently in young people (younger than 35 years of age) who are asymptomatic or mildly symptomatic. However, the risk is not limited to this age-group. Researchers continue to attempt to predict the HCM population that is at high risk for sudden cardiac death so that ICDs can be implanted (see Box 8-4). As risk criteria continue to be evaluated, most literature agrees that ICDs should be placed in any patient with an episode of sudden cardiac death, sustained ventricular tachycardia, or a family history of sudden cardiac death. Patients with other risk factors should not be eliminated from ICD consideration because multiple risk factors may warrant placement of a device. Medication to treat the ventricular dysrhythmias should be utilized in conjunction with the ICD; amiodarone is the drug of choice.

BOX 8-4: MAJOR RISK FACTORS FOR SUDDEN CARDIAC DEATH IN HCM

- Cardiac arrest (ventricular fibrillation)
- Spontaneous sustained ventricular tachycardia
- Nonsustained ventricular tachycardia
- Family history (one or more first-degree relatives) with an episode of sudden cardiac death
- Left ventricular wall thickness greater than or equal to 30 mm
- Prolonged or repetitive nonsustained ventricular tachycardia on Holter monitor
- Hypotensive blood pressure response to exercise
- Unexplained syncope or near syncope

(Maron et al., 2003)

Clinical Application

Implantation of an ICD is a very emotional process and patients should be provided with emotional support. Many facilities that place ICDs are aware of an ICD support group that can be helpful to patients dealing with the emotions associated with the risk of sudden death and implantation of this device.

Activity Recommendations

Patients with HCM should be restricted from intense competitive sports. HCM is the most common cause of sudden cardiac death in young athletes, especially in football and basketball. Not all sudden cardiac death occurs with intense activity; in fact, sudden cardiac death can occur at rest. However, the incidence of sudden cardiac death increases with the intensity of the activity in the presence of HCM. Patients do not need to restrict activity all together but should avoid "burst" exertion, such as sprinting, and isometric exercises, such as heavy lifting. No evidence supports the exclusion from competitive sports of athletes with a family history of HCM but no personal evidence of the disease.

Patient response to activity provides a guide for determining the level of activity that is acceptable. Development of chest pain, overt shortness of breath, and syncope may indicate that the activity is too strenuous.

Family Evaluation

HCM is largely a genetic disease process. If HCM is diagnosed or an HCM-related death occurs, all first-degree relatives should be screened for the disease and other blood relatives should be encouraged to undergo screening. The ACC/ESC Clinical Expert Consensus Document on Hypertrophic Cardiomyopathy recommends genetic testing if available. If genetic testing is not feasible, a variety of other tests are appropriate for screening (see Box 8-5). These screenings should occur annually from 12 through 18 years of age. Delayed adult onset is also possible; therefore, relatives with normal studies through 18 years of age should have an evaluation every 5 years. Children younger than 12 years of age need not undergo evaluation unless there is a high-risk family profile or the child is involved in intense competitive sports.

BOX 8-5: SCREENING METHODS FOR FAMILIAL HCM

- History and physical examination
- 12-lead ECG
- Echocardiography

Outcomes

Patients who survive past 35 years of age have the best long-term prognosis (Shah, 2009). After the patient is diagnosed with the disease, routine follow up every 12 to 18 months is recommended. Sudden cardiac death continues to be the primary cause of shortened life spans. Prevention and identification of the risk of sudden cardiac death is a major area of focus. Many studies continue to increase the understanding of the genetic code and its impact on the disease process. Hopefully, these studies will provide the key to successful treatment in the future.

ARRHYTHMOGENIC RIGHT VENTRICULAR CARDIOMYOPATHY

Definition

The 1995 report of the WHO/International Society and Federation of Cardiology Task Force on the Definition and Classification of Cardiomyopathies defines ARVC as a progressive fibrofatty replacement of right ventricular myocardium (Richardson et al., 1996). AVRC is also referred to as *arrhythmogenic right ventricular dysplasia*. In relation to the other types of cardiomyopathy, this is a relatively new type of cardiomyopathy that was first identified in the literature in the late 1970s (Corrado et al., 2000). Over the past 30 years a great deal of information has been learned about this type of cardiomyopathy, but much is still being learned. AVRC is characterized as an inherited muscle disorder that is characterized by the replacement of normal myocardial tissue with fibrofatty infiltrates. The resultant effect is right ventricular and, eventually, left ventricular dysfunction that mimics dilated cardiomyopathy. Patients with AVRC are prone to ventricular dysrhythmias that place them at great risk for sudden cardiac death.

Prevalence

The actual number of patients with AVRC is difficult to quantify because many times the disease is diagnosed on autopsy after an episode of sudden cardiac death. Some older adult patients are wrongly diagnosed with DCM when they present with signs of heart failure. Screening tests for AVRC are still being developed. With this lack of a diagnostic test, the diagnosis may be missed. More males than females experience AVRC (McRae, Chung, & Asher, 2001). The onset of the disease is most often after puberty and, usually, in the late 20s or early 30s (Richardson et al., 1996).

Causes

The cause of AVRC in more than 50% of the patients is an autosomal dominant genetic disorder (McRae et al., 2001). Research continues in an attempt to identify the causes of this relatively new disease process.

Pathophysiology

In AVRC there is a progressive loss of the normal cardiomyocytes. Fibrofatty tissue replaces the cardiomyocytes. A similar type of fibrofatty infiltration is also observed in some types of muscular dystrophies. The dysplasia that results first affects the right ventricle. The right ventricular wall thins and dilation occurs. Eventually, the left ventricle may become affected as well. As a result of the ventricular thinning and dilation, mechanical function of the ventricle is impacted and symptoms of right-sided heart failure and, ultimately, left-sided heart failure occur. The mechanical dysfunction is the same as the dysfunction that occurs with DCM, with a decrease in ejection fraction due to loss of contractility. The development of right-sided heart failure is a later sign of this progressive disorder. Right ventricular dysrhythmias develop because of the fibrofatty infiltrates. Sudden cardiac death is most commonly the first sign of AVRC (Zipes et al., 2006).

Clinical Presentation

In many cases, the first presentation of AVRC is an episode of sudden cardiac death. In one study in Italy, 20% of the sudden cardiac deaths in those younger than 35 years of age was attributed to AVRC (McRae et al., 2001). Several presentations in young adults may lead to a suspicion of AVRC, including presyncope, syncope, palpitations, premature ventricular contractions (PVCs), ventricular dysrhythmias, and right-sided heart failure (McRae et al., 2001). Some patients are identified through screening when

a family member experiences an episode of sudden cardiac death.

The literature identifies four phases of the disease process that can explain some of the symptoms. These phases include:

1. The concealed phase, which is characterized by subtle changes to the structure of the right ventricle. This phase is often without symptoms. Occasionally, a young athlete may experience an episode of sudden cardiac death during intense exertion or a competitive sport.

2. An overt electrical disorder demonstrated by symptomatic dysrhythmias that originate from the right ventricle, causing an episode of sudden cardiac death. Functional and structural abnormalities of the right ventricle are obvious during this phase.

3. Right ventricular failure characterizes the third phase of the disease process and causes dysfunction of the right ventricle.

4. Biventricular failure characterizes the fourth and final phase of the disease process. At this point the disease process has moved beyond the right ventricle. It now also impacts the left ventricle and congestive heart failure occurs.

(Corrado et al., 2000)

Physical Examination

The findings during the physical examination will be consistent with right ventricular failure in the early phases and right and left ventricular failure in the fourth phase of AVRC. These findings are those identified with right- and left-sided heart failure discussed in Chapter 7.

Diagnosis

ARVC is difficult to diagnose in the early stages of the disease process. The diagnosis of AVRC is accomplished with a variety of tools including the ECG, echocardiography, magnetic resonance imaging (MRI) and myocardial biopsy. Differentiating between AVRC and DCM is key in the diagnosis. Those with AVRC develop ventricular dysrhythmias and sudden cardiac death without any significant left ventricular dysfunction (Sen-Chowdhry, Syrris, & McKenna, 2005). Although sudden cardiac death and ventricular dysrhythmias are also present in those with DCM, those with DCM have significant left ventricular dysfunction.

Electrocardiogram

There are several changes on the ECG that lead to the diagnosis of AVRC. However, a normal ECG does not rule out AVRC. The abnormal findings may include:

1. T wave inversion in leads V_1 through V_4

2. Incomplete right bundle branch block

3. Ventricular dysrhythmias with a left bundle branch configuration

4. Epsilon waves.
(McRae et al., 2001)

Echocardiogram

The echocardiogram provides information about the structural disease found in AVRC. Right ventricular cardiomyopathy has a specific pattern of dysplasia that can be identified on an echocardiogram. Diffuse right ventricular enlargement seen on an echocardiogram supports a diagnosis of AVRC. It is important to make sure that other causes of right ventricular disorder are also ruled out before a diagnosis of ARVC is made (McRae et al., 2001).

MRI

An MRI, in most cases, provides definitive evidence of ARVC. Thinning of the right ventricular wall and the fatty infiltrates can be visualized with this test. There are normally fatty infiltrates in all hearts, but the pattern of infiltration with AVRC is specific to the disease process and different from normal fatty infiltration.

Endomyocardial Biopsy

Over the years, the definitive diagnosis of ARVC occurred with transmural biopsy of the myocardium at transplantation or during autopsy (McRae et al., 2001). Endomyocardial biopsy is less sensitive than transmural biopsy but may provide information that leads to a diagnosis of AVRC. This type of diagnostic test is not without risk. Traditionally, during myocardial biopsy, tissue samples are taken from the right ventricular septal wall. The fatty infiltrates with AVRC affect the free wall of the right ventricle. Myocardial biopsy of the right ventricular free wall are more prone to myocardial perforation and subsequent cardiac tamponade. A biopsy that is free from fibrofatty infiltrates does not completely rule out a diagnosis of AVRC. There are instances when the specific site of tissue removal demonstrates no evidence of the disease process because of the patchy pattern of infiltrate.

Treatment

Treatment of AVRC continues to remain controversial because long-term researched clinical outcomes data are not in abundance. The focus initially is the prevention of sudden cardiac death. Therapy for dysrhythmia management begins with medical therapy, with sotolol being the most effective medication to control sustained ventricular dysrhythmias. Amiodarone may also be used, but it has not demonstrated the same success rate in controlling these dysrhythmias as sotolol (McRea et al., 2001). If ventricular dysrhythmias become refractory to medical treatment, radiofrequency ablation may be indicated. Finally, with the risk of sudden cardiac death, implantation of an ICD is often warranted. When the patient develops signs of biventricular failure, routine treatment options for heart failure are initiated, including an ACE inhibitor, digoxin, and diuretics (Corrado et al., 2000).

TAKOTSUBO CARDIOMYOPATHY

Definition

Takotsubo cardiomyopathy was first described in 1991 by Dote et al., who described a transient contractile abnormality of the left ventricle that resembled the shape of a jar used to catch an octopus. The term takotsubo comes from the Japanese terms "tako," which means octopus, and "tsubo," which means jar (Derrick, 2009). Takotsubo is also referred to as *broken heart syndrome* because the disease is associated with an excessive release of catecholamines that occurs with stress. Characteristic with this disease process is a sudden loss of contractile function, resulting in low ejection fractions. Patients with takotsubo present as an acute MI; however, during cardiac catheterization, no significant coronary occlusion is present.

Prevalence

Akashi et al. (2003) reports that takotsubo accounts for approximately 1% of all acute MIs. Takotsubo is primarily a disease of postmenopausal women (Derrick, 2009). In a review by Gianni et al. (2006), 89% of the patients reviewed were female.

Causes

Much is still being learned about this process, however, it is currently believed that exposure to excessive catecholamine release, such that occurs with stressful situations, is the cause of the left ventricular apical ballooning and loss of left ventricular function that occurs with no appreciable coronary artery disease (CAD).

Pathophysiology

Although the pathyphysiologic mechanism that occurs with takotsubo is still not fully understood, most patients with this phenomenon have abnormally high levels of catecholamines. Wittstein et al. (2005) demonstrated that patients presenting with takotsubo had catecholamine-related levels 7 to 34 time higher than normal. This was compared to acute patients with MIs who demonstrated levels 2 to 3 times normal.

A patient with takotsubo experiences a sudden loss of contractile function of the myocardium. This process mimics an acute MI with loss of ven-

tricular function. Left ventricular ejection is decreased, resulting in a decrease in forward ejection of ventricular contents. This process is the same as the one that occurs with systolic dysfunction and dilated cardiomyopathy.

Clinical Presentation

Patients with takotsubo present symptoms similar to those with MI including chest pain. The symptoms associated with takotsubo tend to be moderate to mild (Kurisu et al., 2002). Depending on the extent of the left ventricular dysfunction, patients may present in acute pulmonary edema or cardiogenic shock.

The ECG findings are also similar to those with acute MI, including ST segment elevation, most frequently in leads V_3 through V_6 (Kurisu et al., 2002). However, in some patients there may be T wave changes.

Cardiac biomarkers that provide diagnostic information for MI, specifically cardiac troponin levels, are usually elevated in patients presenting with takotsubo.

Physical Examination

The physical examination findings in the patient with takotsubo are indistinguishable from the patient with acute MI. Please see Chapter 5 for a full discussion of the physical findings.

Diagnosis

Diagnosis of takotsubo is generally made in the cardiac catheterization laboratory. It is during cardiac catheterization that the absence of significant CAD is discovered. Also during cardiac catheterization, a left ventriculogram is completed. During the injection of dye into the left ventricle, the left apical ballooning is observed, a finding that can be confirmed with echocardiography.

Treatment

Treatment is supportive, based on the patient's symptoms and presentation, and similar to the treatment for an acute MI with left ventricular dysfunction (see Chapter 5 for a full discussion). Stress reduction is an important aspect of treatment for this patient population, and nursing care should focus on helping the patient through this stressful time. Medications that reduce anxiety may be helpful.

Outcomes

Left ventricular function generally returns to normal within 2 to 3 weeks after takotsubo (Akashi et al., 2003). After the acute phase has passed, long-term outcomes are good. The literature reports a low reoccurrence rate of 10% (Prasad, 2007). However, these rates may be higher than once thought because of a better understanding of the disease itself. Before this disease process was fully understood, many patients with takotsubo were diagnosed with coronary spasm or acute myocarditis because no significant occlusions of the coronary arteries were found and many were low risk for CAD. Now that there is a better understanding and awareness of takotsubo, the diagnosis is occurring more often.

Long-term medications that are used for MI such as beta-blockers, ACE inhibitors, and aspirin, are not indicated when ventricular function returns to normal.

An important aspect in the long-term care of a patient with takotsubo is understanding the role stress plays in the disease process. Developing good coping mechanisms is important in this population. Bedside clinicians can guide patients to develop adequate coping skills to prevent recurrences of takotsubo.

Occasionally, mild to moderate coronary artery occlusion may also be discovered during a cardiac catheterization that reveals takotsubo. Although the occlusion is not the cause of the takotsubo, the patient still needs to participate in cardiac risk factor modification.

Clinical Application

Although it is always important to provide a quiet calm healing environment for hospitalized patients, it is most important for the patient with takotsubo. Those caring for such patients should assure adequate rest for the patient and assist with stress reduction. Medication to assist with decreasing anxiety may be indicated. A careful assessment of family dynamics can assist in determining the importance of family presence. Many times, an incidence of takotsubo results from a traumatic event such as the death of a spouse or child. In these situations, family at the bedside may be very important to the comfort of the patient. The nurse should assist the patient in developing stress reduction tools that meet the patient's needs. In-hospital referrals may include a clinical nurse specialist consultation, and out-of-hospital referrals may include Phase II cardiac rehabilitation or another formal stress management program. Specific complimentary strategies that may be used in stress reduction include deep breathing, visualization, and guided imagery.

CONCLUSION

Cardiomyopathy impacts millions of people, including those who are diagnosed with these diseases and many more who are related to them and care for them during debilitating years. Early recognition of the disease process, in conjunction with good medical follow-up care and patient compliance with treatment strategies and risk factor adjustments, can improve long-term outcomes. Every healthcare professional caring for patients will come in contact with someone with cardiomyopathy at some point in his or her career. A good knowledge base of these disease processes helps with early recognition and improves outcomes for these patients.

EXAM QUESTIONS

CHAPTER 8
Questions 64-70

Note: Choose the one option that BEST answers each question.

64. Cardiomyopathy is a group of disorders caused by dysfunction of the

    a. pericardium.
    b. endocardium.
    c. myocardium.
    d. epicardium.

65. The primary types of cardiomyopathy are dilated, restrictive, and

    a. alcoholic.
    b. hypertrophic.
    c. peripartum.
    d. dysrhythmogenic.

66. The primary pathophysiological change associated with DCM is

    a. decreased ventricular filling.
    b. decreased ventricular chamber size with decreased ventricular filling.
    c. obstruction of the left ventricular outflow tract.
    d. ventricular dilation with decreased ventricular contraction.

67. The most useful diagnostic tool in all cardiomyopathies is

    a. chest X-ray.
    b. echocardiography.
    c. cardiac catheterization.
    d. ECG.

68. One of the primary treatment goals for DCM includes

    a. reducing contractility.
    b. decreasing afterload.
    c. increasing the left ventricular afterload.
    d. increasing the heart rate to greater than 100 beats per minute.

69. HOCM occurs when there is obstruction of the

    a. left atrial outflow tract.
    b. right atrial outflow tract.
    c. left ventricular outflow tract.
    d. right ventricular outflow tract.

70. Medications that should be avoided when obstructive cardiomyopathy has developed include medications that

    a. increase contractility.
    b. decrease contractility.
    c. decrease heart rate.
    d. decrease impulses from the atrium to the ventricle.

CHAPTER 9

AORTIC VALVE DISEASE

CHAPTER OBJECTIVE

After completing this chapter, the learner will be able to recognize aortic valve disease and identify its impact on the body.

LEARNING OBJECTIVES

After completing this chapter, the learner will be able to

1. identify the pathophysiology that occurs with aortic stenosis.

2. describe key signs and symptoms of aortic stenosis.

3. explain the medical and surgical treatment options available for patients with aortic stenosis.

4. identify the pathophysiology that occurs with aortic regurgitation.

5. describe key signs and symptoms of aortic regurgitation.

6. define the key differences between acute and chronic aortic regurgitation.

7. explain the medical and surgical treatment options available for patients with aortic regurgitation.

INTRODUCTION

The aortic valve is the gateway to the circulatory system of the body. Proper functioning of the valve allows blood to flow from the left ventricle to the aorta when open, and prevents backflow of blood from the aorta to the ventricle when closed. Valve dysfunction occurs when the valve does not open properly or close completely. Blood flow from the left ventricle to the aorta is key in delivering the required oxygenated blood to the body.

AORTIC VALVE FUNCTION

The normal aortic valve consists of an annulus and three cusps (see Figure 9-1). The aortic valve functions by pressure changes in the left ventricle and the aorta. During diastole, the aortic valve is closed while the left ventricle fills with blood from the left atrium. As the left ventricle fills, the pressure in the left ventricle rises. When the pressure in the left ventricle becomes greater than the pressure in the left atrium, the mitral valve closes between the left atrium and left ventricle, ending diastole. The left ventricle begins to contract as systole begins. When the pressure in the left ventricle is greater than the pressure on the other side of the aortic valve, the valve is forced open and blood is ejected out of the left ventricle into the aorta. After ejection is complete, the pressure in the left ventricle becomes

FIGURE 9-1: AORTIC VALVE SHOWING THE THREE CUSPS

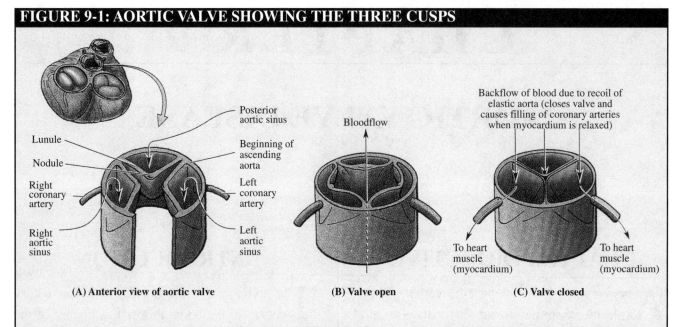

(A) Anterior view of aortic valve

Posterior aortic sinus

Beginning of ascending aorta

Lunule

Nodule

Right coronary artery

Right aortic sinus

Left coronary artery

Left aortic sinus

(B) Valve open

Bloodflow

(C) Valve closed

Backflow of blood due to recoil of elastic aorta (closes valve and causes filling of coronary arteries when myocardium is relaxed)

To heart muscle (myocardium)

To heart muscle (myocardium)

Note the right coronary artery arises from the right aortic sinus (cusp) and the left coronary artery arises from the left aortic sinus (cusp).

Note. From *Clinically Oriented Anatomy* (4th ed.), by K.L. Moore and A.F. Dalley, 1999, Philadelphia, PA: Lippincott Williams & Wilkins. Reprinted with permission from Lippincott Williams & Wilkins (http://lww.com)

less than the pressure in the aorta and the aortic valve snaps shut. The aortic valve closes tightly to prevent the backflow of blood from the aorta to the left ventricle, and the cycle begins again. Normal aortic valve function is essential for normal cardiac output. Impedance of forward flow of blood, or backflow of blood that should be moving forward, can greatly affect cardiac output. A more detailed description of the cardiac valves is can be found in Chapter 1.

Abnormal Valve Function

Basically, two functional valve alterations are responsible for valvular heart disease: stenosis and regurgitation. Valve stenosis occurs when a constriction or narrowing of the valve opening impedes the free flow of blood across the valve. Regurgitation occurs when the valve leaflets do not close completely to form a tight seal, resulting in backward flow of blood. Other terms used to refer to backward blood flow include prolapse, insufficiency, and incompetence. Although these terms refer to differences in the anatomical process, they all represent a valve that does not close properly.

AORTIC STENOSIS

Definition

Aortic stenosis is said to exist when there is obstruction of flow at the level of the aortic valve. Opening of the aortic valve leaflets is usually restricted.

Causes

Aortic valve stenosis is classified as congenital or acquired. Congenital valve disease occurs when an abnormal number of valve cusps (unicuspid or bicuspid) are present. Most commonly, there is a fusion of one or more of the commissures (Bonow et al., 2008). It is the most common cause of aortic stenosis in patients younger than 70 years of age. Congenital aortic stenosis occurs four times more often in men then in women (Moons et al., 2008). Only 1 in 50 children born with this type of valve abnormality will have significant valve stenosis or regurgitation in their lifetime (Bonow et al., 2008).

Acquired aortic stenosis, caused by rheumatic heart disease or degenerative calcification, accounts for most symptom-producing aortic stenosis in patients older than 70 years of age (Schoen & Mitchell, 2010). Aortic stenosis affects 2% to 4% of persons older than 65 years old and affects more men than women (Lauck, Mackay, Galte, & Wilson, 2008). Aortic disease that is secondary to rheumatic heart disease is almost always accompanied by mitral valve disease (Bonow et al., 2008; Darovic, 2002). Aortic stenosis without the presence of mitral valve disease is generally considered nonrheumatic in origin. The incidence of rheumatic aortic valve disease has decreased appreciably with the decrease in the incidence of rheumatic heart disease in this country.

The most common cause of aortic stenosis in adults is senile degenerative calcification (Schoen & Mitchell, 2010). Degenerative calcification is a disease process involving lipid accumulation, inflammation, and calcification of the valve leaflets (Bonow et al., 2008). As the disease progresses, the valve leaflets retract and stiffen (Weigand, Pruess, & Hambach, 2008) and the leaflets become non-compliant (see Figure 9-2). Aortic stenosis resulting from degenerative calcification has been associated with male gender, elevated lipoprotein and elevated low-density lipoprotein cholesterol levels, hypertension, smoking, diabetes, elevated serum calcium levels, and elevated serum creatinine levels (Ledoux, 2010).

Pathophysiology

The primary process occurring with rheumatic heart disease is progressive fibrosis of the valve leaflets with fusion of the commissures (points where the valve leaflets connect) and, occasionally, calcification. In senile degenerative calcification, the valve leaflets thicken and develop calcified nodules that restrict their movement, resulting in valve leaflets that do not open easily or fully (see Figure 9-2).

As the aortic valve opening narrows (because of damaged valve leaflets), blood flow through the valve becomes turbulent and less efficient. The left

FIGURE 9-2: DEGENERATIVE AORTIC VALVE DISEASE

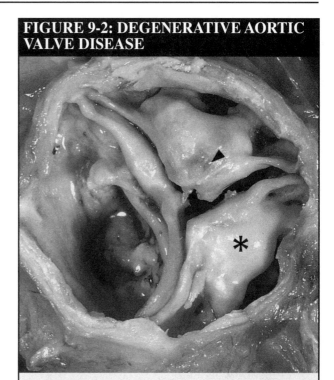

This photo shows severe stenosis of the aortic valve with marked calcific deposits on the left (*) and the posterior noncoronary (▲) cusps, without commissural fusion.

Note. From *Atlas of Heart Diseases: Valvular Heart Disease* by R. Virmani, A. Burke, & A. Farb. Edited by E. Braunwald (series editor) & S.H. Rahimtoola. Copyright 1997, by Current Medicine. Used with permission from Images.MD.

ventricle must work harder to eject blood across the stiff, noncompliant valve. As valve compliance decreases, afterload increases. Afterload is the pressure the left ventricle must overcome to eject blood. In an effort to compensate for the increase in afterload, the left ventricular wall mass (myocardial wall thickness) increases in size, resulting in progressive concentric left ventricular hypertrophy. Concentric hypertrophy is characterized by increasing left ventricular wall mass with no increase in ventricular chamber size. In fact, the increasing muscle mass may begin to encroach on the chamber and actually decrease the size of the intraventricular chamber. As the left ventricular wall becomes thicker, an associated decrease occurs in the ability of the ventricular wall to expand normally during ventricular filling. Referred to as *diastolic dysfunction,* this inability to expand results in decreased ventricle filling during diastole. With less volume entering the ventricle, there is less volume available for ejection during systole. The ventricle normally ejects 50% to 60% of its contents with each beat. Now, however, the thickened myocardium compensates with a stronger contraction and ejects a larger percentage of the decreased volume, thereby maintaining good cardiac output. As the disease progresses, the left ventricle's attempt to compensate ultimately fails and left ventricular contractile function begins to decrease. This decrease in contractile function results in decreased stroke volume, leaving the ventricle with an excess volume at the end of each contraction. This overload is transferred to the left atrium and ultimately the lungs, as signs of heart failure begin.

Clinical Application

Intravascular fluid balance in patients with severe aortic stenosis is critical because the left ventricular chamber is no longer able to expand during filling; to produce an adequate stroke volume, complete filling of the ventricular chamber is essential.

Clinical Application

The development of atrial fibrillation results in the loss of atrial kick, which results in a decrease in ventricular preload (ventricular filling) and an associated decrease in stroke volume.

Clinical Presentation

As the obstruction to flow from the left ventricle continues to increase, so does left ventricular mass. This ability to compensate can last many years before symptoms appear. Symptoms generally begin to appear when the valve opening is one third of its normal size. When symptoms appear, mortality rates rise greatly. After the onset of symptoms, the average survival rate without surgical correction is 2 to 3 years. (Bonow et al., 2008,). Generally, after the sixth decade of life, a trio of classic symptoms occurs:

1. angina pectoris
2. syncope
3. heart failure.

(Bonow et al., 2008; Carabello & Crawford, 2009)

Angina

Increased left ventricular wall mass (hypertrophy) increases left ventricular myocardial oxygen demand. While the patient is at rest, blood supply may be adequate to meet the body's needs. However, with stress or exercise, the increased myocardial oxygen demand of the thickened ventricular wall can no longer be met, resulting in angina. Commonly, angina during exercise is the first presenting symptom in aortic stenosis. Angina can, of course, be caused by coronary heart disease (CHD) in addition to increased wall mass. Approximately one half of aortic stenosis patients presenting with angina also have CHD (Bashore, Granger, Hranitzky, & Patel, 2010).

Clinical Application

Patients with little or no significant CHD may still have angina as a result of a thickened myocardial wall. These patients benefit from the same measures that increase oxygen supply to the myocardium, such as supplemental oxygen and adequate hemoglobin levels.

Syncope

During exercise, total systemic vascular resistance (ventricular afterload) normally decreases to allow for a better flow of blood out of the ventricle. This decrease in systemic vascular resistance results in decreased blood pressure. The normal compensatory mechanism of the heart is to increase cardiac output to compensate for decreased pressure. This system keeps blood pressure in a normal range and allows patients to tolerate exercise while providing the body with an increased flow of oxygenated blood. However, with a narrowed valve opening, it is essentially impossible to increase cardiac output because the restriction of the valve does not allow for increased blood flow. Patients with severe aortic stenosis experience decreased blood pressure during exercise, resulting in light-headedness, dizziness, and blackout spells. In patients with aortic stenosis, exercise may also cause ventricular or atrial dysrhythmias, resulting in syncopal episodes.

Clinical Application

Patients should be reminded not to make any sudden position moves. They should be taught to move from a lying to standing position slowly as well as to be aware that exercise may result in syncope.

Clinical Application

Patients with mild aortic stenosis are not restricted in activity levels or exercise. Patients with moderate aortic stenosis should avoid strenuous activities and competitive sports. Patients with severe aortic stenosis should be advised to limit their activities to low levels.

Heart Failure

Patients with severe aortic stenosis develop diastolic and, ultimately, systolic failure. Left ventricular hypertrophy results in diastolic dysfunction as the thick-walled ventricle becomes noncompliant and loses its ability to expand during filling. This inability to expand decreases the amount of blood that can enter the left ventricle from the left atrium, and results in a back up of blood into the left atrium. The subsequent overload in the left atrium is transferred back to the pulmonary veins, and pulmonary edema results.

Additionally, over time, the hypertrophy that has been compensating for the increased afterload causes the myofibrils to stretch beyond the point of returning to a normal state. The ability of the ventricle to contract decreases and ejection fraction begins to decline (systolic dysfunction). This decrease in ejection fraction again results in a state of extracellular fluid (ECF) overload because the ventricle is unable to empty properly. The patient experiences dyspnea on exertion, orthopnea, and

paroxysmal nocturnal dyspnea as well as other signs of volume overload.

Physical Examination

A stenotic aortic valve may produce a murmur before causing any noteworthy hemodynamic changes. The systolic ejection murmur of aortic stenosis is best heard over the second intercostal space, left of the sternal border. The murmur is described as a medium-pitched murmur heard equally with the bell or diaphragm of the stethoscope (Buss & Thompson, 2010). It is described as rough and may become harsh as stenosis worsens. The murmur radiates to the right shoulder and both carotid arteries. In older adults with calcific aortic stenosis, the murmur may also radiate to the apex (fifth intercostal space, left midclavicular line), resulting in a misinterpretation of mitral regurgitation. The intensity of the murmur does not correspond with the severity of the stenosis. As aortic stenosis increases in severity, the murmur actually decreases in intensity.

In addition to the murmur and normal first and second heart sounds (S_1 and S_2, or "lub" and "dub" respectively), a fourth heart sound (S_4) may be audible just prior to the S_1. As left ventricular mass increases, the compliance of the ventricle decreases along with the ventricle's ability to expand during diastolic filling. With this decrease in compliance, the S_4 can be heard late in ventricular diastole, when atrial kick ejects blood into the already full ventricle. When aortic stenosis is advanced and systolic failure occurs, a third heart sound (S_3) can also be heard.

The normal pulse is sharp and quick. As aortic stenosis worsens, it becomes more difficult for the left ventricle to quickly push the valve open. As the valve slowly opens, the rush of blood through the valve is delayed, resulting in a decrease in the sharpness of the upstroke of the pulse.

Clinical Application

When assessing for an S_4 listen at the 5th intercostal space, left midclavicular line with the bell of the stethoscope. Normal S_1 and S_2 sound like "lub dub." When the S_4 is added, it will sound like "da lub dub," "Believe Me," or "Tennessee."

Diagnosis

The best method of screening for valvular heart disease is through cardiac auscultation. The murmur of aortic stenosis is usually recognized long before the patient presents with symptoms. Whereas some systolic murmurs may result from conditions other than aortic stenosis, a cardiac echocardiogram is a useful tool in determining the presence of valvular heart disease after a murmur is identified.

Echocardiography

The cardiac echocardiogram is the primary tool utilized to confirm the diagnosis of aortic stenosis and quantify its severity. During echocardiography, pressure gradient difference from one side of the valve to the other can be assessed. As valve stenosis worsens, the pressure gradient increases. Additionally, the aortic valve area is calculated. Normal valve area ranges from 3 to 4 cm^2. It is not until the valve area is approximately one fourth of the normal size that any changes in flow occur. A valve area of less than 1.0 cm^2 indicates severe stenosis (Bonow et al., 2008). Left ventricular mass, valve leaflet mobility, and systolic and diastolic function can also be assessed using echocardiography.

Cardiac Stress Testing

Exercise stress testing is contraindicated in the patient with aortic stenosis who is having symptoms (Bonow et al., 2008) because of the high risk of complications. In the patient without symptoms, exercise stress testing may be utilized to elicit symptoms of aortic stenosis. Patients with asymptomatic aortic stenosis undergoing exercise stress testing should be observed carefully for symptoms

of severe aortic valve disease, especially for signs of syncope.

Cardiac Catheterization

Patients with symptomatic aortic stenosis require cardiac catheterization to determine the extent, if any, of CHD. If valve replacement is questionable, the presence of treatable CHD answers the question and moves the patient toward surgery. A valve area of less than 0.8 cm^2 on cardiac catheterization indicates critical aortic valve stenosis and supports a decision for valve replacement (Carabello & Crawford, 2009).

Electrocardiogram

An electrocardiogram (ECG) demonstrates an increased QRS voltage with associated ST-segment and T-wave abnormalities when the patient has aortic stenosis. The increased QRS voltage is due to the increase in myocardial mass. Atrial abnormalities (demonstrated by abnormal P waves) indicate atrial enlargement. These ECG changes are neither sensitive nor specific to aortic stenosis and always require other testing for confirmation.

Chest X-ray Film

On chest X-ray film, the heart with stenosis usually appears normal in size. The shape, however, demonstrates a rounded left ventricular border, representing concentric hypertrophy. The aortic shadow may become enlarged and, occasionally, calcification of the valve is visible on the lateral view.

Clinical Application

Any clinician in any practice environment should assess for cardiac murmurs. Murmur detection is the key to early recognition of valvular heart disease. When the patient is aware of the presence of valvular heart disease, routine follow up can be established to assure the successful long-term treatment of the disease process.

Medical Therapy

There are no current medical treatment strategies that have demonstrated a slowing of the disease progression with calcific aortic stenosis. There have been some studies evaluating the effect of statins on slowing the progression of calcific aortic stenosis, but these studies have failed to demonstrate a significant benefit. (Bonow et al., 2008). Medical treatment beyond the occasional need for rate control with atrial fibrillation is rarely needed early in the disease process. Medication temporarily resolves heart failure; however, if the valve is not replaced, failure worsens and death is the end result.

Clinical Application

Severe aortic stenosis complicates the treatment of heart failure and often leaves the patient who is not a surgical candidate with limited treatment options. Referral to palliative care is important to offer the patient and family as much psychosocial support and as many options for symptom management as possible.

Routine Follow Up

The patient without symptoms should understand the importance of routine follow up with the physician. Periodic echocardiograms along with a physical assessment allow the physician to monitor the progression of the valvular stenosis. The patient should be aware to report any signs and symptoms of angina, heart failure, or syncope, which would indicate the presence of severe or worsening aortic stenosis.

Physical Activity and Exercise

Physical activity is not restricted in the patient with asymptomatic aortic stenosis. Patients with moderate to severe aortic stenosis should not participate in competitive sports. When in doubt about the ability to exercise, an exercise stress test can be preformed to assess activity tolerance.

ACE Inhibitors

Although indicated for heart failure, angiotensin-converting enzyme (ACE) inhibitors are generally contraindicated in patients with severe aortic stenosis. ACE inhibitors decrease systemic vascular resistance, which decreases blood pressure (Carabello & Crawford, 2009). The normal response to this change is an increase in heart rate to compensate for the decrease in blood pressure. A stenotic valve prevents large volumes of blood from being forced through, resulting in an inability to increase cardiac output. The patient develops hypotension and, ultimately, syncope could result.

Nitroglycerin

Nitrates should be used cautiously in patients with severe disease. It is important to remember that low-dose nitroglycerin decreases preload. With the hypertrophy that has developed, preload is already decreased because of the ventricle's inability to expand during filling. Any further loss of filling would result in a decrease in stroke volume. Nitroglycerin at high doses could further complicate the issue by causing a decrease in systemic vascular resistance similar to the effects of ACE inhibitors

Beta-blockers

Beta-blockers are contraindicated in severe aortic stenosis because they block the normal adrenergic response that has been occurring to compensate for decreased cardiac output (increased heart rate and contractility) and lessen the ability of the ventricle to overcome the pressure gradient that has developed (Carabello & Crawford, 2009).

Clinical Application

Vasodilators and other medications that can cause hypotension must be used with great caution in patients with severe aortic stenosis, because aortic stenosis is a mechanical obstruction that results in a fixed cardiac output and inability of the heart to compensate for hypotension. However, in a patient with significant hypertension, these medications may be used to lower blood pressure and reduce left ventricular afterload.

Endocarditis Prophylaxis

Antibiotic prophylaxis for endocarditis was considered essential in all patients with aortic stenosis, regardless of age or symptoms, until the American Heart Association (AHA) published the new Prevention of Infective Endocarditis Guidelines in April 2007. With these new guidelines, the prophylactic use of antibiotics for patients with native valve disease is no longer recommended. (Nishimura et al., 2008; Wilson et al., 2007). The AHA notes:

> The maintenance of optimal oral health and hygiene may reduce the incidence of bacteremia from daily activities and is more important than prophylactic antibiotics for a dental procedure to reduce the risk of infective endocarditis (Wilson et al., 2007, p. 3).

Surgical Intervention

With the onset of symptoms, mortality rates dramatically increase. When symptoms appear, the need for surgical repair becomes imminent. Additionally, the risk of sudden death increases with the onset of symptoms, further adding to the urgency of valve replacement surgery (Bonow et al., 2008). Surgical outcomes improve with early detection. Therefore, close follow up of patients with aortic stenosis, with an early decision to treat when symptoms begin, is imperative. Several options are available after the patient becomes symptomatic.

Percutaneous Balloon Valvuloplasty

A balloon inflated in the valve orifice can be used to fracture calcium deposits in the leaflets and stretch the aortic annulus. This procedure is considered palliative and should be reserved for patients who are not surgical candidates but are seeking relief from symptoms. The American College of Cardiology (ACC) and AHA recommendations for aortic balloon valvuloplasty in adults with aortic stenosis are reviewed in Box 9-1. This procedure has no effect on long-term mortality rates. Six months after the procedure, about one half of the

---

BOX 9-1: ACC/AHA RECOMMENDATIONS FOR AORTIC BALLOON VALVULOPLASTY

• A bridge to surgery in hemodynamically unstable patients with severe aortic stenosis who are too unstable to undergo surgery.

• Palliative care in patients with aortic stenosis who are too high risk for surgery because of serious comorbid conditions.

(Bonow et al., 2008)

---

patients have developed restenosis of the valve (Ledoux, 2010). Before the procedure, patients should be evaluated for aortic regurgitation. Aortic regurgitation is an expected postoperative result after valvuloplasty. The procedure should not be performed if the patient has 2+ or greater aortic valve regurgitation.

Aortic Valve Replacement

Surgery to replace the valve is the treatment of choice in most adults with aortic stenosis after symptoms develop (see Box 9-2). There has been no demonstrated benefit from surgery for patients with mild to moderate aortic stenosis who do not have symptoms (Carabello & Crawford, 2009). Therefore, surgery is not indicated until symptoms appear. However, there is controversy regarding the timing of surgery for the patient with asymptomatic severe aortic stenosis noted on echocardiogram. Surgery is usually recommended for such patients with ejection fractions less than 50%.

Before surgery, the mitral valve is also evaluated because, quite frequently, mitral regurgitation also exists and mitral valve replacement may also be necessary. Cardiac catheterization should also be performed to determine the need for coronary artery bypass surgery. A preoperative assessment of left ventricular function determines systolic and diastolic dysfunction. Surgical mortality risk is lowest in those with normal left ventricular function and increases as systolic function decreases (Darovic, 2002).

BOX 9-2: ACC/AHA RECOMMENDATIONS FOR AORTIC VALVE REPLACEMENT

- Patients with severe aortic stenosis who are symptomatic

- Patients with severe aortic stenosis (with or without symptoms) undergoing coronary artery bypass surgery

- Patients with severe aortic stenosis (with or without symptoms) undergoing surgery on the aorta or other heart valves

- Patients with severe aortic stenosis (without symptoms) and one of the following:

  - left ventricular systolic dysfunction (ejection fraction < 50%)

  - abnormal response to exercise

  - high likelihood of rapid disease progression

  - extremely severe aortic stenosis (valve areas < 0. 6 cm^2, mean gradient > 60 mm Hg, jet velocity > 5.0 m/sec) when operative mortality is expected to be 1% or less

(Bonow et al., 2008)

Clinical Application

Patients with aortic valve disease should be aware of signs of decompensation. With early recognition, the appropriate treatment can take place before any systolic dysfunction occurs.

The type of valve prosthesis used is determined by the anticipated longevity of the patient and the patient's ability to tolerate anticoagulants. Mechanical valves have better durability than tissue valves that come from human or pig donors (bioprosthetics). Mechanical valves require lifelong anticoagulation with warfarin, which is not necessary for tissue valves. Patients with tissue valves are usually required to take an aspirin daily, but no further anticoagulation is necessary. Mechanical valves are generally best suited for young patients with no contraindications to anticoagulation. However, young female patients who wish to become pregnant require tissue valves because the utilization of anticoagulation during pregnancy increases fetal mortality (Carabello & Crawford, 2009). Older adult patients with a life expectancy less than that of the tissue valve (7 to 10 years) are better suited for tissue valves and can avoid the need for anticoagulation and its associated complications.

Some centers also perform the Ross procedure, which involves placing a patient's pulmonic valve in the aortic valve position and placing a tissue valve in the pulmonic valve location. It has been noted that tissue valves last longer in the lower pressure right heart and the need for anticoagulation is avoided (Carabello & Crawford, 2009). There are advantages and disadvantages to this approach. Although there are some advantages in children (valves grow with the child), overall in adults, the deterioration of the tissue valve offsets the potential advantages (Bonow et al., 2008).

Transcatheter/Transapical Aortic Valve Replacement

As the prevalence of aortic valve stenosis will most likely increase as the population ages, there are attempts at treatment that will avoid an open heart procedure. Unlike traditional valve replacement, this procedure does not require the removal of the native valve. A bioprosthetic valve is attached to a stent. The stent is expanded at the site of the native valve with the stent holding the new valve in place. There are several approaches with minimally invasive aortic valve replacement. The transcatheter approach utilizes either the femoral artery directly to the aortic valve or reaches the aortic valve through the femoral vein with a puncture through the septum. The transapical approach requires a small left-sided incision about the location of the sixth intercostal space, with a small puncture of the left ventricle to reach the aortic valve. This procedure is currently in clinical trials and experience is limited; however, the preliminary results are encouraging and demonstrate that these minimally invasive procedures will be feasible alternatives to valve replacement surgery in the future (McRae, Rodger, & Bailey, 2009).

Outcomes

After successful aortic valve replacement, decreased left ventricular systolic pressure and decreased afterload result in improved ejection fraction and increased cardiac output. Left ventricular hypertrophy actually regresses, with most of that regression occurring in the first year, but continuing to improve for up to 10 years (Rahimtoola, 2008). However, diastolic function most likely never returns to normal because of the increase in collagen content in the myocardial tissue. After the damaged valve has been replaced with either a tissue or mechanical valve, the risk for endocarditis increases and patients with prosthetic valves do benefit from endocarditis prophylaxis with antibiotics prior to dental procedures (Bonow et al., 2008; Nishimura et al., 2008; Wilson et al., 2007). Patients with a mechanical valve are placed on lifelong warfarin therapy. Those with a tissue or bioprosthetic valve may be placed on warfarin for 3 months postoperatively, then switched to lifelong aspirin therapy.

AORTIC REGURGITATION

Definition

Aortic regurgitation occurs when the valve cusps do not close tightly and blood is allowed to travel retrograde, or backward, through the valve during ventricular systole. A variety of processes can affect the valve cusps, the aortic root, or both, resulting in aortic regurgitation (see Figure 9-1).

Causes

Aortic regurgitation occurs in about 5% of the general population and is more common in men

than in women (Leeper, 2009). Aortic regurgitation can be classified as acute or chronic. Symptoms depend on the severity and rapidity of onset. With the decreased incidence of rheumatic valve disease in the United States, chronic non-rheumatic causes now account for the majority of isolated cases of aortic regurgitation. Causes of non-rheumatic valve disease include congenital bicuspid valve, systemic hypertension, myxomatous degeneration, infective endocarditis, and connective tissue diseases as well as calcifications that affect the valve's cusps. Many patients with chronic aortic regurgitation have processes that affect the aortic root, including Marfan's syndrome, aortic dissection, inflammatory diseases, collagen vascular disease, and syphilitic aortitis (Ledoux, 2010). Acute aortic regurgitation is seen with trauma, acute bacterial endocarditis, and acute aortic dissection (Bonow et al., 2008). Because the presentation of acute aortic regurgitation is entirely different than that of chronic aortic regurgitation, the two are discussed separately.

CHRONIC AORTIC REGURGITATION

Pathophysiology

Normally, as the ventricle ejects blood through the aortic valve, the aorta expands to accept the volume. When the pressure in the ventricle becomes less than the pressure in the aorta, the aortic valve closes. The aorta relaxes and blood is dispersed to the area of least resistance. This expansion and relaxation of the aorta are known as the elastic and recoil properties of the aorta. With a competent aortic valve, blood moves forward. The closed valve stops blood from moving backward toward the aortic valve (see Figure 9-3).

In aortic regurgitation, blood enters the left ventricle normally from the left atrium. Blood also enters the left ventricle from the aorta because the valve does not close properly, and backflow occurs from the aorta through the aortic valve into the left

FIGURE 9-3: NORMAL FUNCTIONING OF THE AORTA DURING SYSTOLE AND DIASTOLE

Note. From *Critical Care Nursing: Diagnosis and Management* (2nd ed.), by L.A. Thelan, J.K. Davie, L.D. Urden, & M.E. Lough, 1994, St. Louis, MO: Mosby, ©Elsevier. Reprinted with permission.

ventricle. This results in a larger-than-normal volume in the left ventricle. To compensate, left ventricular chamber size increases to allow for the additional volume. Left ventricular wall thickness also increases to help maintain normal wall stress. The enlarged left ventricular chamber size maintains a normal or near-normal preload and the increase in wall thickness helps to increase stroke volume. This increased stroke volume is necessary because a portion of the blood ejected to the aorta with each beat returns to the left ventricle during ventricular diastole through the regurgitant valve. If the ventricle can eject a larger-than-normal volume with each beat, the cardiac output needs should be met. While maintaining preload, normal wall stress, and contractility, ejection fraction remains the same. This phase of the disease process is considered the chronic compensatory phase and lasts for many years or even decades. As with aortic stenosis,

patients remain asymptomatic for years with very low morbidity.

Eventually, however, the compensatory mechanisms begin to fail and the enlarged heart begins to show signs of decompensation. As dilation of the left ventricle continues, contractility eventually decreases because the myocardium has been over-stretched. Left ventricular ejection fraction also decreases, resulting in decreased cardiac output (systolic dysfunction). As ejection fraction decreases, left ventricular volume (preload) increases because of the inability of the ventricles to empty appropriately. Additionally, afterload increases to compensate for decreased cardiac output. Heart rate also increases to compensate for the decrease in cardiac output; however, this increased rate is often ineffective. After decades without any difficulties, patients begin to develop symptoms of ECF overload.

Clinical Presentation

Although patients commonly remain asymptomatic for years, the initial symptoms noted most frequently are exertional dyspnea and fatigue due to the failing left ventricle. As the disease progresses, patients can also develop paroxysmal nocturnal dyspnea and orthopnea with pulmonary edema. Angina can result from an inability of the coronary arteries to supply the volume of oxygenated blood needed for the increased myocardial mass. Patients with aortic regurgitation commonly experience ischemia without associated CHD. The incidence of concurrent CHD with aortic regurgitation is less common than with aortic stenosis.

Physical Examination

A variety of signs can lead a healthcare professional toward a diagnosis of aortic regurgitation. A diastolic murmur, displaced left ventricular impulse, wide pulse pressure, and specific peripheral findings, are characteristic signs of chronic aortic regurgitation. The characteristic murmur of aortic regurgitation is a soft, diastolic murmur best heard at the third intercostal space to the left of the sternum. The murmur is loudest at end-expiration and is better recognized with the patient sitting and leaning forward (Wiegand et al., 2008). If the patient has aortic root disease (Marfan's syndrome), then the murmur is best heard to the right of the sternum (Bonow et al., 2008; Buss & Thompson, 2010). Occasionally, the murmur is described as a diastolic rumble heard best at the apex; in this case, it is referred to as an *Austin Flint murmur* (Zoghbi & Crawford, 2009). The apical impulse (normally at the apex of the heart) is displaced leftward and downward because of the hypertrophy and is forceful because of increased stroke volume.

As regurgitation progresses, diastolic blood pressure decreases, resulting in a widened pulse pressure (difference between the systolic and diastolic pressure). Diastolic blood pressure decreases as more blood is returned to the left ventricle; it is generally less than 60 mm Hg (Wang, 2010) and may be as low 0 mm Hg. Additionally, systolic pressure increases as a result of increased stroke volume. Pulse pressure is commonly greater than 50 mm Hg (Wiegand et al., 2008). The same physiological changes that are responsible for widened pulse pressure also result in a variety of peripheral signs that have been associated with chronic aortic regurgitation (see Table 9-1).

Clinical Application

If the Korotkoff sound is heard down to zero when auscultating a blood pressure, note the point at which muffling of the Korotkoff sound occurs. This point correlates with the diastolic pressure (Leeper, 2009).

Diagnosis

Echocardiography

When the characteristic signs of aortic regurgitation are detected, echocardiography is again the test of choice to confirm the diagnosis. During echocardiography, an assessment can be made of the severity of regurgitation, morphology of the valve, left ventricular size and function, and the aortic root. The severity of regurgitation is determined by a variety of methods and calculations. Generally, the regurgitation is expressed as a number from 1 to 4 (see Table 9-2).

Cardiac Catheterization

Cardiac catheterization should be completed in patients with symptomatic aortic regurgitation who are having aortic valve replacement surgery to determine the extent, if any, of CHD. As with aortic stenosis, if valve replacement is questionable, the presence of treatable CHD can answer the question and move the patient toward surgery. Cardiac catheterization is also indicated to assess the severity of regurgitation and the extent of left ventricular function if noninvasive tests are inconclusive.

TABLE 9-1: PERIPHERAL SIGNS OF CHRONIC AORTIC REGURGITATION

Sign	Description
Water-hammer pulse (Corrigan's pulse)	A rapid rise and collapse of the pulse upon palpation of the peripheral pulse
de Musset's sign	Bobbing of the head with each heart beat
Traube's sign (pistol-shot sounds)	Booming systolic and diastolic sounds heard over the femoral artery
Duroziez's sign	Systolic bruit heard over the femoral artery when compressed proximally and diastolic murmur heard over the femoral artery when compressed distally

(Zoghbi & Afridi, 2003)

TABLE 9-2: AORTIC REGURGITATION SEVERITY

1+	Mild aortic regurgitation
2+	Moderate aortic regurgitation
3+	Moderately severe aortic regurgitation
4+	Severe aortic regurgitation

(Hilkert & Yoo, 2002)

Chest X-ray Film

A chest X-ray film shows left ventricular hypertrophy (enlarged heart) and pulmonary congestion, as would be expected in a patient with heart failure.

Electrocardiogram

A 12-lead ECG demonstrates the increased QRS voltage that is seen with left ventricular hypertrophy. These ECG changes are neither sensitive nor specific to aortic regurgitation and always require other testing for confirmation.

Stress Test

Stress testing can be useful in patients with mild symptoms but is not indicated in the patient who is symptomatic. The test provides an evaluation of exercise tolerance, with an assessment of both symptomatic response and hemodynamic effects. This test assists in determining the need for surgical intervention in the patient who is asymptomatic.

Medical Therapy

Patients may remain asymptomatic for many years. If patients with mild aortic regurgitation remain asymptomatic and have normal left ventricular function, no treatment is necessary.

Routine Follow Up

The patient who is asymptomatic should understand the importance of routine follow up with the physician. Periodic echocardiograms, along with a physical assessment, allow the physician to monitor the progression of the valvular regurgitation. The patient should be aware of the signs and symptoms indicating severe aortic regurgitation.

Vasodilator Therapy

Vasodilators (hydralazine, nifedipine, and ACE inhibitors) can be helpful by decreasing left ventricular afterload. A decrease in afterload decreases regurgitant volume by making it easier for blood to move forward through the aorta and less apt to move backward through the malfunctioning valve. According to the ACC and the AHA valve guidelines, there are three potential uses for vasodilator therapy in patients with severe aortic regurgitation (does not apply to mild or moderate disease):

1. Vasodilator therapy is indicated for chronic therapy in patients with severe aortic regurgitation who have symptoms of left ventricular dysfunction when surgery is not recommended because of additional cardiac or noncardiac factors.

2. Vasodilator therapy may be considered for short-term therapy to improve the hemodynamic profile of patients with severe heart failure symptoms and severe left ventricular dysfunction before proceeding with aortic valve replacement.

3. Vasodilator therapy may be considered for long-term therapy in patients who are asymptomatic with severe aortic regurgitation and who have left ventricular dilation but normal systolic function (Bonow et al., 2008).

Vasodilator therapy has not proven beneficial in patients with mild to moderate disease who are asymptomatic, so is not utilized in these situations.

Physical Activity and Exercise

Physical activity is not restricted in the patient with asymptomatic aortic regurgitation. Patients with moderate aortic regurgitation who are asymptomatic may be able to participate in competitive sports. When in doubt about the ability to exercise, an exercise stress test can be preformed to evaluate activity tolerance.

Endocarditis Prophylaxis

Antibiotic prophylaxis for endocarditis was considered essential in all patients with aortic regurgitation, regardless of age or symptoms, until the AHA published the new Prevention of Infective Endocarditis Guidelines in April 2007. As noted with aortic stenosis, the publication of these new guidelines eliminated the need for prophylactic use of antibiotics for patients with native valve disease (Bonow et al., 2008; Nishimura et al., 2008; Wilson et al., 2007).

Surgical Intervention

Because mortality with valve replacement worsens as ejection fraction worsens, careful assessment of left ventricular function is essential. Patients with chronic aortic regurgitation should have regular follow-up serial testing. When patients develop left ventricular dysfunction, with or without symptoms, with an ejection fraction less than 50%, valve replacement surgery should be considered (Bonow et al., 2008). (See Box 9-3). As the severity of left ventricular dysfunction increases, so does the mortality rate with surgery; therefore, early intervention is indicated (Bonow et al., 2008; Darovic, 2002).

Surgical options for replacement of the aortic valve in patients with aortic regurgitation are the same as those for aortic stenosis. Older adults commonly have aortic stenosis and CHD in addition to the aortic regurgitation. According to the ACC/AHA guidelines, the determination for surgery should be based on quality of life and not longevity. Symptom relief should be the most important guide in making the decision for aortic valve replacement.

Outcomes

Left ventricular function generally improves for up to 2 years after surgery, with a gradual decline in ventricular hypertrophy (Zoghbi & Crawford, 2009). These results vary depending on the preoperative condition of the left ventricle. An echocardiogram should be performed shortly after surgery. If the initial echocardiogram shows improvement, then serial echocardiograms are not necessary. Patients who continue to demonstrate left ventricular dysfunction should be treated, as are others with left ventricular dysfunction, including with the use of ACE inhibitors. After valve replacement with either a tissue or a mechanical valve, all patients are at high risk for endocarditis and do benefit from endocarditis prophylaxis before dental procedures (Wilson et al., 2007). Patients with mechanical valves are placed on lifelong warfarin therapy. Those with tissue or bioprosthetic valves may be placed on warfarin for 3 months postoperatively, then switched to lifelong aspirin therapy.

ACUTE AORTIC REGURGITATION

Pathophysiology

Acute aortic regurgitation is most noted with trauma, aortic dissection, and acute cases of infective endocarditis (Bonow et al., 2008). When acute aortic regurgitation occurs, a volume of blood suddenly returns to the left ventricle from the aorta. This acute regurgitation occurs with no ability of

---

BOX 9-3: ACC/AHA RECOMMENDATIONS FOR AORTIC VALVE REPLACEMENT IN PATIENTS WITH AORTIC REGURGITATION

- Symptomatic patients with severe aortic regurgitation irrespective of left ventricular systolic function.

- Asymptomatic patients with chronic severe aortic regurgitation and left ventricular systolic dysfunction (ejection fraction 50% or less) at rest.

- Patients with chronic severe aortic regurgitation while undergoing coronary artery bypass grafting or surgery on the aorta or other heart valves.

(Bonow et al., 2008)

the left ventricle to make adjustments to the sudden increase in volume. The volume overload is transferred backward to the left atrium and, ultimately, the pulmonary veins. This results in the development of acute pulmonary edema. The left ventricle is unable to increase stroke volume because it has no time to adapt. Stroke volume dramatically decreases because much of the blood is returned to the ventricle with each cardiac cycle. The body attempts to compensate for this decrease in cardiac output by increasing heart rate; however, this compensation is generally ineffective. Additionally, peripheral vasoconstriction occurs to compensate for the decrease in cardiac output. Volume travels to the area of least resistance, therefore, vasoconstriction only increases afterload and results in a worsening of the acute aortic regurgitation.

Clinical Presentation

Patients with acute aortic regurgitation generally present with acute pulmonary edema and possibly cardiogenic shock. They experience severe dyspnea, orthopnea, and weakness. The onset of symptoms is generally abrupt.

Physical Examination

Examination of the lungs reveals bilateral rales indicative of pulmonary edema. The patient is tachycardic and hypotensive. Because the long-term compensatory mechanisms have not had time to occur, not all of the peripheral signs associated with chronic aortic regurgitation are present.

Clinical Application

Patients with acute aortic regurgitation are acutely ill and generally in a life-threatening situation, especially in the presence of aortic root dissection.

Diagnosis

Cardiac echocardiography is utilized to quickly confirm the diagnosis of aortic regurgitation as well as to determine the extent of the problem. A transesophageal echocardiogram may be done if aortic dissection is suspected. Cardiac catheterization may be done, if there is time, to further evaluate the aortic regurgitation and aortic dissection.

Medical Therapy

Early surgical treatment is necessary because patients with acute aortic regurgitation often die of pulmonary edema, ventricular dysrhythmias, or cardiogenic shock (Bonow et al., 2008). While patients are being prepared for surgery, sodium nitroprusside (Nipride) is helpful because it decreases preload and afterload (Zoghbi & Crawford, 2009). Dobutamine assists with ventricular contractility and helps increase cardiac output. If the patient has developed acute aortic regurgitation as a result of infective endocarditis, 48 hours of antibiotics are preferred if the patient can tolerate the delay in surgery (Ledoux, 2010). However, surgery should not be delayed if the patient is hemodynamically unstable.

Clinical Application

Although utilized in acutely ill patients, intra-aortic balloon pumping is contraindicated in patients with aortic regurgitation because it grossly increases aortic regurgitation. As the balloon inflates in the aorta during ventricular diastole, blood in the aorta is forced to return to the ventricle through the regurgitant valve.

Surgical Replacement

For an unstable patient, surgical intervention resolves the instability. Valve replacement with a mechanical or bioprosthetic valve should be done as quickly as possible. If the patient has aortic dissection, repair of the aorta is also necessary.

Outcomes

When a patient with acute aortic regurgitation has the valve successfully replaced, outcomes are very good. If left ventricular function was normal prior to the acute event, there should be no long-term effects on the ventricle. Follow up is the same as with all valve surgeries.

CONCLUSION

The aortic valve is the gateway to the body from the left ventricle. If this gate does not function correctly, it can have long-term effects on the body as the structures surrounding the valve attempt to compensate. Healthcare professionals should assist the patient in understanding the disease progression associated with aortic valve disease. With a full understanding, the patient can recognize symptoms of decompensation early and intervention can take place in a timely manner.

EXAM QUESTIONS

CHAPTER 9
Questions 71-78

Note: Choose the one option that BEST answers each question.

71. Fibrosis of the valve leaflets with fusion of the commissures is the primary pathophysiologic change that occurs in which type of aortic stenosis?

    a. Congenital valve disease
    b. Rheumatic heart disease
    c. Senile degenerative fibrosis
    d. Senile degenerative calcification

72. The classic trio of symptoms noted in patients with aortic stenosis who are symptomatic is

    a. angina, syncope, and heart failure.
    b. hypotension, palpitations, and angina.
    c. murmurs, hypotension, and palpitations.
    d. palpitations, syncope, and angina.

73. The primary tool used for diagnosing valvular heart disease is

    a. echocardiography.
    b. chest X-ray.
    c. cardiac catheterization.
    d. cardiac stress testing.

74. The class of medications that is contraindicated in patients with severe aortic stenosis because of its effect of decreasing systemic vascular resistance is

    a. beta-blockers.
    b. ACE inhibitors.
    c. low-dose nitrates.
    d. aspirin.

75. In patients with chronic aortic regurgitation, a physiological change that is the direct result of the heart compensating for the regurgitation is

    a. left atrial enlargement.
    b. left ventricular enlargement.
    c. aortic enlargement.
    d. decreased contractility.

76. The most frequently noted first symptoms of chronic aortic regurgitation include

    a. hypotension, syncope, and angina.
    b. systolic murmur and head bobbing with each heart beat.
    c. exertional dyspnea and fatigue.
    d. edema and systolic murmur.

77. Surgical replacement of the aortic valve for aortic regurgitation should occur when the patient develops left ventricular dysfunction with an ejection fraction less than

    a. 65%.
    b. 60%.
    c. 55%.
    d. 50%.

78. Signs and symptoms specific to patients with acute aortic regurgitation include

    a. decreased activity tolerance.
    b. bradycardia.
    c. water-hammer pulse.
    d. abrupt onset of shortness of breath.

CHAPTER 10

MITRAL VALVE DISEASE

CHAPTER OBJECTIVE

After completing this chapter, the learner will be able to recognize mitral valve disease and identify its impact on the body.

LEARNING OBJECTIVES

After completing this chapter, the learner will be able to

1. identify the pathophysiology that occurs with mitral stenosis.

2. describe key signs and symptoms of mitral stenosis.

3. explain the medical and surgical treatment options available for patients with mitral stenosis.

4. identify the pathophysiology that occurs with mitral regurgitation.

5. describe key signs and symptoms of mitral regurgitation.

6. explain the medical and surgical treatment options available for patients with mitral regurgitation.

INTRODUCTION

The mitral valve is the gateway between the left atrium and left ventricle. Proper function of the valve allows blood to move from the atrium to the ventricle. Its normal function plays a key role in the volume in the left ventricle before ejection. This volume is essential for systemic perfusion. A dysfunctional valve can alter left ventricular preload and, consequently, perfusion.

MITRAL VALVE FUNCTION

The mitral valve opens passively during the beginning of diastole, allowing blood to flow passively from the atrium to the ventricle. At the end of diastole, the atrium contracts (atrial kick) and sends an additional volume to the ventricle. As the pressure in the ventricle increases, the mitral valve begins to close. Isovolumic contraction begins and further pressure in the ventricle builds, forcing the mitral valve to snap shut. The papillary muscles contract, preventing the mitral valve leaflets from prolapsing into the left atrium during systole. The closed mitral valve forms a tight seal to assure that the blood being ejected from the ventricle flows forward through the aortic valve and not backward into the left atrium. When ventricular ejection is complete and the pressure in the left ventricle becomes lower than the pressure in the left atrium, the mitral valve opens and the cycle begins again (see Figure 10-1). A more detailed description of the cardiac valves is covered in Chapter 1. Definitions of stenosis and regurgitation are provided in Chapter 9.

FIGURE 10-1: NORMAL MITRAL VALVE

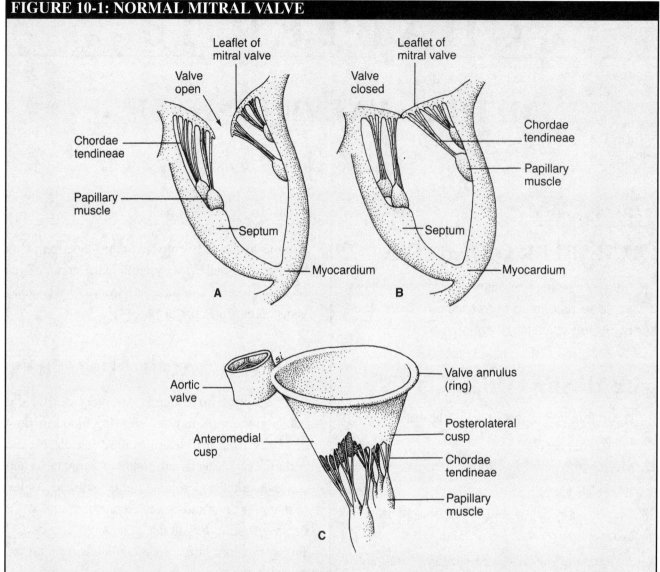

A) The valve leaflets are widely open in ventricular diastole. B) The valve leaflets close during ventricular systole. C) The mitral valve annulus and cusps form a funnel-like structure when the mitral valve is open.

Note. From *Hemodynamic Monitoring: Invasive and Noninvasive Clinical Application* (3rd ed.), by G.O. Darovic, 2002, Philadelphia, PA: Saunders, ©Elsevier. Reprinted with permission.

MITRAL STENOSIS

Definition

Mitral stenosis occurs when the mitral valve no longer opens normally, causing an obstruction of blood flow from the left atrium to the left ventricle (see Figure 10-2).

Causes

The number one cause of mitral stenosis is rheumatic fever (Darovic, 2002). As the incidence of rheumatic fever decreases in the United States, so does the incidence of mitral stenosis. Congenital mitral stenosis, atrial myxoma, systemic lupus erythematosus, and bacterial endocarditis can also cause mitral stenosis, but these causes are rare (Ledoux, 2010). Mitral stenosis is twice as common in women than in men. Forty percent of all patients with rheumatic heart disease develop mitral stenosis, and this accounts for 60% of all cases of mitral stenosis (Bonow et al., 2008). Many patients with rheumatic mitral stenosis have no recollection of having rheumatic fever.

FIGURE 10-2: MITRAL VALVE STENOSIS

Note. From Cleveland Clinic Heart Center. Reprinted with permission, Cleveland Clinic Center for Medical Art & Photography ©2005-2011. All rights reserved. Retrieved January 16, 2005, from http://www .clevelandclinic.org/heartcenter/pub/guide/disease/valve/balloon_ valve.htm

Pathophysiology

The rheumatic mitral valve develops fibrosis and calcification of the valve leaflets. The valve commissures fuse together, and the chordae tendineae thicken and shorten. The combination of some or all of these changes results in a valve orifice that is much smaller than normal. The normal mitral valve area is 4 to 5 cm^2 (Bonow et al., 2008). As the valve opening becomes smaller, it becomes more difficult for blood to flow passively from the atrium to the ventricle. Because the ventricle depends on diastolic filling to maintain stroke volume, left atrial pressure must rise in an attempt to maintain normal flow across the valve. This increase in left atrial pressure is transferred back to the pulmonary vascular bed, as pulmonary pressure subsequently increases. As the obstruction worsens, the chronic increase in left atrial pressure results in pulmonary hypertension and, ultimately,

right ventricular failure. The left atrium dilates and hypertrophies in response to the increased pressure and volume, and it becomes increasingly more difficult to empty the atrium. The enlarged left atrium puts the patient at risk for the development of thrombi in the atrium.

Clinical Presentation

The development of symptoms could begin as long as 20 to 40 years after the development of rheumatic fever (Bonow et al., 2008). After the onset of initial symptoms, another 10 years may pass before symptoms occur that change the patient's lifestyle. Symptoms that occur with activity usually appear when the valve area has narrowed to less than 2.5 cm^2. Symptoms that occur at rest usually appear when the valve orifice is less than 1.5 cm^2 (Bonow et al., 2008). When symptoms begin, they develop slowly and patients make adjustments in activity levels to compensate for the changes, often without being aware that they are doing so. Dyspnea with exertion, with no symptoms at rest, is the most common initial finding. Conditions that increase heart rate, such as pregnancy, new-onset atrial fibrillation, hyperthyroidism, or fever, commonly result in symptoms that alert the physician to the possibility of mitral stenosis. An increased heart rate shortens diastole and, therefore, decreases ventricular filling time. Decreased filling time results in decreased stroke volume, which contributes to decreased cardiac output. When cardiac output is insufficient, symptoms of dyspnea and fatigue occur.

As valve dysfunction increases and the valve orifice decreases, symptoms increase. Pulmonary symptoms, such as orthopnea and paroxysmal nocturnal dyspnea, develop. With the development of severe mitral stenosis (valve orifice less than 1 cm^2), the patient develops dyspnea at rest and is essentially confined to a bed or chair, as the complications of pulmonary hypertension worsen. Cough and hemoptysis develop as the disease progresses. Ultimately, the failure of the system affects the right side of the heart, and signs of right ventricular failure appear.

Clinical Application

Patients with severe mitral stenosis may develop acute pulmonary edema with exercise because the narrowed mitral opening cannot handle the increased blood flow produced by the normal increase in heart rate and venous return that occurs with exercise.

Clinical Application

Although patients with mild to moderate mitral stenosis should be counseled to avoid unusually stressful exercise, they should be encouraged to maintain a low-level aerobic exercise program to maintain cardiovascular fitness. The limits of this exercise should be determined by individual patient tolerance.

With the atrium enlarging and cardiac output decreasing, the risk of thrombi development in the atrium increases, as does the risk of embolization. Stroke, caused by an embolus, is the first indication of mitral stenosis in many cases. The probability of a stroke exists if the patient is in sinus rhythm; however, the probability increases with the development of atrial fibrillation. Atrial fibrillation is noted in more than one half of patients with mitral stenosis because of atrial enlargement (Bashore et al., 2010).

Clinical Application

Patients with mitral stenosis are dependent on atrial contraction for a large portion of ventricular filling because stenosis slows the passive filling of the ventricle from the atrium. Therefore, the development of atrial fibrillation in patients with mitral stenosis can quickly result in symptoms of decreased perfusion because atrial contraction is lost with the onset of atrial fibrillation.

Physical Examination

On cardiac auscultation, the first heart sound (S_1, or "lub") is louder than normal unless the valve is heavily calcified; then the sound is diminished (Curtin & Griffin, 2009). The second heart sound (S_2, or "dub") is associated with closure of the aortic and pulmonic valves. At the same time, the mitral and tricuspid valves open. Opening of a stenotic mitral valve results in a sound that may be heard immediately after the second heart sound. This sound is called an opening snap and is best heard at the cardiac apex (fifth intercostal space, at the midclavicular line) with the diaphragm of the stethoscope. At the same location, a low-pitched rumbling diastolic murmur can be heard with the bell of the stethoscope. The murmur occurs during ventricular diastole and can be heard after the second heart sound and before the first heart sound. The more severe the disease process, the longer the murmur lasts throughout diastole. The murmur is best heard with the patient lying on the left side and increases with exercise (Buss & Thompson, 2010). Patients may also present with signs of right ventricular failure, including crackles, jugular venous distension, hepatomegaly, and peripheral edema. Mitral facies is a pinkish purple discoloration of the cheeks that is common in patients with severe mitral stenosis (Darovic, 2002).

Clinical Application

Diastolic murmurs are often difficult to hear because of their low pitch. It is important to listen carefully in a quite room. It may take 5 to 10 seconds to recognize a lower grade diastolic murmur. The murmur of mitral stenosis is best heard with the bell of the stethoscope placed lightly over the apex of the heart (5th intercostal space, left midclavicular line).

Diagnosis

The best method of screening for valvular heart disease is through cardiac auscultation. The murmur of mitral stenosis is usually recognized long before the patient presents with symptoms. Although some systolic murmurs may result from conditions other than valve disease, diastolic murmurs most often indicate an abnormal valve.

Echocardiography

Cardiac echocardiography is the method of choice for diagnosing mitral stenosis. With echocardiography, the mitral valve orifice can be measured to assist in the determination of stenosis severity (see Table 10-1). Valve motion, leaflet thickness, and calcification can also be evaluated with echocardiography. In addition to an evaluation of the valve itself, left atrial size and pulmonary artery pressures are measured. Patients with mitral stenosis may also benefit from transesophageal echocardiography to detect valve vegetation or thrombi in the left atrium.

TABLE 10-1: MITRAL STENOSIS STAGES	
> 1.5 cm^2	Mild
1.0 to 1.5 cm^2	Moderate
< 1.0 cm^2	Severe
(Bonow et al., 2008)	

Cardiac Catheterization

Cardiac catheterization allows for assessment of the need for coronary artery revascularization if valve replacement is needed. During cardiac catheterization, left atrial pressure can be measured to assist in the evaluation of the progression of the disease. However, cardiac catheterization is not as useful in determining the severity of the stenosis as is echocardiography.

Chest X-ray Film

The presence of signs of mitral stenosis on chest X-ray film depends on the extent of the disease. As the disease progresses and pulmonary hypertension develops, the pulmonary arteries are more visible on the X-ray film. An elevation of the left mainstem bronchus, with left atrial enlargement, also may be noted. Signs of pulmonary edema are noted if the patient is in a volume overload state.

Electrocardiogram

The electrocardiogram (ECG) demonstrates signs of left atrial enlargement with abnormal P waves (wide, notched P waves in lead II.) If right ventricular hypertrophy is present, a QRS axis shift to the right may be visible. These ECG changes are neither sensitive nor specific to mitral stenosis and always require other testing for confirmation.

The ECG may also show atrial fibrillation. New-onset atrial fibrillation is a treatable rhythm that can be identified by comparing the patient's current ECG to previous ECGs.

Clinical Application

Clinicians should be particularly alert for the development of atrial fibrillation because the incidence of stroke is high with this rhythm. Many patients are unaware of the development of an irregularly irregular heart rhythm, but astute practitioners can recognize the changes of atrial fibrillation and begin appropriate treatment.

Medical Therapy

Endocarditis Prophylaxis

As with aortic valve disease in the new American Heart Association (AHA) American College of Cardiology (ACC) guidelines, the prophylactic use of antibiotics for patients with native valve disease is no longer recommended (Nishimura et al., 2008; Wilson et al., 2007). However, it is important to discuss good oral hygiene practices as a primary strategy for the prevention of endocarditis.

Rhythm Control

Medical management is of limited use in patients with normal sinus rhythm who are asymptomatic. When symptoms begin, treatment is directed to alleviation of symptoms. Atrial fibrillation occurs in 30% to 40% of patients with mitral stenosis who are symptomatic (Bonow et al., 2008). Calcium channel blockers (diltiazem and verapamil), beta-blockers, or digoxin can be useful in the treatment of atrial fibrillation to maintain a ventricular rate of less than 100 beats per minute because these medications slow conduction through the atrioventricular (AV) node. Because atrial fibrillation is poorly tolerated, it is reasonable to attempt to return the patient to normal sinus rhythm with cardioversion, either electrical or chemical (with medications). Continued use of antiarrhythmics after successful cardioversion to sinus rhythm has proven to be helpful in maintaining a normal rhythm.

Anticoagulation

Anticoagulation is necessary for patients with mitral stenosis and either sustained or intermittent atrial fibrillation. There is controversy in the literature over the benefits of anticoagulation in patients with mitral stenosis and normal sinus rhythm. Patients with mitral stenosis and normal sinus rhythm who have a history of embolic events have experienced some benefits on anticoagulation. Currently, no clinical trials support the use of anticoagulants in patients without a history of embolic events (Bonow et al., 2008).

Beta-blockers

By decreasing contractility, beta-blockers can help decrease ventricular pressure and improve filling from the atria. Decreased heart rate can benefit patients experiencing symptoms from high heart rates during activity. The decrease in heart rate provides a longer diastolic time, resulting in better diastolic filling of the ventricle and emptying of the atrium. Beta-blockers may also help to control atrial fibrillation.

Diuretics

Diuretics and sodium restrictions provide symptomatic support for patients who develop symptoms of extracellular fluid (ECF) overload. These measures reduce volume and, ultimately, venous return to the heart (preload).

Physical Activity and Exercise

Patients with mitral stenosis that is considered to be more than mild should be advised to avoid physical stress. The increase of heart rate decreases the diastolic filling time and will decrease the ability to move blood from the left atrium to the left ventricle. Patients with mitral stenosis (especially moderate to severe) should be instructed to seek medical attention if they have a sudden onset of shortness of breath. Acute pulmonary edema can occur suddenly in these patients, especially with the onset of rapid atrial fibrillation (Bonow et al., 2008).

Surgical Intervention

When the valve area becomes less than 1.5 cm^2, most patients with mitral stenosis begin to experience symptoms at rest and lifestyle is affected. When these symptoms occur, surgical options should be considered.

Mitral Valvotomy

Valvtomy of the mitral valve has better long-term results than that of the aortic valve. In this procedure, a balloon is passed through the valve and inflated, causing the fused leaflets to split. Valvotomy is greatly beneficial to patients with only fusion of the valve commissures. If calcification of the valve is present, the results will be suboptimal. The ACC/AHA guidelines recommend valvotomy as described in Box 10-1. Mitral valvotomy should not be performed on patients who also have mitral regurgitation of 2+ or more because the procedure increases the amount of regurgitation (Bonow et al., 2008). The older adult population is more often suited for valve repair or replacement because their valve morphology is not suited for valvotomy.

Mitral Commissurotomy

As stenosis develops, the commissures (points where valve leaflets come together) begin to fuse together. During mitral commissurotomy, commissures are cut apart to allow for increased movement of the leaflets. This procedure is beneficial to patients with pliable leaflets that have no calcification. ACC/AHA recommendations for mitral valve repair are listed in Box 10-2. Mitral commissurotomy can be performed as a closed heart repair or an open heart repair. However, open-heart repair is becoming the preferred method because the surgeon can visualize the valve and remove calcium deposits as well as left atrial clots (Bonow et al., 2008). Open mitral commissurotomy involves an open-heart procedure requiring the use of cardiac bypass.

Mitral Valve Replacement

Patients with extensive calcification and mitral regurgitation, in addition to stenosis and pulmonary hypertension, are candidates for mitral valve replacement. If the valve is replaced with a mechanical valve, lifelong anticoagulation therapy is required. Anticoagulation therapy is not required if the patient in sinus rhythm receives a bioprosthetic valve. (Chapter 9 includes a more in-depth discussion of valve replacement options.)

Outcomes

As cardiovascular technology and skill continue to advance, patients undergoing valvotomy and open heart commissurotomy continue to experience excellent short- and long-term results (Bonow et al., 2008; Bryg, 2009) Patients who have the correct valve anatomy should undergo valvotomy to avoid the risks associated with bypass surgery. The operative risk for surgery increases with age but continues to remain fairly low (Bonow et al., 2008). Patients begin to experience an improvement in symptoms as soon as the valve is replaced or repaired. There is gradual regression of the pulmonary hypertension over time. An echocardiogram should be completed no sooner than 72 hours after the procedure. Patients should follow up yearly with a physical examination, chest X-ray film, and ECG. Further echocardiograms are only indicated if patients develop recurrent symptoms (Bonow et al., 2008).

All patients after valve replacement (with either a tissue or a mechanical valve) are at high risk for endocarditis and do benefit from endocarditis prophylaxis prior to dental procedures (Bonow et al., 2008; Nishimura et al., 2008; Wilson et al., 2007). Patients with a mechanical valve will be placed on lifelong warfarin therapy. Those with a tissue or bioprosthetic valve may be placed on warfarin for 3 months postoperatively, then switched to lifelong aspirin therapy.

BOX 10-1: ACC/AHA RECOMMENDATIONS FOR MITRAL BALLOON VALVOTOMY

- Patient with moderate or severe mitral stenosis who has symptoms, pliable leaflets, and no atrial clot or significant mitral regurgitation.

- Patient with moderate or severe mitral stenosis who has no symptoms, pliable leaflets, no atrial clot or significant mitral regurgitation, and the presence of pulmonary hypertension (pulmonary artery pressure > 50 mm Hg at rest or > 60 mm Hg with activity).

- Patient with moderate or severe mitral stenosis who has symptoms, no atrial clot or significant mitral regurgitation, and nonpliable calcified valve and who is a high-risk surgical candidate.

(Bonow et al., 2008)

BOX 10-2: ACC/AHA RECOMMENDATIONS FOR MITRAL VALVE REPAIR OR REPLACEMENT

- Patients with moderate or severe mitral stenosis who have symptoms, with no valvotomy available.

- Patients with moderate or severe mitral stenosis who have symptoms, and left atrial clot (despite anticoagulants), or if moderate mitral regurgitation is present.

- Patients with moderate or severe mitral stenosis who have symptoms and calcified valves (decision to repair or replace made during surgery).

(Bonow et al., 2008)

MITRAL VALVE REGURGITATION

Definition

Mitral regurgitation (insufficiency) occurs when a backward flow of blood occurs from the left ventricle to the left atrium during ventricular systole. This backward flow of blood is caused by inadequate closure of the mitral valve.

Causes

Mitral valve prolapse is the most common cause of mitral regurgitation. However, not all patients with mitral valve prolapse have mitral regurgitation. Mitral valve prolapse is a billowing of one or both of the mitral valve leaflets into the left atrium during ventricular systole, with or without regurgitation (Bonow et al., 2008). Young women are most commonly affected by mitral valve prolapse. Mitral valve prolapse can be familial and passed from generation to generation. Patients with Marfan syndrome and other connective tissue diseases also have an increased prevalence of mitral valve prolapse (Bonow et al., 2008; Schoen & Mitchell, 2010).

In addition to mitral valve prolapse, rheumatic heart disease, bacterial endocarditis, ischemic heart disease, left ventricular dilation, and hypertrophic cardiomyopathy are some of the primary causes of mitral regurgitation (Ledoux, 2010). As the incidence of rheumatic heart disease in the United States decreases, so does the incidence of mitral regurgitation. However, rheumatic heart disease is still prevalent in underdeveloped countries.

The causes of mitral regurgitation can be classified as organic or functional (Crawford, 2009). Organic processes are considered to be disease processes that involve the structure of the valve itself. The mitral valve is a unique, complex structure. Normal function of the mitral valve depends on normal valve leaflets, chordae tendineae, and papillary muscles that stretch and contract appropri-

ately, as well as normal ventricular tissue where the papillary muscle attaches to the ventricular wall. Functional abnormalities include changes in other structures that result in changes in valve function. These abnormalities can include left ventricular or left atrial dilation.

Mitral valve prolapse occurs when changes in the valve leaflets and chordae tendineae result in lengthening of the chordae tendineae. The papillary muscle (functioning normally during ventricular systole) contracts. This contraction applies pressure to the chordae tendineae. As contraction occurs, the chordae tendineae pull on the valve leaflets to prevent them from prolapsing into the atria as the force of ventricular contraction and ejection pushes against the leaflets (see Figure 10-1). In mitral valve prolapse, the lengthened chordae tendineae cannot keep the valve leaflet in its proper place and the valve leaflets are forced into the left atrial chamber (see Figure 10-3). Mitral valve prolapse that occurs in young, otherwise healthy women may cause either no regurgitation or only mild mitral regurgitation, with little effect on the heart.

In rheumatic heart disease, the valve leaflets become fibrotic and shorten. Inflammation of the valve from the disease process may also lead to calcification. When marked calcification occurs, the leaflets become very stiff and remain in a fixed open position.

Myocardial infarction (MI) can result in impairment or rupture of a papillary muscle. When the myocardial wall becomes damaged, attachment of the papillary muscle to that ventricular wall can become impaired. As the heart continues to pump, the papillary muscle continues to contract. With each contraction of the papillary muscle, the attachment to the ventricle can weaken. If enough damage to the myocardial wall or papillary muscle has occurred, the papillary muscle can disconnect from the ventricular wall (see Figure 10-4). This results in an acute mitral regurgitation state, and emergency measures are necessary to prevent death.

FIGURE 10-3: MITRAL VALVE PROLAPSE

Clinical Application

Inferior wall MIs greatly increase the risk of acute papillary muscle ruptures. Papillary muscle ruptures generally do not occur at the onset of the infarct but may develop 48 to 72 hours later.

Bacterial invasion of the heart, with the development of endocarditis, can cause chordae tendineae or papillary muscle dysfunction or rupture. Vegetation can also develop on the valve leaflets themselves, disrupting their ability to close properly.

Without damage to the valve leaflets, changes in the size of the left atrium or left ventricle can affect the mitral valve annulus. Dilation of the left ventricle or left atrium can stretch the mitral annulus, preventing the leaflets from closing properly.

Mitral valve regurgitation has a variety of causes; however, the pathophysiological results are the same no matter what the cause. Rather, the development of regurgitation, be it acute or chronic,

FIGURE 10-4: RUPTURED PAPILLARY MUSCLE

changes the clinical picture. Therefore, chronic and acute mitral regurgitation are discussed separately.

CHRONIC MITRAL REGURGITATION

Pathophysiology

During ventricular systole, the contracting left ventricle forces blood forward through the aortic valve. In the presence of mitral regurgitation, some of that forward blood flow is diverted retrograde (backward) through the dysfunctional mitral valve. This retrograde flow decreases the normal stroke volume (forward flow) by the percentage of blood that is diverted backward. As the left atrium continues to fill normally from the pulmonary system, the volume of blood returning through the abnormal mitral valve increases the normal volume of blood in the left atrium. This increase in left atrial volume results in an increase in pressure in the left atrium. The left atrium responds to this increased volume and pressure by dilating. If this dilation is not adequate to handle the increased volume and pressure, the effects are transferred backward to the pulmonary system and pulmonary hypertension develops.

Because the left atrium has a larger volume, the left ventricle ultimately receives this larger volume from the atrium during diastole. The ventricle adjusts to this increased volume by enlarging. Additionally, left ventricular contractions actually may become stronger for a period of time. The purpose of these changes (increase in left ventricular filling and an increase in contraction) is to compensate for the volume of blood that is returned to the atrium with each beat. As ejection occurs, normal stroke volume is ejected forward with the additional volume being returned to the left atrium through the regurgitant valve. This compensatory mechanism functions well for many years, until the myocardial fibers have been stretched beyond their physical limitations and systolic ventricular dysfunction occurs.

Clinical Presentation

Patients with chronic mitral regurgitation remain asymptomatic for many years. As symptoms develop, the patient most frequently reports fatigue and dyspnea, initially on exertion. These symptoms progress to include paroxysmal nocturnal dyspnea, orthopnea, and even palpitations from atrial fibrillation. In many cases, the initial diagnosis of mitral regurgitation is made when patients present with new-onset atrial fibrillation. Patients with mitral valve prolapse early on may report symptoms of tachycardia, orthostatic hypotension, or panic attacks.

Clinical Application

Patients with mitral valve prolapse should avoid caffeine and other stimulants because they can increase the incidence of tachycardia and anxiety attacks.

Physical Examination

The classic murmur of mitral regurgitation is a systolic, blowing, high-pitched murmur that is best heard at the apex of the heart with the diaphragm of the stethoscope. Occasionally, due to the leaflet that is prolapsed, the murmur is louder at the aortic area (second intercostal space, right sternal border). The murmur generally radiates to the axillae but may also be heard over the spine, again depending on the leaflet that is defective. In addition to the murmur, an extra heart sound (S_3) is audible due to the increased left ventricular volume.

Increased heart rate is noted in patients with atrial fibrillation or heart failure. As stroke volume decreases, pulse pressure narrows and the carotid pulse volume may decrease. The apical impulse, normally at the apex, becomes displaced due to dilation of the left ventricle. If the patient is in heart failure, assessment findings may include increased respiratory rate with audible crackles. If left ventricular failure has progressed enough to reflect failure on the right side of the heart, then jugular venous distension, hepatomegaly, and edema will be present.

Clinical Application

When assessing for an S_3 listen at the 5th intercostal space, left midclavicular line with the bell of the stethoscope. Normal S_1 and S_2 sound like "lub dub." When the S_3 is added, it will sound like "lub dub da," "I Believe," or "Kentucky."

Diagnosis

Echocardiogram

Echocardiography is the recommended standard for assessment of mitral valve disease. An echocardiogram can determine left ventricular and left atrial volumes, left atrial ejection fraction, and an approximation of the severity of regurgitation. The cause of the mitral regurgitation is commonly determined during this study. The severity of the disease process will be identified as: mild or 1+, moderate or 2+, and severe or 3 to 4+. Echocardiography is a good baseline study that can be utilized for many years to monitor the progression of the disease.

Cardiac Catheterization

Cardiac catheterization is necessary to determine the presence of coronary artery disease in patients facing mitral valve surgery. Ventricular function and ejection fraction can be assessed as well as pulmonary pressures. However, echocardiography remains the gold standard for this diagnosis.

Chest X-ray Film

An enlarged left atrium and left ventricle are noted on chest X-ray film. If pulmonary hypertension has developed, right ventricular and pulmonary artery enlargement are also present. Patients in a volume overload state show signs of pulmonary edema.

Electrocardiogram

The 12-lead ECG shows evidence of left atrial hypertrophy with abnormal P waves (wide, notched P waves in lead II). Left ventricular hypertrophy is also demonstrated by large QRS complexes with associated ST-segment abnormalities. Atrial fibrillation or ectopic beats may be noted. These ECG changes are neither sensitive nor specific to mitral regurgitation and always require other testing for confirmation.

Medical Therapy

For patients with normal ventricular function who are asymptomatic, no treatment has been found to decrease the progression of the disease process (Bonow et al., 2008; Darovic, 2002). When patients have been diagnosed with mitral valve regurgitation, they should be monitored on a regular basis. The ACC/AHA guidelines recommend an initial echocardiogram and yearly physical exams for patients with mild mitral regurgitation, no symptoms, and no evidence of left ventricular dysfunction or enlargement (Bonow et al., 2008). Patients should be instructed to report any signs of physical deterioration to their physicians. When symptoms develop, an annual or biannual echocardiogram should be completed if moderate or severe mitral regurgitation is present (Bonow et al., 2008).

Clinical Application

Regular follow up for patients with mitral regurgitation becomes important in determining the correct timing for valve replacement. Appropriate timing of replacement can prevent irreversible ventricular damage.

Rhythm Control

Digoxin and beta-blockers can provide ventricular rate control for atrial fibrillation (Moser & Riegel, 2008). Attempting to return the patient to a regular rhythm with cardioversion, either electrical or chemical, is reasonable if the normal guidelines are followed regarding anticoagulation.

Anticoagulation

Anticoagulation therapy is the same as with mitral stenosis. There is some evidence in the literature indicating that the occurrence of embolization in patients with atrial fibrillation and mitral regurgitation is lower than in those with mitral stenosis (Bonow et al., 2008). However, this information should not change the normal treatment patterns.

Endocarditis Prophylaxis

As with mitral stenosis, the new AHA/ACC guidelines note the prophylactic use of antibiotics for patients with native valve disease is no longer recommended (Nishimura et al., 2008; Wilson et al., 2007).

Fluid Control

If the patient exhibits signs of heart failure, a low-sodium diet and fluid restriction may be beneficial. However, liberal salt and water intake can benefit mitral valve prolapse patients who are experiencing orthostatic hypotension.

ACE Inhibitors

If patients are not surgical candidates due to increased risk or a desire not to have surgery, vasodilators, especially angiotensin-converting enzyme (ACE) inhibitors, have been found to be helpful in decreasing regurgitation. ACE inhibitors decrease afterload and preload. The decrease in afterload decreases the resistance to ejection, thereby decreasing regurgitation and allowing blood to move forward. There is no definitive evidence that ACE inhibitors provide any benefit in the patient with mitral regurgitation who does not have symptoms.

Physical Activity and Exercise

Physical activity is not restricted in the patient with asymptomatic mitral regurgitation, a normal left ventricle and atrium, and no signs of pulmonary hypertension.

Surgical Intervention

When symptoms of heart failure develop, surgery should be considered. With careful monitoring of the patient to assess for the development of left ventricular dysfunction, the decision for surgery can be made quickly. If surgical intervention occurs before marked damage, the ventricle can be preserved and pulmonary hypertension should improve. As the severity of left ventricular dysfunction increases, so does operative mortality. Therefore, patients with mild to moderate mitral regurgitation who have no symptoms and an ejection fraction less than 60% are also candidates for surgery (Bonow et al., 2008).

The mitral valve can either be replaced or repaired. The mitral valve is a very complex struc-ture, but preservation of as much of that structure as possible results in good long-term outcomes. Repair is more difficult because, in many cases, structures other than the leaflets require repair. Mitral valve repair surgeries take longer than mitral valve replacement and results in longer cardiopulmonary bypass time. Repairs also require very skilled surgeons. Repaired valves offer patients the opportunity to avoid anticoagulants if they are not in atrial fibrillation and prevent the need for future replacements.

If valve replacement is required, the chordae tendineae and papillary muscles may be left in place and attached to the new valve. Mechanical valves are preferred over bioprosthetic valves for their longevity; however, lifelong anticoagulation is required. Bioprosthetic valves may be appropriate for patients who need to avoid anticoagulation.

Outcomes

Patients who have developed mitral regurgitation due to myocardial ischemia or infarction have a poorer prognosis than others (Crawford, 2009). These patients generally have left ventricular dysfunction from the MI. Patients with rheumatic heart disease have better results, but those with mitral valve prolapse have the best outcomes. As noted with aortic valve disease, when the native valve has been replaced with either a tissue or a mechanical valve, the risk for endocarditis increases and these patients do benefit from endocarditis prophylaxis with antibiotics prior to dental procedures (Wilson et al., 2007). Patients with mechanical valves will be placed on lifelong warfarin therapy. Those with tissue or bioprosthetic valves may be placed on warfarin for 3 months postoperatively, then switched to lifelong aspirin therapy. The literature demonstrates a higher risk for thromboembolism in patients with mechanical mitral valves. For this reason, international normalized ratios (INR) in such patients are maintained at levels that are higher (2.5 to 3.5) than with mechanical valves in other locations.

ACUTE MITRAL REGURGITATION

Pathophysiology

In contrast to the progressive development of chronic mitral regurgitation, acute mitral regurgitation occurs when a sudden event causes the immediate development of mitral regurgitation. In many cases, a papillary muscle tears away from the ventricular wall. With the papillary muscle free, the attached valve leaflet does not close, leaving a gaping hole through which blood ejects.

With each ejection of blood from the ventricle, blood moves to the area of least resistance, or lowest pressure. With only a portion of the mitral valve area closing, a very large volume of blood is ejected retrograde into the atrium and stroke volume is greatly decreased. Decreased stroke volume and, subsequently, decreased cardiac output result in increased systemic vascular resistance (afterload). As the vessels constrict in an attempt to compensate for the decreased forward flow of blood, the resistance against which the ventricle must pump increases. With an increase in systemic vascular resistance, even more blood is ejected retrograde into the atrium and less is available for cardiac output (forward flow).

Clinical Presentation

Because of the acute changes that occur during acute mitral regurgitation, the heart has no time to compensate. With no time for the left atrium to dilate, the pulmonary system quickly becomes overloaded. Pulmonary edema ensues and patients present with acute dyspnea. Blood pressure may initially be normal but quickly deteriorates because the body cannot continue to compensate. Heart rate is rapid, with a decreased pulse amplitude. Cardiac dysrhythmias can develop as perfusion decreases. Patients with acute regurgitation have the same murmur as those with chronic regurgitation. However, a new systolic murmur in an acutely ill patient is a key finding because the patient most likely did not have chronic mitral regurgitation before this event.

Diagnosis

With acute mitral regurgitation, there is usually no time for extensive testing. Therefore, the most reliable diagnostic tools should be utilized. Echocardiogram is the key diagnostic tool in this acute situation. This test quickly identifies the primary valve problem. Cardiac catheterization is indicated when ischemia may be causing the problem. However, patients are rarely stable enough to undergo cardiac catheterization. The decision to use cardiac catheterization should be made based on the patient's stability.

Surgical Intervention

Valve replacement is the treatment of choice and is most often performed urgently. While preparing the patient for surgery, vasodilators may prove helpful. Venous vasodilators decrease preload and, therefore, decrease the volume overload state. More importantly, however, arterial vasodilators decrease systemic vascular resistance, allowing more blood to propel forward. This can be accomplished with such medications as nitroprusside, nitroglycerin, or ACE inhibitors (Leeper, 2009). Intra-aortic balloon pumping is also beneficial in assisting to decrease afterload (Leeper, 2009). Antibiotics are necessary in patients with acute regurgitation to prevent endocarditis. It is always beneficial to provide as many days as possible of antibiotic therapy before surgery if the patient can tolerate waiting; however, if the patient cannot be stabilized, surgery should never be held because of antibiotics.

Outcomes

If surgical valve replacement is successful, patients can do well depending on the cause of the acute event. In patients with acute MI, the outcomes are less promising because it is usually a large infarction that results in papillary muscle rupture. Postoperative follow up is the same as with chronic mitral regurgitation.

CONCLUSION

The mitral valve is an essential part of the functioning heart. Abnormal valve function causes the heart to make adjustments in an attempt to compensate. Over time, these adjustments have detrimental effects. In many cases, the first inkling of valve disease comes through the ears of a cognizant healthcare professional. Early recognition of cardiac murmurs can result in the chance to educate patients early in the disease process so intervention can be taken before it is too late.

A major challenge in caring for patients with valvular heart disease is that they are often asymptomatic with a long latent period before the development of lifestyle limiting symptoms. This type of heart disease does not lend itself to the degree of therapeutic nursing interventions and patient counseling associated with such conditions as heart failure and acute coronary syndrome. However, nursing knowledge and skill related to heart sound assessment is important in the identification of murmurs before the development of symptomatic disease. Additionally, valvular heart disease frequently occurs in the presence of other forms of heart disease and can complicate the care of patients with such conditions as heart failure and acute coronary syndrome. Nursing knowledge of the physiological changes associated with valvular heart disease can aide in the effective management of these patients. Finally, valvular abnormalities are mechanical problems that need intervention when the patient reaches the point of symptom development. Educating patients on reportable signs and symptoms is a high priority to assure timely surgical intervention.

EXAM QUESTIONS

CHAPTER 10
Questions 79-85

Note: Choose the one option that BEST answers each question.

79. The heart's compensatory response to the chronic increase in left atrial pressure from mitral stenosis is

    a. increased ventricular contractility.

    b. increased left ventricular wall thickness.

    c. hypertrophy of the left atrium.

    d. loss of atrial kick.

80. Symptoms of mitral stenosis at rest generally occur after the valve orifice is

    a. greater than 2.5 cm^2.

    b. 2 cm^2 to 2.5 cm^2.

    c. 1.5 cm^2 to 1.9 cm^2.

    d. less than 1.5 cm^2.

81. The development of rapid heart rates with exercise in patients with mitral stenosis can be detrimental. The class of medications that can help control heart rate, even with exercise, is

    a. beta-blockers.

    b. ACE.

    c. angiotensin receptor blockers.

    d. class III antiarrhythmics.

82. The most common form of mitral regurgitation is

    a. rheumatic heart disease.

    b. mitral valve prolapse.

    c. mitral valve insufficiency.

    d. bacterial endocarditis.

83. When assessing heart sounds in a patient with symptomatic mitral regurgitation, the examiner can expect to find

    a. diastolic murmur and an S$_4$.

    b. systolic murmur and an S$_4$.

    c. diastolic murmur and an S$_3$.

    d. systolic murmur and an S$_3$.

84. If a patient with mitral regurgitation is not a candidate for surgical valve replacement, the class of medication that can be helpful in decreasing regurgitation by reducing afterload is

    a. beta-blockers.

    b. ACE inhibitors.

    c. diuretics.

    d. digoxin.

85. Forty-eight hours after diagnosis, a hospitalized patient with an inferior wall MI reports that he suddenly started to have difficulty breathing. During your assessment, you notice acute dyspnea and a rapid heart rate. You also discover a new systolic murmur that was not present during an earlier assessment. As you call the physician, you anticipate that, with the timing of the onset of these symptoms, the patient most likely has a

    a. pericardial effusion.

    b. pulmonary embolism.

    c. papillary muscle rupture.

    d. recurrent myocardial infarction.

CHAPTER 11

ATRIAL FIBRILLATION

CHAPTER OBJECTIVE

After completing this chapter, the learner will be able to discuss the implications and current management strategies of atrial fibrillation.

LEARNING OBJECTIVES

After completing this chapter, the learner will be able to

1. describe the difference between atrial fibrillation and the normal heart rhythm of sinus rhythm.

2. list several acute and temporary causes of atrial fibrillation.

3. define paroxysmal, persistent, and permanent atrial fibrillation.

4. contrast the pathophysiology of paroxysmal atrial fibrillation with persistent and permanent atrial fibrillation.

5. describe the major complications associated with atrial fibrillation.

6. define the difference between ventricular rate control and rhythm control in atrial fibrillation.

7. define the unique side effects and special nursing considerations associated with amiodarone therapy.

8. discuss the importance of anticoagulation prior to cardioversion.

INTRODUCTION

Atrial fibrillation is rapid, chaotic activity of the atria, resulting in the deterioration of atrial mechanical activity. This rapid, unorganized atrial activity produces irregular atrial fibrillation waves with an atrial rate greater than 350 beats per minute. Atrial fibrillation is the most common of all sustained cardiac dysrhythmias. The prevalence of atrial fibrillation increases as the population ages. In the United States, atrial fibrillation affects more than 2.2 million people annually (Rosenthal & McManus, 2008).

In a normal rhythm, the sinoatrial (SA) node acts as the heart's pacemaker. The electrical impulse then travels through the right and left atria, depolarizing both atria before it reaches the atrioventricular (AV) node. After conduction passes through the AV node, it passes down both bundle branches to the Purkinje fibers, depolarizing both ventricles. On an electrocardiogram (ECG), sinus rhythm is identified by a P wave, representing atrial depolarization, followed by a QRS complex, representing ventricular depolarization. Figure 11-1 shows a normal sinus beat. Figure 11-2 shows consecutive sinus beats, or a regular sinus rhythm. In atrial fibrillation, the P wave on the ECG is replaced with atrial fibrillation waves (see Figure 11-3).

Atrial fibrillation has variable ventricular conduction, resulting in an irregularly irregular ventricular rhythm (also seen in Figure 11-3). In atrial fibrillation, the AV node is bombarded with atrial depolarization waves and, when AV nodal conduction is intact, a very rapid ventricular response rate can result. A slow ventricular response in the presence of untreated atrial fibrillation is a sign of an underlying conduction abnormality.

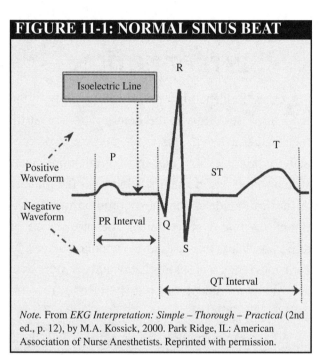

FIGURE 11-1: NORMAL SINUS BEAT

Note. From *EKG Interpretation: Simple – Thorough – Practical* (2nd ed., p. 12), by M.A. Kossick, 2000. Park Ridge, IL: American Association of Nurse Anesthetists. Reprinted with permission.

Clinical Application

It is important to remember that atrial fibrillation is not the only cause of an irregular rhythm, so an irregular pulse alone cannot be used to diagnose atrial fibrillation. Also, a patient in atrial fibrillation with an implanted pacemaker may have a regular ventricular response and, therefore, a regular pulse; however, atrial fibrillation remains the underlying rhythm.

An ECG reading in at least one lead is necessary to confirm the presence of atrial fibrillation waves for proper diagnosis of atrial fibrillation.

CAUSES

There are many acute and temporary noncardiopulmonary causes of atrial fibrillation, including surgery, hyperthyroidism, electrocution, and alcohol use. Acute cardiopulmonary causes include pulmonary embolism, myocardial infarction (MI), myocarditis, pericarditis, and cardiac or thoracic surgery (Fuster et al., 2011; Rosenthal & McManus, 2008).

FIGURE 11-2: REGULAR SINUS RHYTHM

FIGURE 11-3: ATRIAL FIBRILLATION

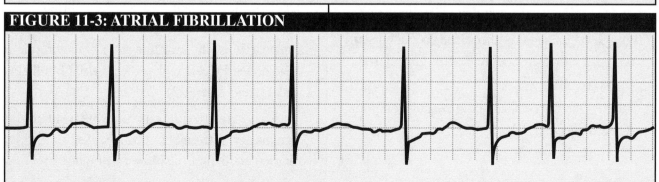

The incidence of atrial fibrillation increases with age, and atrial fibrillation is commonly associated with chronic cardiovascular conditions, including mitral valve stenosis, hypertension, heart failure, cardiomyopathy, coronary heart disease (CHD), and Wolff-Parkinson-White (WPW) syndrome (Fuster et al., 2011; Rosenthal & McManus, 2008). Lung pathology in chronic lung disease is also a common cause of atrial fibrillation because increased pulmonary pressures cause an increase in right ventricular work and right ventricular enlargement. Eventually, the right atrium is also affected, increasing the risk for atrial dysrhythmias.

CLASSIFICATIONS

Atrial fibrillation can be classified by more than one method. The first classification involves determining if the atrial fibrillation is a first occurrence (single episode) or if it is recurrent (two or more episodes). Atrial fibrillation can also be classified as paroxysmal, persistent, or permanent (Fuster et al., 2011). Paroxysmal atrial fibrillation comes on spontaneously and terminates itself. To be classified as paroxysmal, atrial fibrillation cannot last longer than 7 days, and it usually lasts less than 24 hours. Persistent atrial fibrillation is defined by a rhythm that lasts longer than 7 days. Both paroxysmal and persistent atrial fibrillation can be seen with first time presentation. They can also both be recurrent. Permanent atrial fibrillation is diagnosed when the rhythm is accepted as permanent or when it lasts longer than one year. Further attempts to restore sinus rhythm are not indicated in permanent atrial fibrillation.

Classifications of Atrial Fibrillation Based on Pathophysiology

Lone Atrial Fibrillation

Lone atrial fibrillation is defined as atrial fibrillation in patients with normal cardiac and pulmonary function and with no known predisposing factors. Patients must also be younger than 60 years of age and not have hypertension.

Nonvalvular Atrial Fibrillation

Nonvalvular atrial fibrillation refers to atrial fibrillation in patients without rheumatic heart (mitral valve) disease, a prosthetic valve, or history of valve repair.

Rheumatic heart disease results in mitral stenosis, which increases the risk for atrial fibrillation because the left atrium enlarges as a result of contracting against the stenotic mitral valve.

Neurogenic Atrial Fibrillation

Neurogenic atrial fibrillation accounts for atrial fibrillation in a small number of patients. In these patients, either increased vagal tone or increased adrenergic tone triggers the onset of atrial fibrillation.

PATHOPHYSIOLOGY

Atrial fibrillation can start with a premature atrial contraction (PAC), an ectopic beat (beat beginning outside the SA node). This PAC is usually the source of paroxysmal atrial fibrillation. Premature atrial beats are usually caused by trigger beats coming from one or more of the superior pulmonary veins located near the junction of the left atrium (Rosenthal & McManus, 2008). These trigger beats occur because of enhanced automaticity of the tissue. Other sources for ectopic beats triggering paroxysmal atrial fibrillation include the right atrium and, less commonly, the superior vena cava or coronary sinus.

Structural disease of the atria is usually responsible for maintaining atrial fibrillation, such that occurs in persistent and permanent atrial fibrillation. The existence of atrial fibrillation contributes to the development of the structural damage of the atria, with the end result being atrial scarring, fibrosis, and myopathy. Various pathological processes are thought to be involved in the development of these structural changes, including inflammation, fatty infiltration, atrial hypertrophy, and progressive atrial dilation (Fuster et al., 2011). Atrial hypertrophy and progressive atrial dilation can be either a cause or a consequence of atrial fibrillation. Pathological changes, such as fibrosis of the atria, occur with aging and may explain the increased incidence of atrial fibrillation in the older adult population (Folkeringa, Tieleman, & Crijns, 2004). In patients with structural disease of the atria, a reentrant mechanism, rather than a focal ectopic mechanism, is usually responsible for the maintenance of atrial fibrillation. Reentrant mechanisms in atrial fibrillation can involve many microcircuits.

SYMPTOMS

Symptoms of atrial fibrillation are commonly related to the fast ventricular rate. The duration of the episode of atrial fibrillation also impacts the symptoms. If the entricular rate is controlled and the patient is still symptomatic, symptoms are related to the loss of atrial kick. Patients who already have decreased ventricular function experience more symptoms from loss of atrial kick than those with normal left ventricular function. Common symptoms of atrial fibrillation include palpitations, dyspnea, fatigue, light-headedness, diaphoresis, and chest pain. Patients in atrial fibrillation may also experience polyuria due to the increased release of atrial natriuretic peptide from overstimulation of the atria (Fuster et al., 2011).

Many patients with atrial fibrillation are asymptomatic. These patients are at risk for developing tachycardia-induced cardiomyopathy from poor ventricular rate control. These patients may also present for the first time with more serious complications, such as stroke or heart failure.

Clinical Application

Patients who present with symptoms of stroke or transient ischemic attack (TIA) should be assessed for the presence of asymptomatic, undiagnosed atrial fibrillation.

When patients experience hemodynamic compromise due to atrial fibrillation, then more serious symptoms, such as syncope and pulmonary edema, can occur. Syncope is a rare symptom and usually indicates additional underlying pathology compromising cardiac output, such as aortic valve stenosis or hypertrophic obstructive cardiomyopathy (HOCM).

COMPLICATIONS

Atrial fibrillation is rarely immediately life threatening but does cause long-term complications. The two major complications associated with atrial fibrillation are hemodynamic compromise and an increased risk of thromboembolic events, particularly stroke.

Stroke

Patients with atrial fibrillation are at increased risk for thromboembolism because of an increased risk of thrombus formation in the left atrium and left atrial appendage. Embolization of a thrombus in the left atrium or left atrial appendage can cause stroke. Patients in atrial fibrillation may also have other independent risk factors for stroke. Those at highest risk are those with:

- hypertension
- previous stroke or TIA
- diabetes mellitus
- heart failure
- moderate to severe left ventricular systolic dysfunction
- age greater than 65 years.

(Fuster et al., 2011)

Patients in atrial fibrillation who are younger than 60 years of age and who have no existing cardiac or pulmonary disease (lone atrial fibrillation) are at the lowest risk for stroke. Patients with atrial fibrillation with rheumatic heart disease have an even higher risk of stroke than those with nonvalvular heart disease (Fuster et al., 2011).

In patients with atrial fibrillation, thrombi most commonly form in the left atrial appendage and are the source of clots in stroke. In atrial fibrillation, the velocity of blood flow through the left atrium and left atrial appendage is decreased. This decrease in velocity increases the risk of thrombus formation. Atrial fibrillation is commonly diagnosed for the first time in patients presenting with new thrombotic stroke. Prevention of thrombotic complications is a major goal in the treatment of atrial fibrillation.

Patients in permanent atrial fibrillation require lifelong warfarin therapy to decrease the risk of stroke. Warfarin has been shown to substantially reduce the risk of stroke in patients with atrial fibrillation (Rosenthal & McManus, 2008). Dabigatran (an oral direct thrombin inhibitor) is another option for anticoagulation to reduce stroke risk in select patients with non-valvular atrial fibrillation. Antiplatelet therapy alone, such as aspirin or clopidogrel, is not generally used for stroke prevention in patients with atrial fibrillation. In certain young patients with lone atrial fibrillation and no other stroke risk factors, antiplatelet therapy may be used (Dresing & Schweikert, 2009).

Age is an important risk factor for the development of stroke with atrial fibrillation. All patients older than 65 years of age should be anticoagulated with warfarin unless contraindicated (Rosenthal & McManus, 2008). Unfortunately, older adult patients have an increased risk of bleeding complications from oral anticoagulation and are less likely to receive therapy with warfarin. Aspirin therapy should be considered in older patients with contraindications to warfarin therapy.

In patients receiving oral anticoagulation for stroke prevention, the international normalized ratio (INR) should be between 2 and 3. If a patient needs anticoagulation for another reason, such as a prosthetic valve, the INR may need to be higher.

The INR is checked at least weekly during the initiation phase. After the INR is therapeutic and stable, it can be reassessed monthly. Aspirin is used only in young, low-risk patients or as an alternative for patients with contraindications to oral anticoagulation. Patients in atrial flutter have the same antithrombotic prevention strategies as those in atrial fibrillation.

Hemodynamic Complications

Hemodynamic complications of atrial fibrillation are associated with rapid ventricular rate, irregular ventricular response, and loss of atrial contraction (kick). Atrial fibrillation can cause a loss in cardiac output of up to 20% because atrial contraction is lost. People become more dependent on atrial kick with age. Loss of atrial kick can lead to increased left atrial pressure and, in turn, can lead to increased pulmonary pressure. The irregularity of the R-R interval (irregularity of the QRS complexes) within the cardiac rhythm also adversely impacts hemodynamic performance.

Some patients are at high risk for experiencing a substantial decrease in cardiac output with atrial fibrillation. These patients have conditions that impair diastolic filling at baseline, including mitral stenosis, hypertrophic cardiomyopathy (HCM), restrictive cardiomyopathy (RCM), and hypertension with diastolic dysfunction.

Another long-term complication of atrial fibrillation is the development of ventricular dilated cardiomyopathy from an accelerated ventricular rate. This complication is also called tachycardia-induced cardiomyopathy. Control of ventricular rate can lead to complete or partial reversal of this complication.

TREATMENT CONSIDERATIONS

If a patient presents with an initial episode of paroxysmal (self-terminating) atrial fibrillation, no additional treatment may be needed. If paroxysmal atrial fibrillation is recurrent and the patient is symptomatic, then antidysrhythmic therapy may be prescribed to keep the patient in sinus rhythm or to limit the number of episodes. If the patient has continued paroxysmal episodes, then rate control medication and antithrombotic medication may also be given.

Historically, the goal of treatment in atrial fibrillation has been to restore and maintain sinus rhythm; however, this is now controversial. New research compares the benefits of rhythm control (restoration and maintenance of sinus rhythm) and rate control (allowing atrial fibrillation but controlling the rate and treating with antithrombotic therapy). For example, the AFFIRM trial compared rate control to rhythm control in patients with atrial fibrillation and found no survival benefit in the rhythm control treatment arm (Wyse et al., 2002). Ongoing research and current controversy continue regarding the optimum treatment strategies for those in atrial fibrillation.

When patients first present with persistent atrial fibrillation, a decision must be made between these two treatment arms. The maintenance of sinus rhythm generally requires the use of antiarrhythmic pharmacology, so the benefits of sinus rhythm have to be weighed against the adverse or toxic effects of antiarrhythmic medications. For this reason, rate control may be considered acceptable in patients who are not symptomatic. Whether patients with no symptoms benefit from cardioversion is currently a topic of debate. If symptoms of atrial fibrillation are present with effective rate control, then cardioversion is attempted.

Rate Control

It is very important to control the ventricular rate in atrial fibrillation to avoid the development of tachycardia-induced cardiomyopathy. Without proper rate control in atrial fibrillation, ventricular rate can be rapid. Ventricular rate is considered controlled when it is between 60 and 100 beats per minute at rest, and between 90 and 115 beats per minute with moderate exercise (Fuster et al., 2011). Rate control is accomplished by medications that slow conduction through the AV node, including beta-blockers, nondihydropyridine calcium channel blockers (verapamil and diltiazem), and digoxin. Nondihydropyridine calcium channel blockers and beta-blockers are the most commonly used medications for rate control in atrial fibrillation. In patients with heart failure, digoxin or amiodarone can be used to control ventricular rate. In patients with the presence of an accessory pathway (WPW syndrome), special considerations must be taken when using medications to slow ventricular rate. These considerations are discussed at the end of this chapter.

Patients with paroxysmal atrial fibrillation who receive rate-control medications may experience sinus bradycardia or heart block as a complication when they are in a normal sinus rhythm. Other patients may develop too slow of a ventricular response and become symptomatic, even while in atrial fibrillation. These patients may require insertion of a permanent pacemaker to maintain a minimum ventricular rate (prevent sinus bradycardia and heart block) while on sufficient doses of medications to control the ventricular rate.

If medication therapy does not adequately control ventricular rate, the AV node can be ablated. AV node ablation results in complete heart block and requires the placement of a permanent pacemaker. Although this strategy can be helpful in preventing tachycardia-induced cardiomyopathy, it has potential downsides. Because atrial fibrillation remains the underlying rhythm, the patient needs continued anticoagulation. With ablation of the AV node, permanent loss of AV synchrony occurs and the patient has continued pacemaker dependence.

Many patients who have experienced at least one unsuccessful attempt to restore and maintain their rhythm to sinus rhythm (rhythm control) are left in atrial fibrillation with appropriate rate control and continuous antithrombotic therapy.

Clinical Application

Diltiazem is commonly used for rate control in patients with atrial fibrillation and rapid ventricular response. It is important to remember that in decompensated heart failure, diltiazem should not be the drug of choice for ventricular rate control because it may worsen the patient's hemodynamic status.

Rhythm Control

Potential benefits of restoring sinus rhythm include prevention of thrombus formation, prevention of atrial myopathy, and relief of the patient's symptoms. When a patient presents for the first time with persistent atrial fibrillation and the decision is made to restore and maintain sinus rhythm, cardioversion (electrical or pharmacological) is performed. A patient who has been in atrial fibrillation for longer than 48 hours will need special considerations to prevent an embolic complication of the cardioversion. (This is discussed in the section on cardioversion.) For the first cardioversion, antiarrhythmic drug therapy generally is not used unless the patient has been in atrial fibrillation for longer than 3 months (Fuster et al., 2011).

If the first cardioversion is unsuccessful or if there is early recurrence of atrial fibrillation, repeat electrical cardioversion with antiarrhythmic drug therapy is performed. The use of antiarrhythmic drug therapy with electrical cardioversion increases the long-term success rate. However, all antiarrhythmic medications, including those used for pharmacological cardioversion and those used to maintain sinus rhythm, have the potential for toxic side effects.

Antiarrhythmic Medications

Antiarrhythmic agents are used in the treatment of atrial fibrillation. These agents are assessed by their classifications and also by their roles in the pharmaco-

logical cardioversion of atrial fibrillation and the maintenance of sinus rhythm. According to the Vaughan Williams Classification System, antiarrhythmic drugs can be grouped into four classifications.

Class II medications are beta-blockers and class IV medications are calcium channel blockers. These medications have been discussed in Chapter 3. Their role in the treatment of atrial fibrillation is primarily that of rate control by slowing conduction through the AV node. Beta-blockers may also be used to help maintain sinus rhythm in lone atrial fibrillation and prevent recurrence of atrial fibrillation due to adrenergic stimulation. Beta-blockers work by blocking the sympathetic nervous system and are the only group of medications in this classification system that do not affect the cardiac action potential.

Class I antiarrhythmic agents are sometimes called sodium channel blockers because they work in the fast sodium channel of the cardiac action potential. Class I agents have three distinct subgroups: Class Ia, Ib, and Ic. Class III agents are sometimes called potassium channel blockers because they work by blocking the influx of potassium during the cardiac action potential. Both class I and class III antiarrhythmic medications have serious potential side effects and, therefore, require careful nursing assessment and patient education. The term *antiarrhythmic medication* or *antiarrhythmic therapy* refers to medications in class I or III of this system. Table 11-1 outlines antiarrhythmics used in the management of atrial fibrillation.

One of the dangerous side effects of the class I and III medications used in the treatment of atrial fibrillation is the development of ventricular dysrhythmias, such as torsades de pointes, polymorphic or monomorphic ventricular tachycardia, or ventricular fibrillation. Medications with this potential are called *proarrhythmic.*

Torsades de pointes is a particular type of ventricular dysrhythmia that can occur in the presence of a long QT interval. The QT interval is measured from the beginning of the QRS complex to the end

TABLE 11-1: ANTIARRHYTHMICS (BY VAUGHAN WILLIAMS CLASSIFICATION) USED IN ATRIAL FIBRILLATION

Class	Specific Medications	Purpose of Medication	Major Cardiac Side Effects
Class Ia	Disopyramide Procainamide Quinidine	Rhythm control Rhythm control Rhythm control	Torsades de pointes, heart failure Torsades de pointes Torsades de pointes
Class Ib	Not used in atrial fibrillation		
Class Ic	Flecainide Propafenone	Rhythm control Rhythm control	Ventricular tachycardia, heart failure, atrial flutter Ventricular tachycardia, heart failure, atrial flutter
Class II	Beta-blockers	Rate control	
Class III	Amiodarone* Dronedarone* Dofetilide Ibutilide Sotalol* (also contains Dronedarone beta-blocker)	Rhythm control Rhythm control Rhythm control Rhythm control Rhythm control	Torsades de pointes (rare), extracardiac organ toxicity Torsades de pointes Torsades de pointes Torsades de pointes Torsades de pointes, heart failure, beta-blocker side effects
Class IV	Calcium channel blockers	Rate control	

* *Note:* Additional rate control component
(Fuster et al., 2011)

of the T wave. (Figure 11-1 points out the QT interval in a normal beat.) Class Ia and III agents place the patient at particular risk for torsades de pointes due to their potential for increasing the QT interval. Class Ia agents delay depolarization and prolong the QRS, whereas class III agents delay repolarization and prolong the T-wave. Both actions have the end result of prolonging the QT interval. Figure 11-4 illustrates the effect of class I and class III antiarrhythmic agents on the cardiac action potential. For this reason, most of these medications are initiated only in a hospital setting, where the patient can be monitored with a cardiac monitor. Some antiarrhythmic medications also have atrial proarrhythmic effects and can potentially promote conversion of the atrial dysrhythmia to atrial flutter. For example, flecainide and propafenone have the potential to induce atrial flutter when they are used for the pharmacological cardioversion of atrial fib-

rillation (Fuster et al., 2011). Because of the high side effect profile of all antiarrhythmic medications, any reversible causes of atrial fibrillation should be eliminated before medications are initiated.

Amiodarone is a class III antiarrhythmic with unique considerations. Although effective, it has the potential to cause the development of extracardiac organ toxicity, including thyroid dysfunction, polyneuropathy, and liver and pulmonary toxicity (Gold Standard/Elsevier, 2010). One of the most dangerous side effects is a potentially lethal interstial pneumonitis that results in irreversible pulmonary fibrosis (Gold Standard/Elsevier, 2010). Patients taking amiodarone should have a baseline pulmonary function study and chest radiographs every 3 to 6 months. Liver function studies are also monitored on a regular basis. Because the toxic effects are cumulative and dose related, the use of amiodarone is reserved for carefully selected patients who are not

FIGURE 11-4: EFFECT OF CLASS I, III, AND IV ANTIARRHYTHMIA AGENTS ON CARDIAC ACTION POTENTIAL

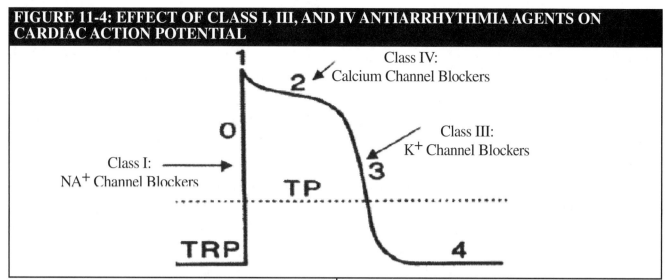

suited for other treatments. Patients who take amiodarone should receive the lowest effective dose.

Patients with heart failure are sensitive to the proarrhythmic effects of drugs; therefore, not all antiarrhythmic drugs are safe in patients with heart failure. Amiodarone is a safer medication in the presence of heart failure or considerable left ventricular hypertrophy because, although it does increase the QT interval, it rarely causes torsades de pointes. Dronedarone, a newer class III antiarrhythmic, is used to decrease hospitalizations in patients with atrial fibrillation. There are less extra cardiac side effects compared to amiodarone (Chan, Nallamothu, & Oral, 2009). It should not be administered to patients with class IV heart failure or those who have had decompensated heart failure in the past 4 weeks, especially if they have depressed left ventricular function (Fuster et al., 2011).

Clinical Application

Amiodarone is generally not used in young patients because the risk of toxicity is cumulative and increases with the length of therapy.

Cardioversion

Most cardioversions are performed electively. (Special considerations for emergency cardioversions are discussed at the end of this chapter.) When the decision is made to restore a patient's rhythm to sinus rhythm, the choice between electri-

cal and pharmacological cardioversion must be made. Pharmacological cardioversion is most effective in patients presenting with their first episode of atrial fibrillation that has lasted 7 days or less. Whether pharmacological or electrical cardioversion is chosen, the patient's heart rate should be controlled prior to elective cardioversion. Patients who are in atrial fibrillation longer than 48 hours require anticoagulation prior to cardioversion to decrease the risk of stroke. If a patient presents with atrial fibrillation of an onset less than 48 hours, then the decision to anticoagulate prior to cardioversion is based on the patient's other risk factors for thrombus formation.

The risk of thrombotic stroke is the same for electrical and pharmacological cardioversion (Rosenthal & McManus, 2008). Two approaches to anticoagulation can be taken prior to cardioversion. Patients can be started on warfarin and wait until the INR is between 2 and 3 for a minimum of 3 consecutive weeks. If waiting for a therapeutic INR for this period of time is not desirable, patients can be anticoagulated with heparin and have a transesophageal echocardiogram (TEE) to rule out thrombi in the left atrium or left atrial appendage. After thrombi are ruled out by TEE, then cardioversion can be performed.

TEE is used to assess for atrial thrombi because the left atrial appendage, a common site for thrombi formation, is not well visualized using transthoracic echocardiography. Patients who have been anticoagulated with heparin prior to cardioversion should remain on heparin until the INR is in a therapeutic range. Anticoagulation with warfarin should continue for a period of time, even after successful cardioversion. After cardioversion (spontaneous, electrical, or pharmacological), the left atrium experiences a period of mechanical dysfunction (stunning) that lasts for several weeks. Thrombi can still form during this period of mechanical dysfunction, and emboli can be released when mechanical function returns to normal (Fuster et al., 2011). Patients need to continue on anticoagulation for a minimum of 4 weeks after cardioversion to prevent thrombus formation. Even patients with no thrombi on TEE prior to cardioversion have the possibility of developing thrombi and emboli after cardioversion.

Direct Current Cardioversion

In direct current (DC) cardioversion, the electrical shock is synchronized with the intrinsic activity of the heart. DC cardioversion is different from the delivery of a desynchronized shock (defibrillation) in the treatment of pulseless ventricular tachycardia or ventricular fibrillation. Most cardioversions are performed with the two paddles placed in the anterior (sternum) and posterior (left scapular area) positions. Defibrillators using a biphasic waveform require lower levels of energy, fewer shocks, and result in better outcomes. Therefore, cardioversion with biphasic waveform is the current standard for cardioversion (Fuster et al., 2011). DC cardioversion is performed with the use of short-acting anesthetic agents or with agents to induce conscious sedation; therefore, the patient must be given nothing by mouth prior to the procedure (Fuster et al., 2011). Personnel skilled in airway management must be present and the patient should be monitored with a cardiac monitor and pulse oximetry. Emergency equipment must be readily available, including oxygen, suction, intu-

bation supplies, and other emergency medications and equipment. Standard hospital policies are followed, as with all patients receiving anesthesia or conscious sedation. Short-term cardiac dysrhythmias are a potential complication of cardioversion. Patients are monitored on a cardiac monitor for a period of time after cardioversion to observe for dysrhythmias. Patients with hypokalemia or digoxin toxicity are at increased risk for developing serious ventricular dysrhythmias after cardioversion. Electrolyte abnormalities should be corrected prior to cardioversion.

Clinical Application

Potassium levels and digoxin levels (for patients on digoxin) should be assessed prior to elective cardioversion.

The initial success rate of cardioversion is much higher than the long-term success rate. If the patient has an early relapse into atrial fibrillation, then repeat cardioversion using preprocedure antiarrhythmic drug therapy can help reduce the rate of recurrent atrial fibrillation. Patients with permanent pacemakers or implantable cardioverter-defibrillators (ICDs) can safely be cardioverted out of atrial fibrillation. The paddles should be placed away from the device to avoid damage, and the device is interrogated before and after the procedure to assure correct functioning.

Pharmacological Cardioversion

The advantage of pharmacological cardioversion is there is no need for sedation of the patient. In addition, some patients are not comfortable with DC cardioversion and prefer pharmacological cardioversion. Medications proven effective in pharmacological cardioversion are listed in Box 11-1. Not all of these medications are approved or labeled for this use in the United States (Fuster et al., 2011). Other antiarrhythmic agents can be used to maintain sinus rhythm after successful cardioversion has occurred.

BOX 11-1: DRUGS PROVEN MOST EFFECTIVE FOR PHARMACOLOGICAL CARDIOVERSION OF ATRIAL FIBRILLATION

Dofetilide

Flecainide

Ibutilide

Propafenone

Note: All of these drugs have a class 1 recommendation for the cardioversion of atrial fibrillation with a duration of less than or equal to 7 days. Dofetilide also has a class 1 recommendation for the cardioversion of atrial fibrillation with a duration greater than 7 days.

(Fuster et al., 2011)

Use of Pharmacological Agents to Maintain Sinus Rhythm

Pharmacology is used to maintain sinus rhythm in patients with recurrent paroxysmal atrial fibrillation or after cardioversion in patients with persistent atrial fibrillation. Because of the chronic nature of atrial fibrillation, most patients are likely to have a recurrence if not treated with antiarrhythmic therapy. Patients who are older, have been in atrial fibrillation longer, and who have underlying heart disease are at risk for increased recurrent episodes. Even with antiarrhythmic therapy, many patients experience a relapse. A relapse does not necessarily indicate treatment failure. Antiarrhythmic therapy that controls the frequency and severity of occurrences may be considered a success.

Before antiarrhythmic drug therapy is used to maintain sinus rhythm, it is important to identify and treat any reversible causes. Due to potential toxic side effects, antiarrhythmic therapy is typically not used in treating the first episode of atrial fibrillation or in treating infrequent episodes of paroxysmal atrial fibrillation that produce tolerable symptoms. Box 11-2 lists medications used to maintain sinus rhythm.

BOX 11-2: MEDICATIONS USED TO MAINTAIN SINUS RHYTHM IN PATIENTS WITH ATRIAL FIBRILLATION

Amiodarone	Procainamide
Disopyramide	Propafenone
Dofetilide	Quinidine
Flecainide	Sotalol

(Fuster et al., 2011)

Listed in Table 11-2 are first-line medications for maintenance of sinus rhythm in special patient populations. Second- and third-line agents are not discussed. All medication decisions are based on individual patient characteristics. In addition, if a single drug therapy fails, combination therapy may be used.

Permanent Pacemaker Insertion

Permanent pacemaker insertion is required after any ablation of the AV node. Implantation of a permanent pacemaker may also be used for more aggressive medication administration for rate control. Pacemakers inserted in patients with atrial fibrillation have mode-switching capability to change modes when the patient enters into atrial fibrillation. The purpose of a mode-switching pacemaker is to avoid a rapid pacing response to the sensing of rapid atrial activity. Ventricular pacing during atrial fibrillation can also provide symptomatic relief by providing a regular ventricular response.

In patients who receive permanent pacemakers for reasons other than atrial fibrillation, atrial pacing (as opposed to ventricular pacing), has reduced the occurrence of atrial fibrillation (Fuster et al., 2011). Atrial pacing was thus thought to be a potential primary strategy for atrial fibrillation prevention. Atrial pacing, however, has not been proven to prevent the development of atrial fibrillation when used as a primary strategy. Pacemaker devices can also be programmed to perform overdrive pacing in response to episodes of atrial fibrillation. The goal

TABLE 11-2: MEDICATIONS USED TO MAINTAIN SINUS RHYTHM IN SPECIAL PATIENT POPULATIONS	
Special Patient Population Description	**Medication Used to Maintain Sinus Rhythm**
Lone atrial fibrillation	Flecainide Propafenone Sotalol Beta-blockers
Neurogenic atrial fibrillation	Disopyramide or flecainide (for vagal induced) Beta-blockers or sotalol (for adrenergic induced)
Atrial fibrillation in heart failure	Amiodarone (less proarrhythmic effects) Dofetilide
Atrial fibrillation in CHD	Sotalol (beta-blocking properties)
Atrial fibrillation in hypertensive heart disease with left ventricular hypertrophy	Propafenone (class Ic - does not prolong QT interval) Flecainide (class Ic - does not prolong QT interval) Amiodarone (with significant hypertrophy)

(Fuster et al., 2011)

of therapy is to override the atrial fibrillation with a paced rhythm.

Atrial Defibrillators

Atrial defibrillators are approved but not widely used. Unlike with ICDs (which shock patients out of life-threatening ventricular dysrhythmias), most patients are not willing to receive a cardioversion shock for non-life-threatening atrial fibrillation. Attempts have been made to find a shock waveform that can successfully cardiovert atrial fibrillation and be tolerated by a conscious patient. Limitations of this technology still prevent it from being frequently used.

Maze Surgical Procedure

The Maze surgical procedure is commonly performed in patients with symptomatic atrial fibrillation undergoing open heart surgery for another reason. The addition of the Maze procedure to another open heart surgical procedure increases the risk of surgery. The Maze procedure involves making a series of incisions in the atria using radiofrequency or some other form of energy. Incisions are made to block reentrant pathways within the atrial tissue and to channel conduction in a more normal fashion. The barriers created by the incisions limit the

amount of myocardium available to sustain the reentrant circuits. The pulmonary veins can also be electrically isolated during the Maze procedure. Because the procedure is so invasive, it is seldom done as a stand-alone surgery. If done alone, the complications of the Maze procedure are similar to other procedures involving a median sternotomy and cardiopulmonary bypass. Less-invasive techniques not requiring a sternotomy are being developed to make this procedure a more attractive option in the treatment of atrial fibrillation.

Catheter Ablation Techniques

Initial catheter ablation techniques in atrial fibrillation used radiofrequency ablation to create linear scars in the atria and mimic the surgical Maze procedure. The next phase in catheter ablation involved targeting foci within or near the pulmonary veins that were often responsible for triggering atrial fibrillation. This technique has evolved from targeting individual foci to doing a circumferential isolation of the entire musculature surrounding the pulmonary vein(s). Subsequent research has shown that triggering foci can originate in multiple areas throughout the right and left atrium. Active research continues in the area of ablation for atrial fibrillation, including techniques such as the use of complex fractionated electrocardiograms to determine the target sites for ablation.

AV Node Ablation

Ablation of the AV node does not cure atrial fibrillation, but rather it permanently prevents any rapid ventricular response. Patients who require AV nodal ablation due to uncontrolled rapid ventricular response also need permanent pacemaker implantation.

Percutaneous left atrial appendage transcatheter occlusion (PLAATO) is performed to prevent thromboembolic stroke in patients with nonvalvular atrial fibrillation. This procedure is done in a cardiac catheterization laboratory. Right cardiac catheterization is done with a transseptal puncture. An occlusive device is placed in the left atrial appendage to prevent embolization of a thrombus (Jacobson, 2010). The atrial appendage can also be sutured during open heart surgery in patients with a history of atrial fibrillation. The goal is to prevent embolization of a thrombus from the left atrial appendage into systemic circulation.

Primary Prevention Strategies

There is currently not enough research to make any recommendations regarding the primary prevention of atrial fibrillation. One strategy that has been suggested as a possibility for primary prevention is the use of atrial or AV synchronous pacing in patients requiring pacing for bradycardia. Other possibilities for primary prevention include the use of pharmacological agents, such as angiotensin-converting enzyme (ACE) inhibitors and statins. At this time, there is not definitive evidence to make recommendations regarding primary prevention of atrial fibrillation with either pacemaker therapy or pharmacological agents (Fuster et al., 2011).

ATRIAL FIBRILLATION IN SPECIAL CIRCUMSTANCES

Atrial Fibrillation in Acute Myocardial Infarction

Atrial fibrillation can be a complication of an acute MI. If a patient develops atrial fibrillation as a complication of acute MI, then the patient is at higher risk for other adverse outcomes (Antman et al., 2004). Immediate cardioversion is commonly indicated. Intravenous (IV) beta-blockers can be used to slow the heart rate if acute heart failure and significant left ventricular dysfunction are absent. IV digoxin or amiodarone can also be used to slow the heart rate. Class Ic antiarrhythmics are contraindicated in acute MI.

Atrial Fibrillation with Hypertrophic Cardiomyopathy

Atrial fibrillation is a common complication of HCM. Patients with HCM are also among the patients most dependent on atrial kick to maintain adequate cardiac output. These patients can experience considerable loss of cardiac output and potential syncope with the development of atrial fibrillation. Disopyramide and amiodarone are the two preferred antiarrhythmics for maintaining sinus rhythm.

Atrial Fibrillation in Wolff-Parkinson-White Syndrome

Patients with WPW syndrome have an accessory pathway that connects the atria to the ventricles. During atrial fibrillation, conduction from the rapidly firing atria can travel over the accessory pathway and cause a faster ventricular response than conduction through the AV node. If this rapidly conducted atrial fibrillation is treated with the typical agents that slow conduction over the AV node, there can be increased conduction over the accessory pathway. The ventricular response can be so rapid that the rhythm can deteriorate to ventricular fibrillation. Long-term treatment involves ablation of the accessory pathway to eliminate conduction over it.

If the patient is hemodynamically unstable, then electrical cardioversion is indicated. IV procainamide or ibutilide is recommended to restore sinus rhythm in patients with WPW syndrome in atrial fibrillation who are hemodynamically stable but who have a wide QRS on the ECG. If the patient is hemodynamically stable, then IV medications that slow conduction over the accessory pathway may be considered for rate control (Fuster et al., 2011). These medications are listed in Box 11-3.

BOX 11-3: MEDICATION OPTIONS FOR RATE CONTROL (SLOW CONDUCTION OVER AN ACCESSORY PATHWAY) IN PATIENTS IN ATRIAL FIBRILLATION WITH WPW SYNDROME

Procainamide	Ibutilide
Disopyramide	Amiodarone

(Fuster et al., 2011)

Clinical Application

It is important to know the history of WPW syndrome in patients with atrial fibrillation. If an accessory pathway is present, patients are at risk for a rapid ventricular response. Patients in atrial fibrillation with known WPW syndrome are treated differently than those without WPW syndrome. Medications that slow conduction through the AV node (including beta-blockers, calcium channel blockers, and digoxin) are not indicated in the treatment of atrial fibrillation in the presence of WPW syndrome.

Acute Hemodynamically Unstable Atrial Fibrillation

If a patient presents emergently with new-onset atrial fibrillation (less than 48 hours in duration), a rapid ventricular rate, and hemodynamic instability, then emergency electrical cardioversion is indicated. Patients should be given unfractionated heparin or low-molecular-weight heparin prior to cardioversion. Immediate cardioversion should also be performed in situations in which rate control in

atrial fibrillation cannot be achieved with pharmacological treatment, including in the presence of acute MI or angina, symptomatic hypotension, and heart failure (Rosenthal & McManus, 2008; Fuster et al., 2011). Rate control is always the first goal in atrial fibrillation with rapid ventricular response. When rate control cannot be achieved through pharmacotherapy, the patient is at risk for becoming hemodynamically unstable and electrical cardioversion should be considered.

CONCLUSION

Atrial fibrillation is a common, chronic cardiac dysrhythmia with no current definitive cure. It can be caused by or can complicate many other cardiac disorders. Patients with atrial fibrillation are at risk for acute decompensation from rapid ventricular response and are also at risk for long-term hemodynamic and thromboembolic complications. The increased risk of stroke is one of the most important potential complications. Long-term anticoagulation is required in most patients with atrial fibrillation to reduce the risk of stroke.

Rate control is an important aspect of treatment for all patients with atrial fibrillation. Patients who are symptomatic also have the option of rhythm control through pharmacological or electrical cardioversion. Most patients require ongoing antiarrhythmic medications to maintain sinus rhythm. Future improvements in ablative techniques may offer more definitive treatment to a larger number of patients with atrial fibrillation, including those who have previously been categorized as having permanent atrial fibrillation.

Nurses outside the cardiac arena are likely to care for patients with atrial fibrillation and play a crucial role in the management of these patients. Assessment of the initial and ongoing rhythm, patient symptoms, and potential complications are key nursing considerations. Patient education regarding compliance with anticoagulation/

antithrombotic medication is critical to the patient in persistent or permanent atrial fibrillation to prevent devastating thromboembolic complications.

EXAM QUESTIONS

CHAPTER 11
Questions 86-93

Note: Choose the one option that BEST answers each question.

86. Atrial fibrillation can be described as a dysrhythmia that

    a. looks the same as sinus rhythm but has an impulse that initiates in the atria instead of the SA node.

    b. is characterized by rapid, irregular atrial activity that produces atrial fibrillatory waves on an ECG and a very variable ventricular response.

    c. is characterized by rapid, irregular atrial activity that produces atrial fibrillatory waves on an ECG and a very predictable ventricular response.

    d. produces atrial and ventricular fibrillation waves on an ECG.

87. Known causes or triggers of atrial fibrillation include

    a. alcohol use and pericarditis.

    b. osteoarthritis and myocarditis.

    c. adolescence and thoracic surgery.

    d. hypertension and hyperglycemia.

88. Paroxysmal atrial fibrillation can be defined as atrial fibrillation that

    a. lasts longer than 7 days.

    b. has only occurred one time.

    c. occurs in patients younger than 40 years of age.

    d. comes on spontaneously and self-terminates.

89. The pathophysiology associated with *persistent* and *permanent* atrial fibrillation is

    a. ventricular septal defect.

    b. structural disease of the atria with a reentrant mechanism.

    c. focal trigger points at the pulmonary veins.

    d. congenital small atria.

90. Common complications of atrial fibrillation include

    a. MI and sudden death.

    b. aortic valve stenosis and outflow tract obstruction.

    c. hemodynamic compromise and thromboembolic complications.

    d. endocarditis and pericarditis.

91. In atrial fibrillation, when rate has been controlled, it may still be necessary to control rhythm when

    a. the patient has reached 75 years of age.

    b. the patient has already been anticoagulated.

    c. paroxysmal episodes have been infrequent.

    d. the patient is symptomatic, despite the rate control.

92. Potential non-cardiac toxicities associated with amiodarone therapy include

    a. liver and pulmonary toxicity.

    b. frequent torsades de pointes.

    c. allergic reaction to aspirin.

    d. development of diabetes mellitus.

93. A true statement about anticoagulation before cardioversion is

    a. anticoagulation is more important for electrical cardioversion.

    b. anticoagulation is more important for pharmacological cardioversion.

    c. anticoagulation can only be achieved by use of IV heparin.

    d. anticoagulation is important before electrical and pharmacological cardioversion.

CHAPTER 12

CARDIAC PACEMAKERS AND IMPLANTABLE DEFIBRILLATORS

CHAPTER OBJECTIVE

After completing this chapter, the learner will recognize the indications for cardiac pacemakers and defibrillators and the impact of these devices on a patient.

LEARNING OBJECTIVES

After completing this chapter, the learner will be able to

1. list three indications for the insertion of a cardiac pacemaker.

2. differentiate between single- and dual-chamber cardiac pacing.

3. identify two potential pacemaker complications.

4. cite two key education topics for the recipient of a permanent cardiac pacemaker.

5. identify the benefit of biventricular cardiac pacing.

6. describe the effect of magnets on an implantable cardioverter-defibrillator.

7. recall the appropriate patient response to a defibrillation received from an implantable cardioverter-defibrillator.

INTRODUCTION

Physicians have been experimenting with electrical stimulation of muscles for many years. In 1788 in London, Charles Kite wrote a paper titled *An Essay Upon the Recovery of the Apparently Dead,* in which he described how he used electrical stimulation to the heart to revive a 3-year-old child (Nelson, 1993). Many devices have been developed over the years in an attempt to stimulate the electrical system of the heart. In the mid-1950s, the first pacemakers were used (Nelson, 1993). Initially, a small wire was placed in the heart. The wire was then connected to an external pacemaker that was the size of a microwave oven. The patient could only travel as far as the power cord could stretch. This drawback was desirable to the alternative, which was death. In 1957, the first battery-powered pacemaker was developed. This device (still an external device) was small enough to be strapped to the patient (Nelson, 1993). In 1960, the first totally implantable human cardiac pacemaker was implanted (Medtronic, Inc., 2010).

Since 1957, the science of cardiac pacing has grown and changed dramatically. Today, 250,000 pacemakers are implanted annually (Akoum, Lowy, & Freedman, 2010). Technology has advanced from a device that was external and the size of a microwave oven to a device that is totally implantable and the size of a half dollar.

Additionally, the field of electrophysiology has become a specialty of its own. As time goes on, the search for a device that mimics the heart's natural electrical system continues. For healthcare professionals, the devices become more complex and intricate. For patients, the implantation and impact on their lives becomes less obtrusive.

CARDIAC PACEMAKERS

Temporary Versus Permanent Cardiac Pacemakers

Pacemakers can be inserted on a temporary or permanent basis. Temporary cardiac pacing is utilized in acute care settings. If a patient presents with a slow rhythm and is symptomatic, a temporary pacemaker wire is inserted into the patient's heart. This wire is connected to an external pacemaker that functions similarly to a permanent pacemaker. If the cause of the slow rhythm is then determined to be permanent, a permanent pacemaker is implanted. Temporary pacemakers are also implanted during cardiac surgery because some patients experience cardiac dysrhythmias that require cardiac pacing after surgery. In most cases, there is no need for permanent cardiac pacing after cardiac surgery.

The development of a totally external temporary cardiac pacing system has decreased the number of temporary pacemaker wires that are inserted. An external temporary cardiac pacing system (transcutaneous pacemaker) involves the placement of two pads on the chest wall at specific locations. These pads adhere to the chest wall as an electrode used for cardiac monitoring would adhere to the chest wall. These pads are connected to a machine (usually a defibrillator) with pacemaker capabilities. The external pacemaker is turned on and an impulse is delivered that stimulates the heart to beat at a rate established by the attached machine. The totally external pacemaker has eliminated the need for a temporary pacemaker in situations when the

patient has a slow rhythm with no symptoms. The external or transcutaneous pacemaker can also serve as a bridge to a temporary pacemaker insertion. The patient is observed and a determination is made regarding the need for a permanent pacemaker. The external pacemaker eliminates the need to subject the patient to the risks associated with inserting a temporary pacemaker wire, which is an invasive procedure. However, this device is not appropriate for patients who require continuous temporary pacing because the delivery of the impulse is uncomfortable and at times painful. The totally external system is best utilized during a cardiac arrest. This chapter focuses only on permanent cardiac pacemakers and does not cover temporary cardiac pacemakers.

Review of the Conduction System

To understand how cardiac pacemakers work, one must understand the cardiac conduction system (see Figure 12-1).

Sinoatrial Node

The sinoatrial (SA) node is the natural pacemaker of the heart. In an adult, this natural pacemaker fires at a rate of 60 to 100 beats per minute. As the natural pacemaker, the SA node begins the electrical cascade of events, which results in organized depolarization and contraction of the heart. When the SA node initiates this cascade, the impulse travels through the right atrium via internodal pathways and the left atrium via Bachmann's bundle. In normal circumstances, this impulse results in contraction of the atria.

Atrioventricular Node

From the internodal pathways, the impulse travels to the atrioventricular (AV) node. The AV node slows conduction from the atria to the ventricles. Conduction is slowed to assure that the ventricles are relaxed at the time of atrial contraction and have time to fill completely before contracting. The AV node is located in the right atrium just above the insertion of the tricuspid valve.

FIGURE 12-1: NORMAL CARDIAC CONDUCTION SYSTEM

Sinoatrial (SA) node

Interatrial conduction tract
(Bachmann's bundle)

Internodal atrial conduction tracts

Atrioventricular
(AV) node

Atrioventricular (AV)
junction

Bundle of His

Left bundle branch

Right bundle branch

Purkinje network

Purkinje fibers

1. Superior vena cava	7. Tricuspid valve
2. Inlet of the superior vena cave	8. Right ventricle
	9. Interatrial septum
3. Right atrium	10. Interventricular septum
4. Inlet of the inferior vena cava	11. Left atrium
	12. Mitral valve
5. Coronary sinus	13. Left ventricle
6. Inferior vena cava	

Note. From *Pass CCRN* (2nd ed.), by R.D. Dennison, 2000, St. Louis, MO: Mosby ©Elsevier. Reprinted with permission.

Bundle of His

From the AV node, the electrical impulse travels along the bundle of His. The AV node and the bundle of His are surrounded by tissue known as the AV junction. In an adult, the AV junction contains pacemaker cells and initiates a heart rate of 40 to 60 beats per minute if no impulse is received from the SA node.

Bundle Branches

The bundle of His divides into the right and left bundles branches. The right bundle branch carries the impulse to the right ventricular myocardium. The left bundle branch divides into the left posterior bundle branch and the left anterior bundle branch. The left posterior bundle branch carries the impulse to the posterior and inferior left ventricle, and the left anterior bundle branch carries the impulse to the anterior and superior left ventricle.

Purkinje Fibers

From the ventricles, the impulse travels to the Purkinje fibers, where the depolarization is carried through to the endocardial layers of the heart. The

Purkinje network is the location for the heart's third group of pacemaker cells. In an adult, if no impulse has been received through the normal conduction patterns, the Purkinje system initiates a heart rate of 20 to 40 beats per minute.

Indications for Cardiac Pacing

As pacemakers continue to improve over the years, the indications continue to change. The decision to insert a pacemaker draws the attention of the medical community and also the insurance industry. These devices, especially implantable defibrillators, can be expensive, and many people scrutinize the need for their insertion. The American College of Cardiology (ACC) and American Heart Association (AHA) have worked jointly for more than 20 years to develop guidelines for a variety of disease processes and procedures related to cardiology. In the late 1990s, these two groups, in conjunction with the North American Society of Pacing and Electrophysiology (NASPE), developed a committee on pacemaker implantation (Gregoratos et al., 2002). As a result, the ACC/AHA/NASPE Guidelines for Implantation of Cardiac Pacemakers and Antiarrhythmia Devices were developed. These guidelines were most recently updated in 2008 (Epstein et al., 2008). Since the guidelines were published in 2002, NASPE has been renamed as the Heart Rhythm Society (HRS). The guidelines have become the gold standard for this procedure. It is important to remember that the field of electrophysiology is rapidly changing. Practitioners should make decisions based on each patient. Indications for permanent cardiac pacemaker insertion can appear complex because there are many variables. In this text, we cover the most common indications for cardiac pacemaker insertion (see Box 12-1).

Atrioventricular Block

The most common reason for pacemaker implantation is heart block, or AV block. In AV block, something in the conduction system pre-

vents the impulse from traveling normally from the SA node through the AV node to the ventricles. There are several types of AV block (see Box 12-2). A simple slowing of conduction from the SA node to the AV node is referred to as first-degree AV block. Second-degree AV block occurs when one atrial impulse at a time is not conducted through to the ventricles. There are two types of second-degree AV block: type I and type II. The block in type I occurs at the level of the AV node; type II occurs below the level of the AV node. Type II is generally more serious. High-grade (or advanced) AV block occurs when more than one impulse in a row from the atrium fails to conduct to the ventricle. A complete loss of communication between the SA node and the ventricles is referred to as complete heart block, or third-degree AV block. Patients are generally unaware of first-degree block; second-degree block can cause symptoms;

BOX 12-1: INDICATIONS FOR PERMANENT CARDIAC PACING

Note: This is a greatly abbreviated listing of the complex indications for pacemakers.

AV blocks (third-degree, high-grade, and type II second-degree AV blocks)

> With symptomatic bradycardia
>
> With heart rate less than 40 beats per minute in awake, asymptomatic patients
>
> As the result of necessary drug therapy in patients with a heart rate less than 40 beats per minute
>
> Asymptomatic third-degree AV block with awake heart rates of 40 or more, especially if left ventricular dysfunction is present

Bifascicular block

> With third-degree block
>
> With type II second-degree block
>
> With alternating bundle branch blocks

SA node dysfunction

> With symptomatic bradycardia, including pauses in heart beat
>
> As the result of necessary drug therapy with a heart rate less than 40 beats per minute
>
> With chronotropic incompetence

Hypersensitive carotid sinus and neurocardiogenic syncope

> With recurrent syncope caused by carotid sinus stimulation resulting in more than 3 seconds of ventricular asystole (cardiac standstill)
>
> Significantly symptomatic and recurrent neurocardiogenic syncope associated with bradycardia documented spontaneously or at the time of tilt-table testing

(Gregoratos et al., 2002)

BOX 12-2: TYPES OF AV BLOCK

First-degree AV block

Second-degree AV block

    Type I (Wenckebach) block

    Type II block

Advanced (high-grade) block

Third-degree AV block

and high-grade blocks and third-degree heart blocks usually result in symptoms, ranging from dizziness to complete unresponsiveness.

Any type of AV block with symptomatic bradycardia is an indication for cardiac pacing. If patients do not have symptoms but have documented heart rates of less than 40 beats per minute, they too are candidates for cardiac pacing. Occasionally, aggressive disease treatment with medications may result in AV blocks and low heart rates. Because many of the medications that lower rates or cause blocks are important to patient welfare, a pacemaker may be implanted instead of stopping the medication. Finally, any patient with third-degree AV block may be a candidate for pacing, even if no symptoms are present. Studies show that placing pacemakers in patients with third-degree AV block, with or without symptoms, can decrease mortality rates (Epstein et al., 2008). The presence of left ventricular dysfunction with AV block further supports the need for a pacemaker.

Bifascicular Block

The next group of patients requiring pacemakers is those with bifascicular blocks, or bundle branch blocks. The right bundle branch has one fascicle, and the left bundle branch has two fascicles: the anterior and posterior fascicles. One or more of these fascicles can become blocked. When the right bundle branch and one of the left bundle branch fascicles become blocked, the patient has a bifascicular block. Many people with bundle branch blocks do not require cardiac pacemakers; however, those with certain conditions do require pacing. The bundle branches supply the impulse to the ventricles. If the

right fascicle and both fascicles of the left bundle branch become blocked, no message is sent to the ventricles to contract. The ACC/AHA/HRS guidelines have identified that patients with bifascicular block and intermittent third-degree AV block or type II second-degree AV block are at high risk for death and require permanent pacing (Epstein et al., 2008).

Sinoatrial Node Dysfunction

When the SA node fails, a variety of dysrhythmias may result. SA node dysfunction is referred to as sick sinus syndrome (SSS). These dysrhythmias include bradycardia (slow heart beat), sinus arrest (no heart beat), SA block (no impulse initiated in the SA node), and paroxysmal supraventricular tachycardias (very fast heart rates alternating with very slow heart rates). Patients with SSS experience very fast and very slow heart rates and are commonly symptomatic. They may actually have a pause in the heartbeat and experience momentary dizziness. All of these dysrhythmias occur intermittently, and 24-hour monitoring is very helpful in documenting rhythm irregularities.

SA node dysfunction may also be demonstrated as chronotropic incompetence. During exercise, heart rate increases as a normal response to meet the body's increased needs. This rate increase is referred to as a chronotropic response. In some patients with SA node dysfunction, this response is no longer present, resulting in symptoms of activity intolerance. Although this response is essential for exercise, it is also important for any increase in activity.

Hypersensitive Carotid Sinus and Neurocardiogenic Syncope

Syncope that is the result of carotid sinus stimulation can be caused by a hypersensitive carotid sinus or neurocardiogenic syncope. All other causes of syncope should be ruled out prior to implanting a permanent pacemaker. Hypersensitive carotid sinus reflex is the result of increased parasympathetic (vagal) response, resulting in a variety of types of slowing of the heart rate when pressure is applied to the carotid sinus. The normal vagal response can produce a normal pause of the heartbeat for up to 3 seconds. In patients with hypersensitive carotid sinus, the pause is longer, resulting in syncope.

The reflex response in neurocardiogenic syncope is caused by a reduction in sympathetic activity that results in hypotension. This type of syncope accounts for 10% to 40% of all syncopal episodes (Epstein et al., 2008). Situations that normally increase stimulation of the sympathetic nervous system may result in syncope in patients with this condition. Normally, such situations as extreme fright, emotional upset, crowded rooms, and pain result in increased heart rate and cause vasoconstriction to increase blood pressure. When this occurs, the normal sympathetic response is reduced, resulting in bradycardia and hypotension.

Concepts of Permanent Cardiac Pacing

As discussed in Chapter 1, the action potential is a series of events that results in a change of the electrical charge inside the cell from negative (resting) to positive (stimulated) and back to negative. This action potential consists of depolarization (stimulation of cardiac muscle cells) and repolarization (return of cells to their resting state). Depolarization is conducted in a systematic method through the electrical system of the heart, as described earlier in this chapter. As depolarization occurs, healthy cardiac muscle cells respond by contracting the muscle. Patients requiring permanent pacemakers no longer have a systematic method for sending the message to the cardiac muscle. Rather, the implanted pacemaker takes over and stimulates the cardiac muscles to contract.

Components of a Permanent Cardiac Pacemaker

The standard cardiac pacemaker that is implanted to regulate heartbeat has several compo-

nents: the pacemaker generator, the pacemaker lead wire, and the pacemaker electrode (see Figure 12-2).

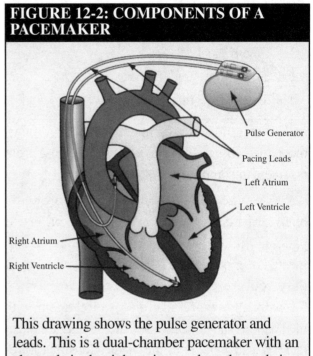

FIGURE 12-2: COMPONENTS OF A PACEMAKER

Pulse Generator

Pacing Leads

Left Atrium

Left Ventricle

Right Atrium

Right Ventricle

This drawing shows the pulse generator and leads. This is a dual-chamber pacemaker with an electrode in the right atrium and an electrode in the right ventricle.

Permission to reproduce this image granted by St. Jude Medical, Inc.

The Pacemaker Generator

The pacemaker generator is also referred to as the pacemaker battery or pacemaker can. It usually consists of a lithium battery and electrical microcircuitry necessary for the cardiac pacemaker to function. The pacemaker generator is usually placed in a subcutaneous pocket in the chest wall. The preferred site is the shoulder (left shoulder of a right-handed person and the right shoulder of a left-handed person). The battery is the only part of a pacemaker system that is removed and replaced.

Clinical Application

It is important to take the patient's lifestyle into consideration prior to insertion. For example, if a patient is a hunter and uses a rifle, the pacemaker generator should be placed in the shoulder that is not used when aiming the gun.

The Pacemaker Lead

The pacemaker lead is an insulated wire that is connected to the pacemaker battery. For a ventricular pacemaker, the lead is threaded through a vein to the superior vena cava and into the right atrium, then through the tricuspid valve and into the right ventricle. The end of the lead wire is left in contact with the wall of the right ventricle. The lead contains a conducting wire that carries the impulse from the pacemaker battery to the wall of the heart. It is insulated to protect against fracture. If the lead fractures, the electrical stimulus no longer reaches the heart and the pacemaker fails. If a lead fractures, a new lead is placed and the old lead is disconnected from the battery, but usually left in place. When pacemaker batteries are replaced, the leads are routinely left in place. It is not unusual to leave a nonfunctioning lead in place and simply add a new functional lead beside it. Removal of a lead may result in a tear in the myocardial wall. If a lead does need to be removed – for example, if it becomes infected – it should only be done by a physician well trained in lead removal.

The Pacemaker Electrode

At the end of the lead is an electrode. The electrode is the device that delivers the stimulus to the cardiac wall. The ability of the electrode to have good contact with healthy cardiac tissue is critical. Many types of "fixation" devices are available to assist with a good connection. Some leads naturally adhere to the wall over time, whereas others can be screwed into the myocardial wall. Different devices are utilized, depending on the ease or difficulty of establishing a good connection. Over time, the electrode at the end of the lead in the heart becomes covered over with fibrous tissue, which helps keep the electrode in place.

Types of Permanent Cardiac Pacing

Single-chamber Pacing

With single-chamber pacemakers, one lead is placed in one chamber of the heart. When pace-makers were first developed, a single lead was placed in the right ventricle. These are called right ventricular pacemakers. Now, a single lead can also be placed in the right atrium, for example, when the SA node does not fire on its own. If an impulse is initiated by the pacemaker in the atrium (simulating the SA node), the rest of the conduction system responds normally.

Right ventricular pacemakers are programmed to stimulate the right ventricle if no other stimulus is received by the ventricle within a preset time frame. This system completely ignores atrial activity and there is loss of atrial kick. Atrial kick contributes 25% of cardiac output. Over time, patients with single-chamber right ventricular pacemakers developed what was referred to as "pacemaker syndrome," primarily as a result of the loss of atrial kick. Pacemaker syndrome is discussed in detail later in this chapter. As a result of the negative effects (or less-than-optimal effects) of single chamber right ventricular pacemakers, researchers strived to develop a pacemaker that better mimicked the normal activities of the heart and dual-chamber pacemakers were developed.

Dual-chamber Pacing

Dual-chamber pacing involves two leads placed in the heart, one in the right atrium and one in the right ventricle. A dual-chamber pacing system is the typical pacemaker configuration that is implanted today. With a lead in the right atrium and a lead in the right ventricle, the pacemaker can sense the activity in both chambers and respond to activity that is present or not present. This configuration mimics the heart's normal conduction system and provides the patient with better cardiac output. As patients present for pacer battery replacement, dual-chamber systems may replace single-chamber pacemakers that were originally placed. Replacing a single-chamber pacemaker with a dual-chamber pacemaker is only done if a cardiologist determines that the patient would benefit from dual-chamber pacing.

Biventricular Pacemakers

Placing pacing leads in both the right and left ventricles is a newer technology that has been developed. This therapy is reserved for a very specific population of patients and will be discussed in more detail later in this chapter.

Cardiac Pacing Modes

Once implanted, cardiac pacemakers are programmed to function in a manner that is determined by a cardiologist to be best for that specific patient. Today, pacemakers can be programmed noninvasively and painlessly in a cardiologist's office. They can be reprogrammed and changed as the patient's needs dictate.

The Pacer Code

When referring to a pacemaker and its function, a series of letters are used to assist healthcare professionals in determining how the pacemaker should function. NASPE and the British Pacing and Electrophysiology Group (BPEG) developed the NBG generic pacemaker code (Bernstein et al., 2002) to establish a system for identifying pacemaker functioning that would be utilized and recognized internationally. The first four letters of this code are consistently utilized to identify pacing modes, whereas the fifth one is not yet used consistently (see Table 12-1). Discussion of the fifth position is beyond the scope of this text.

VVI Pacing Mode

The original pacemakers were ventricular pacemakers only and were designated as VVI pacemakers. Some patients continue to have pacemakers programmed in the VVI mode. In the VVI mode, the first position indicates that the pacemaker electrode in the right ventricle can pace the right ventricle if necessary. The second position indicates that the electrode in the right ventricle senses the patient's own electrical activity in the ventricle. The third position indicates that, upon sensing normal activity in the ventricle, the pacer will not fire (inhibits pacing activity). If there is no normal activity from the heart, the pacemaker will fire. The most common reason for the VVI mode is atrial fibrillation. In atrial fibrillation, communication between the atrium and the ventricle is not normal, and there is little ability to set up a communication system with a dual-chamber pacemaker. It is becoming more common to find patients with a dual-chamber pacemaker in atrial fibrillation to have a pacer mode of DDI. This is a more technologically complex configuration that is beyond the scope of this text, but is mentioned because it is one of the many configurations. A few patients still have old single-chamber pacemakers that were placed many years ago; these systems only function in VVI mode (see Figure 12-3).

DDD Pacing Mode

The most common configuration seen is the DDD mode. When the pacemaker is programmed

TABLE 12-1: REVISED NASPE/BPEG GENERIC CODE FOR ANTIBRADYCARDIA PACING				
Position I	**Position II**	**Position III**	**Position IV**	**Position V**
Chamber(s) paced	Chamber(s) sensed	Response to sensing	Rate modulation	Multisite pacing
O = None	O = None	O = None	O = None	O = None
A = Atrium	A = Atrium	T = Triggered	R = Rate modulation	A = Atrium
V = Ventricle	V = Ventricle	I = Inhibited		V = Ventricle
D = Dual (A+V)	D = Dual (A+V)	D = Dual (T+I)		D = Dual (A+V)
(Bernstein et al., 2002)				

for DDD, an electrode in the right atrium and one in the right ventricle are both utilized for the pacing mode. The DDD mode is commonly referred to as AV sequential pacing (see Figure 12-4). The D in the first position indicates that the electrode in the atrium and the electrode in the ventricle are programmed to pace the atrium and the ventricle if there is no normal electrical activity. The D in the second position indicates that the device can sense any normal electrical activity (depolarization) in the atrium or ventricle. The D in the third and final position refers to the pacemaker's response as it senses the activity of the heart. The best situation in most patients is to allow the heart to function as normally as possible and only utilize the pacemaker if the heart is unable to do so. Therefore, the

atrial electrode is set up to allow a preset period of time for the atrium to contract naturally. If normal contraction occurs, the atrial electrode is inhibited and does not fire. The atrial electrode then sends a message (trigger) to the ventricular electrode. The message to the ventricular electrode is the same as if a message was coming through the AV node to the ventricles via the bundle branches. This message sets up another cycle. The ventricular electrode, while triggered by the atrial system, waits a preset amount of time for the patient's own system to function, causing the ventricle to contract. If natural contraction occurs, then the ventricular electrode senses this and is inhibited and does not fire. Then the cycle repeats itself in the atrium. Any time that the atrium or ventricle does not depolarize naturally, the pacemaker sends an impulse to that part of the heart (see Figure 12-4).

FIGURE 12-3: VVI PACING MODE

V̲VI

Paces the ventricle

VV̲I

Senses the ventricle

VVI̲

Ventricular sensing inhibits ventricular pacing

FIGURE 12-4: DDD PACING MODE

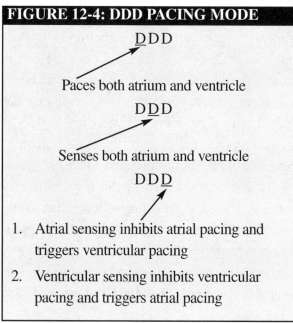

D̲DD

Paces both atrium and ventricle

DD̲D

Senses both atrium and ventricle

DDD̲

1. Atrial sensing inhibits atrial pacing and triggers ventricular pacing
2. Ventricular sensing inhibits ventricular pacing and triggers atrial pacing

Rate Responsiveness

The fourth position noted with pacemaker modes is an R. This stands for rate responsiveness. The body's natural ability to increase heart rate in response to physiologic needs is called a chronotropic response. Rate responsiveness provides the chronotropic response when the patient's body does not. A pacemaker with rate-responsive pacing increases the pacemaker rate based on the physiologic needs of the body. A wide variety of methods are available for detecting the physiologic needs of the body. Motion sensors and minute ventilation sensors are the most common methods of determining chronotropic needs (Jacobson, Marzlin, & Webner, 2007). With the setting of rate variability, the patient will have an upper rate and lower rate programmed. These will be the fastest and the slowest rates that the pacemaker will fire.

Clinical Application

Patients who have rate modulation programmed in their pacemakers may have a wide variability of heart rates when pacing, depending on their physiological needs.

Other Pacemaker Modes

Multiple combinations can be programmed into pacemakers. Pacemaker systems have become very complex, and a physician trained in the complex physiology of cardiac pacing is required to configure the pacemaker functions to best meet the physiologic needs of the patient. Those needs may change as the patient changes, and the pacemaker is reprogrammed to meet those needs.

Paradigm Shift in Permanent Pacing

With advances in technology and knowledge, technology that was once straightforward has become quite complex. Dual-chamber pacemakers were developed in an attempt to mimic the normal AV conduction pattern that was missing with single-chamber ventricular pacemakers. Within the past decade, the literature has demonstrated that there may be an increased incidence of heart failure hospitalization and new onset atrial fibrillation with continuous right ventricular pacing (Sweeney & Prinzen, 2006). The studies further suggest, "there may be deleterious effects from even the modest amount of ventricular pacing" (Epstein et al., 2008 p.e24). This is most likely occurring because right ventricular pacing creates a pattern of left bundle branch block and dyssynchrony between the right and left ventricle. With this in mind, pacemaker programming has become quite sophisticated in an attempt to minimize right ventricular pacing. The goal today with pacemaker programming is to allow the patient's native conduction system to predominate over the pacemaker. Atrial pacing is not related to the deleterious effects, only ventricular pacing. The less right ventricular pacing that occurs, the better for the patient, as long as the patient's own rhythm provides adequate perfusion and the patient is without symptoms. The newer programming modes (not discussed here) make it much more difficult for the untrained practitioner to determine appropriate pacemaker function during bedside cardiac monitoring.

Clinical Application

It is important to understand the reason the patient has a pacemaker, because dual chamber pacemakers are programmed differently than biventricular pacemakers (discussed later in this chapter). When questioning if the pacemaker is functioning normally on a rhythm strip, always assess the patient. The patient's stability should be the first concern. A stable patient allows time for further evaluation of the pacemaker.

Pacemaker Insertion

Pacemaker Insertion

Previously inserted in the operating room by a thoracic surgeon, permanent pacemakers are now commonly inserted in cardiac catheterization or electrophysiology laboratories by cardiologists who specialize in the field of electrophysiology. The procedure itself is conducted in a room with the same physical requirements as an operating room. Patients are usually awake during the procedure, with light medication to keep them comfortable. A local anesthetic is used at the site of insertion. A small incision, 2" to 3" in length, is made for pacemaker generator insertion in the left or right shoulder area, over the location of the subclavian vein. The leads are fed through the subclavian vein into the heart and connected to the pacemaker generator. The pacemaker is programmed and tested. When accurate pacing is assured, the incision is closed. The procedure is relatively quick, usually less than 2 hours. If a patient is only having a generator or battery replaced, even less time is required because the leads remain in place. The old incision is opened and the old generator is disconnected from the old leads and removed. The new generator is connected to the old leads and inserted into the pocket. The pacemaker is programmed and, when functioning is confirmed, the incision is closed. As stated earlier, if a new lead is required, the old lead is usually left in place to avoid the possibility of a myocardial tear or bleeding that can be associated with removal of a lead.

Recovery After Insertion

Patients may go to a recovery room after pacemaker placement, but most often return to a nursing unit that has cardiac monitoring capabilities. With a routine new pacemaker insertion, the patient is often hospitalized overnight. If only the generator has been replaced, the procedure is typically done on an outpatient basis. It is important that the leads remain at the location of placement in the operating room. Over time, fibrous tissue grows around the electrode and keeps the lead in place. The patient initially has some limitation of movement, until there is assurance that the lead is secure. Specifically, the patient should avoid raising the arm above the head on the side where the pacemaker was inserted for approximately 2 weeks after implantation (Ellenbogen & Wood, 2008). These restrictions are only used when a new lead has been implanted – not for generator replacement only. The patient is also instructed to limit the movement of the affected shoulder and not to lie on the affected side for the first 12 to 24 hours.

As with any surgical procedure, it is not uncommon for patients to experience discomfort at the site for the first several days. Generally, over-the-counter pain relief medications ease the discomfort, and discomfort should lessen as the wound heals. The incision may also be discolored. The incision is often closed with internal sutures that do not require removal. If external sutures are used, they are removed in 7 to 10 days. The site should be kept dry for 5 to 7 days (Ellenbogen & Wood, 2008).

After discharge, most activity is resumed quickly, with full recovery in 2 weeks. During the recovery period, which can last up to 3 months depending on the physician's preference, the patient should avoid heavy pushing, pulling, and lifting (10 pounds) with the arm and shoulder where the pacemaker is placed. The patient should be reminded that he or she can use the arm on the affected side during this restricted period, within the guidelines of the restriction. Driving is also limited for a period of 1 to 4 weeks, again according to the physician's preference (Ellenbogen & Wood, 2008).

Clinical Application

Limiting movement of the arm on the affected side is important in the immediate postoperative period when a new pacemaker lead has been implanted. The simple activity of using the elbows to move from a cart to the bed can dislodge some leads.

Pacemaker Complications

Pneumothorax

Pacemaker implantation is not without complications. During the procedure, the physician may puncture the lung while attempting to obtain vein access. A punctured lung may not be initially evident and all pacemaker implant patients should have a chest X-ray after the procedure to assess for pneumothorax. Respiratory distress during or after the procedure should raise the suspicion of pneumothorax. Treatment of pneumothorax depends on the size and symptoms. In more severe cases, insertion of a chest tube is required.

Hemothorax

Bleeding into the thoracic cavity may also occur if an artery is nicked or lacerated by a needle during the procedure. If this occurs, pressure can be applied and the situation resolves. If the artery penetration is large, a hemothorax may result and surgical repair of the artery is required.

Myocardial Perforation

During lead placement, the lead may perforate the heart wall. The lead can go through the heart wall to another chamber or, in the worst case, may traverse the entire heart wall to the pericardium. A full-thickness perforation can occur when myocardial tissue is old, steroid therapy has been used, or there was recent infarction of the right ventricular wall (Ellenbogen & Wood, 2008). Cardiac tamponade (bleeding into the pericardial sac) may occur quickly, requiring pericardiocentesis to remove the fluid in the pericardial sac or surgery to repair the damage. Perforation of the tissue may occur without this severe complication in healthier cardiac muscle tissue. Anticoagulated patients should have anticoagulants held for 8 to 12 hours after the procedure, until there is an assurance of no bleeding (Ellenbogen & Wood, 2008).

Infection

Pacemaker infection can occur in the early postoperative stage or months to years after implantation. *Staphylococcus aureus* is typically the infecting organism in early infections, whereas *S. epidermidis* is found with late-developing infections (Wohl, Peters, Carliner, Plotnick, & Fisher, 1982). Patients with diabetes mellitus and patients who develop postoperative hematomas tend to have a higher incidence of pacemaker site infection (Ellenbogen & Wood, 2008). Bacteria actually adhere to the pacing generator and leads, making removal of the pacing system necessary regardless of the patient's response to antibiotic therapy (Lowy & Freedman, 2004). When an infection is noted, intravenous antibiotic therapy is initiated. The pacemaker generator and leads are then removed and a new system is placed after the antibiotic therapy has had time to take effect and resolve the active infection (Ellenbogen & Wood, 2008). The new pacemaker system usually is placed in a new location to avoid possible reinfection of the new system. If the active infection cannot be successfully treated with the infected pacing system in place, the infected system may be removed and a temporary pacing system may be placed until the infectious process is resolved with antibiotic therapy.

Twiddler's Syndrome

Twiddler's syndrome results from a patient manipulating the pacer generator under the skin. The "twiddler" actually turns the device over and over and over again under the skin. As the device is turned, the leads twist to the point of actual damage to the lead. Usually, the damage is discovered after the pacemaker fails to function properly. The twisted wires are readily seen on chest X-ray film. Surgical intervention is required to open the incision and replace the leads. It is only shortly after the implantation of a device that one can turn it over. Over time, the device becomes attached to its surroundings, making twiddling difficult.

Clinical Application

Instruct patients to ignore the urge to touch their pacemaker in the early, postoperative setting to avoid the possibility of twiddler's syndrome.

Other Complications

Other complications include pacemaker generator migration, which involves actual movement of the pacemaker generator from its original location to a new location in the chest wall. This migration may be of little consequence if there is no malfunction of the pacemaker due to lead displacement or if there is no patient discomfort at the new location of the device. The pacemaker may also erode through the skin, usually due to pressure on the site. Early recognition of pressure on the pacemaker generator by tight skin allows the physician to intervene before the skin is penetrated. After the skin is penetrated, the entire system is considered contaminated and requires replacement (Ellenbogen & Wood, 2008).

Clinical Application

Car seatbelts may irritate a pacemaker site in some patients. Suggest the patient place a thick soft fabric (lambs wool) around the seatbelt strap to provide a soft surface at the site of the pacemaker.

Postoperative Follow Up

Most patients with new implants return to their physicians' offices within the first 4 weeks after insertion. This follow-up appointment allows the physician to observe the insertion site and assess pacemaker function. After this initial visit, patients can have pacemaker function assessed over the telephone.

Telephone Electrocardiogram Transmission

Pacemaker function should be assessed on a regular basis, depending on physician preference. Telephone assessment allows the physician to determine if the pacemaker is functioning as it should and if the pacemaker battery is ready for replacement. Patients with pacemakers are given transmitting devices that allow them to transmit the needed information. There is usually a prescheduled time for the patient to make the phone call to the office. When the call is made, the patient is given instructions on how to transmit. This transmission involves utilizing the phone with the transmitting device over the pacemaker. If the patient is not pacemaker dependent (not utilizing the pacemaker all of the time for a heart rate), the patient needs to transmit using a magnet. A magnet placed over the pacemaker generator causes the pacemaker to function without sensing any of the heart's normal activity. The office receives the transmittal in the form of an electrocardiogram (ECG). The ECG allows the physician to determine if the pacemaker is functioning normally and determines battery life. After the office has received the information, the "appointment" is over. The physician reviews the information and calls the patient if there are any concerns regarding pacemaker function.

Many patients can successfully transmit over the phone without any difficulty. Some patients may require help from a second person. It is usually during the first office visit after insertion that transmission instructions are reviewed and an assessment of the patient's ability to use this method is made.

The need for battery replacement is usually discovered during one of these transmittals. The lithium-iodine pacemaker batteries have a "staged" level of functioning. Staged functioning means that the battery functions at full level of voltage for a period of time. When the battery reaches about 90% depletion, the battery decreases the voltage to a lower level (Ellenbogen & Wood, 2008). This is referred to as the "elective replacement interval" (ERI). This change is detected with the phone transmission. When a transmission indicates that the battery is at the ERI, the patient is notified that a replacement will be necessary in the near future. This replacement is not an emergent situation but should be done soon after ERI is reached. The procedure is usually scheduled as an outpatient procedure.

Clinical Application

It is important to assure patients that by completing pacemaker checks over the phone and following up with the physician according to the scheduled time frames, there will be plenty of warning regarding battery ERI. Patients who are not well informed about battery ERI and battery replacement may think that they will die when the battery is depleted.

Clinical Application

If the patient does not follow up as scheduled by the physician, he or she may miss the ERI warning. When the battery reaches "end of life" (EOL), the battery needs to be replaced immediately in those patients who rely on the pacemaker on a regular basis.

Pacemaker Reprogramming

Occasionally, the original settings on a pacemaker may require adjusting to better meet the physiologic needs of the patient or to optimize the pacemaker function and preserve the battery. During an office visit, a pacemaker programmer is used to assess all functions of the pacemaker. Pacemakers have multiple parameters that may be adjusted at any time with the programmer. Reprogramming a pacemaker involves placing a programmer device over the pacemaker generator. The size and shape of the device varies from one manufacturer to another, but most devices are no larger than the size of a man's hand. The device is a handheld device that is connected to a computer. When it is over the pacemaker, the device transmits information to the computer. A variety of information can be obtained from the pacemaker. Once the information is obtained, the physician can make adjustments on the computer that are transmitted back to the pacemaker. After all of the necessary changes have been made, the reprogramming is over. Reprogramming is a painless, short procedure that should result in improved functioning of the pacemaker.

Patient Education

As pacemakers become more sophisticated, the restrictions for the patient decrease. However, patients should be aware of some specific instructions after they have had a pacemaker inserted. A variety of patient education materials are available. Because of the complexities of permanent pacemaking, patient education should be focused on priority information regarding safety, prevention of infection, and follow up. As with all patient education, healthcare literacy needs to be considered when planning educational interventions.

The patient education information listed below is adapted from the AHA patient education information:

1. Every patient should receive a pacemaker card identifying the type of pacemaker, leads, and date of insertion. Patients should always carry their cards.

2. Patients should always inform physicians and dentists that they have pacemakers prior to receiving care. Dental equipment should not negatively affect pacemakers.

3. A pacemaker may trigger airport metal detectors, but the metal detectors will not harm the pacemaker. Even so, patients should not linger around metal detectors. Patients should inform security personnel of their pacemakers and ask them not to hold metal detectors near their pacemakers longer than necessary.

4. Microwave ovens no longer affect pacemakers. Neither do most typical household electrical appliances, including CB radios, HAM radios, power tools, television remote controls, heating pads, or home metal detectors.

5. Cellular phones less than 3 watts (most typically used in the United States) have not been shown to interfere with pacemaker function. However, as phone technology continues to change, patients should be instructed to keep cell phones 6" away from their pacemakers. This allows patients to hold cell phones to their ears on the sides opposite the pacemakers. Patients should not keep their cell phones in shirt pockets on the same sides as the pacemakers.

6. Portable media players (IPOD etc.) may be a source of electromagnetic interference. Certain brands of headphones and earbuds contain strong magnets in the ear pieces. Patients should be cautioned to not keep these devices in their shirt pockets on the sides of the implanted devices. Patients should also be cautioned not to hang the earpieces around their necks dangling over the pacemakers. These devices need to be kept 6" from a pacemaker (Boston Scientific, 2009).

7. Patients with pacemakers should not undergo magnetic resonance imaging (MRI) because it can damage the pacemaker. The magnet in the MRI will cause the pacemaker to pace asynchronously, without regard for the patient's own rhythm. In some instances, some reprogramming may be done to allow for MRI. However, this is limited to very specific instances. Currently there are studies looking at the viability of MRI in patients with pacemakers, utilizing shielding materials. Other radiology procedures have not been show to affect pacemakers.

8. Radiation equipment used for treating cancer can damage pacemakers. Patients with pacemakers should not have radiation treatments until arrangements have been made with the physicians managing the pacemakers. The pacemaker should be shielded as much as possible, because as radiation dosing increases, so

does the risk to the pacemaker. In some situations, the pacemaker may be moved to another location in the body to avoid direct radiation. The pacemaker should be checked after each radiation treatment. If the patient is pacemaker dependent (fully dependent on the pacemaker for a heart rate), a temporary pacemaker may be inserted during treatment to assure there is no loss of heart rate. The temporary pacemaker battery can be placed away from the body and shielded during the procedure.

9. Lithotripsy (hydraulic shocks to dissolve kidney stones) may cause changes in a pacemaker. Patients with pacemakers may have lithotripsy, but they require close follow up after the procedure, and some reprogramming may be necessary.

10. Power-generating equipment, arc welding equipment, and powerful magnets (such as those found in some medical equipment and motors) can inhibit a pacemaker from functioning properly. Patients should avoid being near this type of equipment. If a patient becomes dizzy around questionable equipment (such as a power station) or while working on a running engine, he or she should back away from the equipment and the pacemaker should resume normal functioning.

11. After the initial recovery period, no restrictions to arm movement are necessary.

12. Patients should report any dizziness or syncope to their physicians. If they are able to learn to take their own pulses, they can be instructed to notify their physicians if their pulses are slower than the programmed low rate on their pacemakers. This may be difficult for some patients. The best indicator for patients with pacemakers is how they are feeling.

13. Patients should be reminded of the importance of keeping appointments for routine pacemaker checks.

CARDIAC RESYNCHRONIZATION THERAPY

Cardiac resynchronization therapy (CRT) is a nonpharmacological treatment strategy for heart failure. Dyssynchrony of contraction of the right and left ventricles contributes to a poor prognosis in patients with advanced heart failure (Bradley et al., 2003). This dyssynchrony occurs most often with left bundle branch block. Cardiac dyssynchrony in patients with advanced heart failure results in poor hemodynamic functioning. These patients have decreased ejection fraction, decreased cardiac output, an increase in myocardial oxygen consumption, and an increase in signs and symptoms of congestion. Additionally, QRS duration on an ECG wider than 120 ms (normal is 100 ms or less) is associated with an increase in mortality in patients with advanced heart failure (Bradley et al., 2003). In left bundle branch block, the right ventricle contracts first, followed by the left ventricle. Generally, the lateral wall of the left ventricle is the last wall to contract in left bundle branch block. CRT is a therapy aimed at eliminating the dyssynchrony and involves the utilization of a pacemaker lead in both the right and left ventricles to resynchronize the ventricles. This therapy is also referred to as "biventricular pacing."

Clinical Application

It is important to remember that CRT is a therapeutic treatment used in heart failure. These devices are not placed because of heart rate issues. With this in mind, when ventricular pacing occurs, therapy is delivered. If there is no ventricular pacing, then there is no synchrony between the right and left bundle. It is important to differentiate this patient population from the patient population with pacemakers implanted to maintain normal heart rates.

Indications

CRT can be costly, so the guidelines for device implantation are strict. Currently, the U.S. Food and Drug Administration (FDA) has approved CRT for a specific group of patients (see Table 12-2). This population includes patients who are symptomatic on full medical therapy for heart failure, they must fall into New York Heart Association (NYHA) class III or IV (Table 12-3), and they must also meet strict criteria for ejection fraction and QRS duration on an ECG.

Biventricular Pacemaker Insertion

Like other pacemakers, the biventricular pacemaker generator is placed in a pocket in the chest wall. Pacemaker leads are placed in the right atrium and right ventricle in the normal method. A third lead is attached to the left ventricle in the location of the left lateral ventricular wall. The right atrial and ventricular leads are placed inside the chambers, whereas the left ventricular lead is threaded through the coronary sinus and into the left ventricular cardiac vein. This approach results in a lead that is pacing from the outer surface of the heart. The left lateral wall placement of the lead is effective because the left lateral wall of the left ventricle is the part of the heart that contracts last. Implantation of this lead may be difficult because the ventricle is typically quite dilated. Occasionally, the lead cannot be placed percutaneously and must be placed in the operating room through a surgical incision in the chest wall (see Figure 12-5).

After the leads are in place, the goal of therapy is to have both ventricular pacemaker leads stimulating the respective ventricles at the same time; this is achieved though extensive programming efforts. Then the procedure is over. Today, almost all patients who are candidates for biventricular pacing are also candidates for implantable carioverterfefibrillators (ICDs), which are placed at the same time as biventricular pacing leads.

Postoperative Care

Postoperative care differs little from that for standard pacemaker implantation. However, patients with CRT are likely to require more frequent in-office follow up, as their pacemakers are adjusted and reprogrammed to best meet their physiologic needs.

Patient Education

The standard education that was reviewed for traditional pacemaker insertion is the same for CRT because it is pacemaker technology. It is important for patients with CRT to realize that this therapy does not eliminate the need for continued medical

TABLE 12-2: INDICATIONS FOR CARDIAC RESYNCHRONIZATION THERAPY

Severity of illness	Moderate to severe heart failure Symptomatic on full medical therapy
NYHA functional class	Class III or class IV
Ejection fraction	≤ 35%
QRS duration	≥ 130 ms
Left ventricular size	Diameter at end of diastole > 55 mm
(Epstein et al., 2009)	

TABLE 12-3: NEW YORK HEART ASSOCIATION CLASSIFICATION OF HEART FAILURE

Class I	Patients with no limitation of activities who suffer no symptoms from ordinary activities.
Class II	Patients with slight, mild limitation of activity who are comfortable with rest or with mild exertion.
Class III	Patients with marked limitation of activity who are comfortable only at rest
Class IV	Patients who should be at complete rest and confined to a bed or chair; any physical activity brings on discomfort and symptoms occur at rest.
(Dolgirin, Fox, Gorlin, & Levin, 1994)	

FIGURE 12-5: TYPICAL LEAD PLACEMENT FOR CRT THERAPY

Note. From *Atlas of Heart Diseases: Arrhythmias: Electrophysiologic Principles* by J. Cockrell & A. Siu. Edited by E. Braunwald (series editor) & M. Scheinman. Copyright 1996, by Current Medicine. Used with permission from Images.MD.

therapy. In fact, medications used for mortality benefit (angiotensin-converting enzyme inhibitors and beta-blockers) may actually be increased to higher therapeutic levels that the patient was unable to tolerate without biventricular pacing. Patient symptoms of heart failure may improve, resulting in an ability to decrease medications utilized for symptom relief (diuretics).

Outcomes

Many studies continue to evaluate the long-term effectiveness of CRT. The preliminary studies are positive. For example, in the Comparison of Medical Therapy, Pacing and Defibrillation in Chronic Heart Failure (COMPANION) study, preliminary reports demonstrated a reduction in deaths and hospitalizations in those who received CRT (Bristow & Feldman, 2003). Studies have reported a mortality benefit with CRT and an approximately 30% decrease in hospitalizations (Bradley et al., 2003; Epstein et al., 2008). Patients also report increased

activity tolerance and an improvement in quality of life (Bradley et al., 2003; Epstein et al., 2008).

IMPLANTABLE CARDIOVERTER-DEFIBRILLATORS

In 1980, the first implantable defibrillator was implanted in a human being (Ganz, 2004). In 1985, the FDA approved their use in a limited population (Ganz, 2004). Over the past 26 years, the technology for ICDs has changed dramatically. The initial devices were large and bulky, requiring thoracic surgery for implantation. The generators were implanted in the abdomen, with patches applied to the heart. Currently, implantation of the device is similar to that of a pacemaker, with the generator (which is slightly larger than that of a pacemaker) implanted in the shoulder.

Indications

The indications for implantation of an ICD are very specific. These devices are very expensive and have quite an impact on the patient. As technology and research continue, the indications for ICDs increase. Originally developed to prevent sudden cardiac death from ventricular tachycardia and ventricular fibrillation, these devices now also treat bradycardia and atrial tachycardias (Gregoratos et al., 2002). Initially, ICDs were indicated (with few exceptions) in patients who had sustained ventricular tachycardia or resuscitated cardiac arrest (Beyerbach, 2009). The indications continue to increase as more and more research becomes available. The Multicenter Automatic Defibrillator Implantation Trial II opened the door for further expanded indications for ICDs. This trial demonstrated a measurable decrease in mortality for patients with prior myocardial infarction and ejection fractions less than 35%. These patients are not required to have the ventricular tachycardia component to qualify for an ICD (Beyerbach, 2009). Criteria for ICD implantations are many. The

ACC/AHA/HRS guidelines (Epstein, 2008) identify 22 different situations that warrant the implantations of an ICD. The *most common* indications for ICD implant are listed in Box 12-3. These indications are the Class I indications, meaning that there is clear evidence that the benefit outweighs the risk and the recommendation should be implemented.

Functions

Like pacemakers, ICDs are multiprogrammable, with a large variety of technical options for treating dysrhythmias. The ultimate goal of therapy is to avoid the dysrhythmias completely. Appropriate administration of antiarrhythmic medications controls the dysrhythmias. It is preferred that the ICD never fires, but firing is available in the event that the medications do not totally suppress the dysrhythmia.

Clinical Application

Patients with ICDs should be instructed to continue taking their medications. ICDs do not eliminate the development of dysrhythmias; they only terminate the dysrhythmias once they have occurred. Antiarrhythmic medications control the development of dysrhythmias.

Clinical Application

Not all patients with ICDs are on antiarrhythmic medications because some of them have not demonstrated any dysrhythmias. These patients are at high risk for the development of a dysrhythmia, but will not be placed on any medication until they have demonstrated evidence of a dysrhythmia.

The ICD generator includes technology for permanent cardiac pacing as well as cardiac defibrillation. The device is programmed to sense

---

BOX 12-3: CLASS I INDICATIONS FOR IMPLANTABLE CARDIOVERTER DEFIBRILLATORS

1. Patients who are survivors of cardiac arrest due to VF or hemodynamically unstable sustained VT after evaluation to exclude any completely reversible causes. *(Level of Evidence A)*

2. Patients with structural heart disease and spontaneous sustained VT, whether hemodynamically stable or unstable. *(Level of Evidence B)*

3. Patients with syncope of undetermined origin with clinically relevant, hemodynamically significant sustained VT or VF induced at electrophysiological study. *(Level of Evidence B)*

4. Patients with LVEF less than or equal to 35% due to prior MI who are at least 40 days post-MI and are in NYHA functional Class II or III. *(Level of Evidence A)*

5. Patients with nonischemic DCM who have an LVEF less than or equal to 35% and who are in NYHA functional Class II or III. *(Level of Evidence B)*

6. Patients with LV dysfunction due to prior MI who are at least 40 days post-MI, have an LVEF less than or equal to 30%, and are in NYHA functional Class I. (Level of Evidence A)

7. Patients with nonsustained VT due to prior MI, LVEF less than or equal to 40%, and inducible VF or sustained VT at electrophysiological study. *(Level of Evidence B)*

Key:

VF = ventricular fibrillation

VT = ventricular tachycardia

LVEF = left ventricular ejection fraction

NYHA = New York Heart Association

DCM = dilated cardiomyopathy

MI = myocardial infarction

(Epstein et al., 2008)

ventricular tachycardia through a variety of sophisticated methods that are programmed to the specific patient when the device is inserted. It is then determined which method is utilized to terminate the dysrhythmia once it occurs. Several options are available.

Antitachycardia Pacing

Antitachycardia pacing is also referred to as overdrive pacing. When a rapid dysrhythmia is detected, the pacemaker paces at a rate higher than the patient's rate in an attempt to override the rapid rhythm. This method has proven to be an effective method to control some ventricular tachycardias. In one study, 96% of all detected episodes of ventricular tachycardia were terminated with antitachycardia pacing (Gregoratos et al., 2002). This option is a nice alternative for the patient because no shock is involved. Patient sensitivity to pacing varies. Some patients do not notice when overdrive pacing is occurring, whereas others do.

Defibrillation

Defibrillation is utilized as needed to terminate dysrhythmias. The shock administered can be either a cardioversion shock or a full defibrillation shock. The cardioversion shock uses less energy than the defibrillation shock. If the cardioversion shock is programmed into the device as a therapy, it is attempted before the defibrillation shock. If cardioversion does not terminate the dysrhythmia, a defibrillation shock is administered. The administration of a shock to the heart is not as strong as those seen with external defibrillators. However, they are most definitely felt by patients and are painful. The lowest amount of energy needed to terminate the dysrhythmia is determined when the device is implanted. The shock administered should be strong enough to take control of the heart and eliminate the dysrhythmia as the controlling rhythm.

Implantation

An electrophysiologist who is trained in ICD insertion should implant the device. Occasionally, an ICD is placed in the operating room by a heart surgeon in conjunction with open-heart surgery. The defibrillator is located on the lead that is placed in the right ventricle. The pacemaker functions as a normal pacemaker. In many cases, the pacemaker is only needed after a shock is delivered and a brief pause in the patient's own rhythm occurs as the heart resets itself after the shock. During implantation of the device, the patient is awake. However, after implantation, it is necessary to test the device to assure it will fire. During this portion of the procedure, conscious sedation or anesthesia is utilized to protect the patient from discomfort associated with defibrillation. The electrophysiologist programs the device to the most effective settings. After the procedure, the patient is returned to a recovery room or a nursing unit capable of cardiac monitoring. Patients are commonly discharged the next day if no complications occur and ventricular dysrhythmias are under control.

Postoperative Follow Up

Postoperative care is similar to the postoperative care necessary for patients with pacemakers. However, ICD patients are generally restricted from driving. These limitations vary somewhat by physician. The ACC/AHA/HRS guidelines recommend no driving for 6 months after device implantation in those patients who have known ventricular arrhythmias. In the patients receiving ICDs as primary prevention (no evidence of treatable ventricular dysrhythmia) the ACC/AHA/HRS guidelines recommend no driving for 7 days after implantation to allow healing (Epstein et al., 2008). Most literature supports varied driving restrictions based on the reason for the implant (Epstein et al., 2008). The goal is to prevent the possibility of developing a dysrhythmia that incapacitates the driver while behind the wheel. Many patients find this restriction very difficult to adhere to.

Office Visits

Follow-up visits after ICD implantation may occur more frequently than with permanent pacemaker insertion. Patients may have office visits rather than phone transmissions, because electrophysiologists want to assess the function of the device. However, most manufacturers have remote device interrogation capabilities, decreasing the need for frequent office visits. This remote monitoring is accomplished through radio frequency transmission via a telephone system. These remote monitoring systems have the ability of notifying the electrophysiologist's office if the device fires or if the device is inadvertently deactivated. In the office, with a programmer similar to the one used for pacemakers, electrophysiologists can determine the number of therapies that have been delivered by the device, including the success of the therapy. During this time, the battery level is also checked. Battery life depends on the frequency of the therapy as well as the energy utilized with those therapies. As with pacemakers, it is predetermined when battery ERI is reached so replacement of the battery can be scheduled. These pacemaker checks are essential in maintaining good function of the ICD.

Magnet Function with an ICD

As noted earlier in the text, a magnet placed over the pulse generator in a normal pacemaker causes the pacemaker to pace without sensing any of the heart's normal activity. An ICD does not function in the same manner. A magnet placed over an ICD disables the device while the magnet is in place. When the magnet is moved away from the device, the device should function in the normal manner. All device companies have specific functionality and each device may function with some differences. It is important for healthcare workers to be aware that a magnet over an ICD disables the device and no treatment will occur if the patient develops dysrhythmias. The best practice is not to utilize magnets near these devices unless instructed to do so by a qualified physician.

Patient Education

Emotional Impact

Patient education for the recipient of an ICD involves technical aspects of care as well as emotional aspects. Implantation of an ICD is generally emotionally difficult because the patient realizes that his or her life may depend on the device. The emotional impact extends beyond the patient to the family. There is a fear of death as well as a fear that the device may not function. Additionally, patients may also experience fear and anxiety related to the anticipation of an actual shock. Patients have reported sleeplessness due to this fear and anxiety. Families may also become overprotective because they worry about the device. Thorough patient education and support is essential to help patients and families understand the device. If an ICD support group is available, the patient and the significant other should be encouraged to attend

Device Activation Education

As stated earlier, the goal of therapy is to have a medication regimen that prevents dysrhythmias from occurring. However, dysrhythmias may occur, so the patient and family should be aware of the proper response. Physicians may vary in preference regarding notification of a shock, but the following is basic information regarding patient response to device activation:

1. All patients with ICDs should have a well-thought-out plan for obtaining emergency medical assistance. Close family and friends should be aware of the plan in the event that the device does not work properly. Close family and friends should all be trained in cardiopulmonary resuscitation (CPR).

2. Patients describe the feeling of a full defibrillation shock as being "kicked in the chest." A cardioversion shock is less intense. The patient should not notice normal cardiac pacing, but

may notice antitachycardia pacing (Heart Rhythm Society, n.d.).

3. Family and friends should be aware they are in no danger if they come in contact with the patient when the defibrillator discharges (Yeo & Berg, 2004). If a shock occurs during sexual intercourse, the partner may experience a tingle or buzz. This shock is not harmful to the partner (Steinke et al., 2005).

4. When a shock occurs, the patient should notify the physician who is handling the ICD that the shock occurred. The physician does not need to be called immediately, but should be notified when the office is next open. The physician needs to be aware of device firing so adjustments can be made as needed.

5. If the device fires multiple times and the patient returns to normal, the physician should be called at that time.

6. If the device continues to fire without success, the family should place a call to the emergency medical system (EMS) and begin CPR if the patient becomes unconscious.

7. If at any time the ICD fires and the patient does not return to normal (awake and appropriate) after the shock, even if only one shock was delivered, the patient should be taken to the nearest emergency department via EMS.

Note: The above are general recommendations. Each electrophysiologist has specific instructions based on the patient's indications for the device and the specific device that was implanted.

Electromagnetic Interference

On rare occasions (less than 1% per patient per year), electromagnetic interference may cause an ICD to fire (Yeo & Berg, 2004). All precautions noted with pacemakers apply to ICDs. It is important for patients to notify security personnel of ICDs. Patients should not allow handheld metal detector wands to be held over the device for more than a few seconds. These contain magnets that can

disable the device if left in place too long (Yeo & Berg, 2004). Again, carrying the manufacturer's identification card is a must.

ICDs present an additional set of concerns for the patient undergoing surgery or procedures such as endoscopy with polyp removal. The patient should make sure those involved with the procedure are well aware that he or she has an ICD. Special precautions are necessary that are beyond the scope of this discussion.

Other Educational Considerations

The surgical complications, postoperative considerations, and patient education discussed for permanent pacemakers also apply to patients with an ICD or CRT because these devices also have pacemaker technology.

Clinical Application

Many patients meeting criteria for CRT therapy also meet criteria for an ICD. It is important to know what therapy your patient has implanted. If the patient has CRT therapy with an ICD, it is often referred to as a CRT-D pacemaker.

CONCLUSION

The field of cardiac pacemakers has grown dramatically over the past 50 years. Research allows for devices that more closely mimic the heart's natural pacemaker. The development of biventricular pacing to resynchronize the ventricles is proving to be a life-prolonging strategy that improves quality of life for many patients with heart failure. Most patients who undergo CRT are also candidates for ICDs. As technology becomes more complex, the cost of these therapies continues to rise. Many decisions are made as to the appropriate candidates for these expensive therapies. Ethical dilemmas come into play, and determinations need to be made about replacement of defibrillators in older adult patients who are reaching the end of life. These defibrillators may prevent what is the natural progression to death as someone ages.

EXAM QUESTIONS

CHAPTER 12
Questions 94-100

Note: Choose the one option that BEST answers each question.

94. The most common reason for pacemaker implantation is

    a. hypersensitive carotid sinus syncope.

    b. bifascicular block.

    c. SA node dysfunction.

    d. AV block.

95. A true statement about dual-chamber cardiac pacemakers is

    a. dual-chamber pacemakers eliminate atrial kick by controlling the atrium and ventricle.

    b. dual-chamber pacemakers most closely mimic the heart's normal conduction system.

    c. dual-chamber pacemakers are the best therapy for patients with heart failure.

    d. dual-chamber pacemakers can cause pacemaker syndrome.

96. A patient with a permanent cardiac pacemaker implanted 1 year ago presents to the office with a temperature of 99.4° F and concerns about his pacemaker site. Upon examination, the nurse notes a small open area at the pacemaker site and the pacemaker can be seen through the opening. The skin surrounding the open area is red and swollen with some pus noted. The nurse anticipates treatment with

    a. antibiotics, removal of the entire pacemaker system (leads and generator), and implantation of a new pacemaker system in a different location.

    b. antibiotics, removal of the entire pacemaker system (leads and generator), and implantation of a new pacemaker system in the same location.

    c. antibiotics and aggressive wound care.

    d. antibiotics, surgical debridement of the wound site, replacement of the generator in a new site.

97. Devices that can affect the function of permanent cardiac pacemakers include

    a. microwave ovens.

    b. cellular phones more than 6" away from the pacemaker.

    c. MRI and lithotripsy.

    d. television remote controls and home metal detectors.

98. The benefits of pacing the right and left ventricle at the same time (biventricular pacing) include

    a. increased cardiac output due to strong ventricular contraction.

    b. control of atrial fibrillation.

    c. better cardiac output due to resynchronization of the contraction of the right and left ventricles.

    d. the ability to pace and shock the heart simultaneously.

99. Any patient with an ICD should know that a magnet placed over the ICD will

    a. make the ICD defibrillate.

    b. make the ICD revert to antitachycardia mode.

    c. deactivate the ICD.

    d. transmit information to the programmer so the device can be evaluated.

100. A 64-year-old man with an ICD is watching TV at home Sunday evening. His ICD suddenly discharges delivering one defibrillation shock. After the shock, the 64-year-old feels fine. At this point the patient knows he should

    a. call his physician at the next most convenient time during normal office hours to let the physician know the ICD has delivered a shock.

    b. call the physician immediately for further instructions and to have the ICD reset.

    c. drive to the hospital to have the ICD checked with the programmer.

    d. call 911 for immediate transport to the hospital.

This concludes the final examination.

Please answer the evaluation questions found on page vii of this workbook.

GLOSSARY

abdominal obesity: Obesity with a distribution of fat around the abdomen that produces an abnormal waist-to-hip ratio.

acetylcholine: The neurotransmitter of the parasympathetic nervous system.

acidosis: Condition characterized by an arterial blood pH less than 7.35.

activated clotting time (ACT): A test to evaluate coagulation status that can be evaluated at the bedside.

activated partial thromboplastin time (aPTT): Coagulation test used to monitor the therapeutic effectiveness and safety range of heparin.

acute coronary syndrome (ACS): The presentation of coronary artery disease in the form of unstable angina, non-ST-segment elevation MI, or ST-segment elevation MI.

acute respiratory distress syndrome (ARDS): A complex clinical syndrome resulting in acute respiratory failure from hypoxic lung injury.

adenosine: Coronary vasodilator used in chemical stress testing. Also used as an antiarrhythmic to slow conduction through the atrioventricular node during some forms of tachycardia.

adenosine diphosphate (ADP): Substance responsible for activation of glycoprotein IIb/IIIa receptors.

adenosine diphosphate (ADP) inhibitors: Medications that prevent ADP-mediated activation of platelets.

adenosine triphosphate (ATP): An enzyme in muscle cells that stores energy and produces energy when split.

adrenal cortex: Outer layer of the adrenal gland.

adrenergic receptor: Receptor of the sympathetic nervous system.

adventitia: Fibrous outer layer of an artery that is designed to protect the vessel and provide connection to other internal structures.

afterload: Pressure the ventricle must overcome to eject its contents.

aggregation: Clustering or coming together.

albumin: A simple protein widely distributed in tissues that circulates in the blood as serum albumin.

alkalosis: Condition characterized by a pH more than 7.45.

aldosterone: A mineralocorticoid hormone that increases sodium and water reabsorption.

aldosterone antagonist: Medication that blocks the effects of aldosterone.

alpha1 adrenergic receptor: Sympathetic nervous system receptor located in the vessels of vascular smooth muscle.

alveolar membrane: Membrane of the alveoli in the lungs and the site of gas exchange.

aminophylline: Pulmonary vasodilator used as an antidote for adenosine or dipyridamole during chemical stress testing.

amiodarone: A class III antiarrhythmic with vasodilative properties that is generally well tolerated in patients with left ventricular dysfunction; used to treat atrial and ventricular dysrhythmias.

amyloidosis: Disease in which protein fibrils (amyloid) collect in body tissues and impair organ function.

anaphylactic shock: Shock caused by an allergic reaction.

androgen: Hormone that produces male characteristics.

anemia: Reduced hemoglobin level or red blood cell count.

angina pectoris: The clinical symptom resulting from decreased blood flow to the myocardium.

angioedema: Allergic response in which the skin, mucous membranes, and viscera become edematous. Commonly occurs around the eyes or lips. Swelling is deep, extending beneath the skin, and can involve the airways.

angiography: Procedure in which serial radiographs of a blood vessel are taken in rapid sequence after the injection of a radiopaque substance. Used to determine the size and shape of vessels. Coronary angiography is also called *cardiac catheterization.*

angiojet thrombectomy: Atherectomy procedure used for the extraction of visible thrombi within the coronary artery.

angiotensin-converting enzyme (ACE): A proteolytic enzyme that converts angiotensin I to angiotensin II.

angiotensin-converting enzyme (ACE) inhibitor: Medication that prevents the conversion of angiotensin I to angiotensin II.

angiotensin I: Precursor to angiotensin II.

angiotensin II: Potent vasoconstrictor and stimulator of aldosterone secretion.

angiotensin II receptor blocker (ARB): Medication that blocks the effects of angiotensin II.

ankle-brachial index (ABI): Blood pressure in the ankle divided by blood pressure in the arm. A decrease in ABI during exercise is an indication that peripheral arterial disease is present.

annulus: Fibrous ring that forms the opening of the valve and joins the valve cusps (leaflets) together.

anorexia: Loss of appetite.

antagonize: To counteract.

anterior myocardial infarction: Myocardial infarction involving the anterior, or front wall, of the left ventricle.

anterolateral myocardial infarction: Myocardial infarction involving the anterior and lateral walls of the left ventricle.

anteroseptal myocardial infarction: Myocardial infarction involving the anterior wall of the left ventricle and the septum.

antianginal: Medication effective in preventing or decreasing angina.

antibody: A protein substance developed in response to an antigen.

anticoagulant: Medication that interferes with clot formation by disrupting the intrinsic, extrinsic, or common pathway of the coagulation cascade.

antioxidant: An agent that protects against oxidation.

antiplatelet: An agent or medication interfering with the action of platelets in clot formation.

antiproliferative: Blocking of rapid cell reproduction.

antitachycardia pacing: Pacemaker therapy that utilizes the pacemaker to override a fast rhythm with a higher pacemaker rate. When the pacemaker has control of the rhythm, it slows the rate to a normal range. Also known as *overdrive pacing.*

antithrombin III: An agent that opposes the action of thrombin, inhibits the coagulation of blood, and inactivates several clotting factors.

antithrombotic: Agent that counteracts clot formation.

anxiolytic: Medication given to reduce anxiety.

aorta: Main trunk of the arterial system that originates from the left ventricle.

aortic dissection: Separation of the layers of the aorta.

aortic regurgitation: Abnormal aortic valve function in which valve cusps do not close tightly, causing retrograde movement of blood through the valve during ventricular systole.

aortic root: Beginning of the aorta, where the aorta attaches to the aortic valve.

aortic stenosis: Abnormal aortic valve function, resulting in obstruction of flow from the left ventricle to incorrect or incomplete valve opening.

aortic valve: Valve between the left ventricle and the aorta.

apex: The bottom of the heart. Located approximately at the fifth intercostal space, at the midclavicular line.

apical impulse: The area normally near the apex of the heart where the contraction of the heart can be palpated.

apoptosis: Programmed cell death.

aprotinin: A serine protease inhibitor and hemostatic agent used to prevent bleeding in high-risk patients undergoing coronary artery bypass graft surgery. Also an anti-inflammatory agent.

arginine vasopressin: Antidiuretic hormone that can also be used as a vasopressor.

arrhythmia: No heart rhythm.

arrhythmogenic right ventricular cardiomyopathy: A genetic disorder characterized by right ventricular cardiomyopathy caused by an electrical disturbance that produces dysrhythmias.

arterioles: Small arteries with thick muscular walls.

ascites: Accumulation of serous fluid in the peritoneal cavity.

atelectasis: A condition in which a portion of the lung is unexpanded or collapsed.

atherectomy: Interventional procedure utilizing a cutting tool to cut atherosclerotic plaque away from the wall of the coronary artery.

atheroma: Extracellular lipid core of atherosclerotic plaque.

atheromatous: Pertaining to atheroma.

atherosclerosis: The deposit of lipids, calcium, fibrin, and other cellular substances within the lining of the arteries and the progressive inflammatory response that results from the effort to heal the endothelium.

atherosclerotic plaque: A buildup of the deposits of lipids, calcium, fibrin, and other cellular substances that occurs with atherosclerosis.

atrial defibrillator: Implantable defibrillator programmed to shock and cardiovert the rhythm of atrial fibrillation.

atrial fibrillation: Rapid chaotic activity of the atria that results in the deterioration of atrial mechanical activity and produces irregular atrial fibrillation waves with an atrial rate greater than 350 beats per minute. Variable ventricular conduction resulting in an irregularly irregular ventricular rhythm.

atrial kick: Atrial contraction, or systole.

atrial myxoma: A benign tumor located in the upper chamber of the heart on the wall that separates the left chamber from the right (the atrial septum).

atrial natriuretic peptide (ANP): Hormone released by the atria during periods of volume overload. Increased production causes vasodilation and diuresis.

atrioventricular (AV) block: Block of the impulse that normally travels from the sinoatrial node to the AV node, disrupting the normal heart rhythm and conduction of impulses through the heart.

atrioventricular (AV) junction: Tissue surrounding the AV node and bundle of His that contains pacemaker cells capable of firing at a rate of 40 to 60 beats per minute.

atrioventricular (AV) node: A small mass of tissue that slows conduction from the atria to the ventricles and is located in the right atrium, just above the insertion of the tricuspid valve.

atrioventricular (AV) node ablation: Ablation of the AV node that permanently prevents any rapid ventricular response. Patients who require AV node ablation also need permanent pacemaker implantation.

atrioventricular (AV) valves: Valves located between the atria and ventricles.

autoimmune response: Process by which the body produces an immunological response against itself.

autologous transfusion: Transfusion of blood donated by the patient himself or herself.

automated external defibrillator (AED): Defibrillator designed to be used by trained laypeople in the event of cardiac arrest due to ventricular fibrillation. Rhythm recognition and defibrillation are done automatically via a hands-off approach.

automaticity: Intrinsic ability to depolarize spontaneously.

autonomic dysfunction: Dysfunction of the autonomic nervous system.

autonomic nervous system: Nervous system that controls involuntary bodily functions. Consists of the sympathetic and parasympathetic nervous systems.

Bachmann's bundle: Conduction pathway that allows depolarization of the left atrial tissue as conduction travels from the sinoatrial node to the atrioventricular node.

baroreceptors: Specialized nerve tissues functioning as sensors that are located in the aortic arch and carotid sinus (the origin of the internal carotid artery).

base: Top of the heart, which is located at approximately the second intercostal space.

beta1 adrenergic receptor: Sympathetic nervous system receptor located in the heart.

beta2 adrenergic receptor: Sympathetic nervous system receptor located in the lungs and periphery.

beta-blocker: Medication that blocks either beta1- or beta2-adrenergic receptors.

beta radiation: Type of radiation used for in-stent restenosis with less dwell time and less scatter than gamma radiation.

Bezold-Jarisch reflex: Cardiovascular reflex that causes a vasovagal response when triggered.

bifascicular block: A block of the normal conduction system involving simultaneous blockage of the right bundle branch and blockage of one of the two fascicles of the left bundle branch.

bile acid sequestrant: Also called a *resin,* a lipid-lowering drug that combines with bile acids in the intestine to form an insoluble complex that is excreted in feces.

bioprosthetic valve: Tissue valve from a human or animal donor.

biphasic waveform defibrillator: Newer generation of defibrillators that use energy more efficiently, therefore requiring lower amounts of energy for a defibrillation or cardioversion shock.

bisferiens carotid pulse: Characteristic of a patient with hypertrophic obstructive cardiomyopathy in which the initial upstroke of the carotid pulse is brisk; however, as systole progresses, left ventricular outflow tract obstruction can occur. This obstruction results in a collapse of the pulse and then a secondary rise.

biventricular pacing: See *cardiac resynchronization therapy.*

body mass index (BMI): An index used to define overweight and obesity. Calculated by using height, weight, and a constant.

brachial plexus: Network of nerves supplying the arm, forearm, and hand.

brachiocephalic artery: Also called the *innominate artery,* the largest branch off the aortic arch that divides into the right common carotid and right subclavian arteries.

bradydysrhythmia: a dysrhythmia characterized by a ventricular rate less than 50 beats per minute.

bradycardia: Heart rate below 50 beats per minute.

brain natriuretic peptide (BNP): A hormone released from myocytes during heart failure that produces vasodilation. Serum BNP levels are used in the diagnosis of heart failure.

bruit: An adventitious sound heard on auscultation of a vessel.

bundle branch block: Block of either the right or left bundle branch.

bundle of His: Conduction pathway that divides and gives rise to the right and left bundles.

bupropion: Oral antidepressant used for smoking cessation.

calcium channel blocker: Medication that decreases the flux of calcium across the cell membrane.

cannulation: The placement of a tube inside a vessel to allow the escape of blood and other fluids from the body. Used in cardiopulmonary bypass surgery.

capillary: The very smallest vessel that connects the smallest arteries and veins. Also the location of oxygen and nutrient exchange.

carbon monoxide: A poisonous gas that is colorless, odorless, and tasteless.

cardiac biomarker: Substance released into the blood when necrosis occurs as a result of myocyte membrane rupture.

cardiac catheterization: An invasive diagnostic procedure, used to identify blockage of coronary arteries, whereby a catheter is threaded through an artery into the heart, a contrast agent (dye) is injected into the coronary arteries, and angiography is performed.

cardiac myoplasty: Surgery that involves wrapping a muscle from the patient's back around the heart and stimulating it to contract via a pacemaker wire.

cardiac output: The amount of blood ejected by the left ventricle every minute.

cardiac resynchronization therapy (CRT): Pacemaker therapy aimed at eliminating dyssynchrony of the contractions of the right and left ventricles that occurs in severe heart failure. Utilizes a pacemaker lead for each ventricle (biventricular pacing).

cardiac tamponade: Accumulation of excess fluid in the pericardium that prevents ventricular filling.

cardiogenic shock: Failure of tissues to receive an adequate blood supply because of severely decreased cardiac output caused by left ventricular failure.

cardiomyopathy: A disorder caused by dysfunction of the myocardium; heart muscle disease.

cardioplegia: Paralysis of the heart.

cardiopulmonary bypass: Process by which the normal circulation of blood bypasses the heart and lungs during the administration of cardioplegia for coronary artery bypass graft surgery. This is accomplished by rerouting the blood through a cardiopulmonary bypass machine that functions in place of the heart and lungs.

cardioversion: Restoration of a tachydysrhythmia (atrial fibrillation, supraventricular tachycardia, ventricular tachycardia) to a normal sinus rhythm, using electrical stimulation or pharmacotherapy.

carotid endarterectomy: A surgical procedure whereby the fatty buildup of plaque is removed from the carotid artery.

catalyze: To speed up the rate of a reaction.

catecholamines: The sympathetic nervous system neurotransmitters epinephrine and norepinephrine.

cerebral vascular accident (CVA): Also known as *stroke.* Injury to the brain caused by inadequate oxygenated blood supply. Can be caused by thrombus or embolus (ischemic stroke) or by hemorrhage (hemorrhagic stroke).

cephalosporin: Class of antibiotics most frequently used to prevent postoperative infection in coronary artery bypass graft surgery.

chemoreceptors: Receptors located in the aortic arch and carotid arteries that respond to changes in blood chemistry, including arterial oxygen content, arterial carbon dioxide levels, and arterial pH.

cholinergic: Name of response of the parasympathetic nervous system.

chordae tendineae: Delicate strands of fibrous material that attach atrioventricular valve leaflets to the papillary muscles.

chronic obstructive pulmonary disease (COPD): A chronic lung disease characterized by a limitation in airflow during normal breathing.

chronotropic: Affecting the heart rate.

cirrhosis: Chronic disease of the liver involving connective tissue, fatty infiltrates, and degenerative changes.

coagulopathy: Pathology of the coagulation system.

coarctation of the aorta: Malformation resulting in narrowing of the aorta.

collagen: Fibrous protein found in connective tissue.

commissure: Point where the cardiac valve leaflets connect.

commissurotomy: Procedure during which the valve commissures are cut apart to allow for increased movement of the leaflets.

common pathway: Final pathway in clotting cascade in which a fibrinogen is converted to fibrin and a fibrin stable clot is formed.

complete heart block: Complete failure of the atrial impulses to be conducted to the ventricles.

concentric hypertrophy: A change in the walls of the ventricle resulting in thickened walls that are stiff and noncompliant but do not increase the overall size of the ventricle.

conduit: Term used to describe a blood vessel used as a bypass graft during coronary artery bypass graft surgery.

contractility: Ability of the ventricle to pump independent of preload or afterload.

contrast-induced nephropathy: Renal dysfunction caused by the administration of contrast agents during invasive or interventional cardiac procedures.

coronary artery bypass graft (CABG) surgery: Surgery during which blood flow through a coronary artery is rerouted around a blockage or narrowing in the coronary artery utilizing a bypass graft. A variety of veins or arteries from the patient or a donor can be utilized as bypass grafts.

coronary artery disease (CAD): Disease process that results in narrowing or occlusion of the coronary artery.

coronary heart disease (CHD): Term used interchangeably with CAD.

coronary sinus: The vessel that receives blood from the cardiac veins and empties into the right atrium.

creatine kinase (CK): Biomarker present in the heart, brain, and skeletal muscle.

creatine kinase-MB: Biomarker specific to the heart that rapidly rises in the presence of myocardial damage.

cryopreservation: Preservation by subjection to very low temperatures.

cryotherapy: Therapy using cold.

crystalloid solution: Clear intravenous solution with dissolved substances that can diffuse across cell membranes. For example, normal saline solution.

cutting balloon: A device used to make incisions into the plaque prior to dilation during percutaneous transluminal coronary angioplasty.

cyclooxygenase: Chemical substance that performs the first step in the creation of prostaglandins.

cyclosporin: Medication used to suppress the immune system.

cytokine: Protein secreted by cells of the immune system that helps to regulate the immune system.

DDD pacemaker: Dual chamber pacemaker that senses and paces in both the right atrium and right ventricle. Responds to any sensed activity by either triggering an action or inhibiting one.

debridement: Removal of dead or damaged tissue from a wound.

defibrillation: Desynchronized shock delivered to patients in ventricular fibrillation.

depolarization: Stimulation of cardiac muscle cells.

diabetes mellitus: Insulin deficit (type I) or inappropriate response to insulin (type II), resulting in a random glucose level greater than 200 mg/dl or a fasting glucose level greater than 126 mg/dl.

diastole: Relaxation of the heart muscle that permits filling of the chamber.

diastolic dysfunction: Left ventricular dysfunction whereby the ventricle has impaired relaxation and does not fill properly.

Dietary Approaches to Stop Hypertension (DASH) diet: A diet that manipulates potassium, calcium, and magnesium while holding sodium constant.

dilatation: Expansion of an organ or a vessel.

dilated cardiomyopathy (DCM): Cardiomyopathy caused by an enlarged, dilated cardiac chamber that affects the ability of the ventricle to contract, resulting in systolic dysfunction.

dipyridamole: A coronary vasodilator used in chemical stress testing.

direct current cardioversion: Procedure in which an electrical shock is synchronized with the intrinsic activity of the heart to convert an abnormal rhythm back into a normal sinus rhythm.

directional atherectomy: Procedure used to cut and remove plaque in native vessels or in saphenous vein grafts by directing a rotating cutter toward the plaque to be removed.

distensibility: Ability to stretch.

dobutamine: Inotropic agent used for chemical stress testing. Also used in critically ill patients in cardiogenic shock or end-stage heart failure.

dopaminergic receptor: Sympathetic nervous system receptor located in the renal, mesenteric, and coronary blood vessels.

Dressler's syndrome: Pericarditis occurring several weeks after an infarction.

dromotropic: Affecting cardiac conduction.

drug-eluting stent: Stent coated with a pharmacological agent aimed at decreasing restenosis.

dual-chamber pacemaker: Pacemaker that has an electrode for pacing in two chambers of the heart; traditionally, the right atrium and the right ventricle.

Duroziez's sign: Systolic murmur heard over the femoral artery when compressed proximally or diastolic murmur heard over the femoral artery when compressed distally.

dyslipidemia: An abnormal amount of lipids in the blood.

dysrhythmia: Abnormal heart rhythm.

eccentric hypertrophy: Hypertrophy caused by volume overload and resulting in ventricular dilation. Wall thickness is in proportion to chamber size.

echocardiogram: Cardiac ultrasound.

ectopic beat: Beat originating outside the sinus node.

ejection: The second phase of systole, during which blood is ejected.

ejection fraction: The percent of volume ejected with each beat.

electrocautery: Cauterization (destruction of tissue) by means of a device heated by a current of electricity.

electromechanical interference: Electrical signals external to a pacemaker that may be sensed by the pacemaker, making it difficult for the pacemaker to sense the heart's activity in the normal manner. This can lead to a dysfunctional pacemaker.

electrophysiology: Field of cardiology dedicated to the study and treatment of disorders of the heart's rhythm.

embolus: A particle of undissolved matter in the blood (can be solid, liquid, or gas; for example, a piece of a clot or fat or an air bubble).

emergency medical system (EMS): Community response system where paramedics and other trained personnel respond to medical emergencies. Activated by dialing "911" in most parts of the country.

endocarditis: Inflammation of the endocardium (the inner lining of heart), including the heart valves.

endocardium: The inner surface of the heart chambers and valves that also covers the walls of the vessels of the entire vascular system.

endomyocardial biopsy: Tissue biopsy obtained from the septal wall of the right ventricle using an invasive catheter-based approach. Used in the diagnosis of restrictive cardiomyopathy.

endomyocardial fibrosis: Fibrosis of the ventricular endocardium and subendocardium that extends to the mitral and tricuspid valves and greatly decreases the functioning of the ventricular chambers.

endothelin: Endogenous hormonal vasoconstrictor released by the endothelium.

endothelium: Layer of epithelial cells that lines the heart, blood vessels, and other body cavities.

endovascular: Minimally invasive techniques using catheter-based treatments, as opposed to full, open surgeries.

epiaortic imaging: Ultrasound imaging directly over the aorta that is used in coronary artery bypass graft surgery.

epicardium: The smooth outer layer of the heart that contains the network of coronary arteries and veins, the autonomic nerves, the lymphatic system, and fat tissue.

epigastric: Referring to the area over the pit of the stomach.

epinephrine: Also called *adrenaline,* a neurotransmitter of the sympathetic nervous system.

epistaxis: Bleeding from the nose.

ergonovine maleate: Arterial vasoconstrictor that can be given during cardiac catheterization to assist in the diagnosis of vasospastic angina.

erythropoietin: A hormone that regulates red blood cell production.

estrogen: Female sex hormone.

external counterpulsation: Nonpharmacological treatment option for debilitating angina in which a series of cuffs are wrapped around the patient's legs and compressed air is used to apply pressure in the cuffs in synchronization with the cardiac cycle, resulting in increased arterial pressure that increases retrograde aortic blood flow into the coronary arteries during diastole.

extrinsic pathway: Pathway in the clotting cascade activated by injured tissue.

extubation: Removal of an endotracheal tube.

Fabry's disease: A lipid storage disorder caused by the deficiency of an enzyme involved in the biodegradation of fats.

fibric acids: A group of lipid-lowering medications most noted for their ability to lower triglycerides. Also called *fibrates.*

fibrin: Fine protein filaments formed by the action of thrombin on fibrinogen that entangle red and white blood cells and platelets and form a clot.

fibrinogen: A protein that is converted to fibrin through the action of thrombin in the presence of calcium ions.

fibrinolytic: Fibrin-specific medication used to break down clots.

fibrous atheroma: Atheroma characterized by the accumulation of fibrous connective tissue within the intima.

fibrous cap: Fibrous tissue, mainly collagen, that covers the lipid core.

fibrous pericardium: External cover of the pericardium.

foam cell: Macrophage (scavenger cell) that is engorged with lipids.

free graft: Graft where both ends of the vessel are removed from their original locations and reattached elsewhere.

gamma radiation: Type of radiation used to treat in-stent restenosis. Has a longer dwell time than beta radiation and is used to treat more difficult lesions.

glomerular filtration rate (GFR): A calculation to determine how well the blood is filtered by the kidneys. It is calculated using a mathematical formula that compares a person's age, sex, and race to serum creatinine, albumin, and blood urea nitrogen levels. Normal GFR in adults is 120 to 125 ml/min.

glycoprotein (GP) IIb/IIIa receptor: Receptor site on platelet surface where platelets and fibrinogen bind to form a fibrin mesh.

graft: A portion of a vessel taken from another part of the body that is used to bypass a coronary artery blockage during coronary artery bypass graft surgery.

great vessels: The aorta, the pulmonary artery, the inferior vena cava, and the superior vena cava.

gynecomastia: Enlarged mammary glands in a male.

glutaraldehyde: Chemical that is used as a cold sterilant and a tissue fixative.

heart block: Condition that arises because of a cardiac conduction system disturbance, resulting in the lack of coordination of the atrial and ventricular activity of the heart.

heart failure: Disorder in which the heart is unable to pump enough oxygenated blood to meet the metabolic needs of the body.

heart rate: Number of times the heart beats in a minute.

hematoma: Mass of blood within the tissue caused by bleeding from a blood vessel.

hemochromatosis: Condition in which the body stores excess iron, causing organ damage.

hemodynamics: Forces influencing the circulation of blood throughout the body.

hemoglobin A1c (HbA1c): Glycosylated hemoglobin, a reflection of the average blood sugar level for 2 to 3 months prior to the test.

hemoptysis: Coughing or spitting up blood that is the result of bleeding from the respiratory system.

hemostasis: Cessation of bleeding.

hemothorax: Collection of blood in the pleural cavity.

hepatojugular reflux: Response of jugular venous pressure when firm pressure is applied to the midepigastric region. This response is exaggerated in right-sided heart failure.

hepatomegaly: Enlargement of the liver.

high-degree atrioventricular (AV) block: The true block of two or more atrial impulses (not in atrial flutter). Also called *advanced AV block.*

high-density lipoprotein cholesterol (HDL-C): A high-density lipoprotein that contains small amounts of cholesterol and triglycerides. Usually associated with a decreased risk of heart disease.

hirudin: Direct thrombin inhibitor.

HMG-CoA reductase: Key enzyme in the synthesis of cholesterol.

HMG-CoA reductase inhibitor: Also called a *statin,* the most widely used lipid-lowering medication in the treatment of cardiovascular disease. Inhibits HMG-CoA reductase during cholesterol synthesis.

holosystolic murmur: A murmur that can be heard throughout systole.

homocysteine: An amino acid that has toxic effects on the endothelium when elevated.

homologous: Similar in both structure and source.

high sensitivity C-reactive protein (hs-CRP): A marker of inflammation. Elevated levels increase cardiovascular risk.

hydrogenated oil: Oil that has hydrogen added to it to make it solid at room temperature.

hydrostatic pressure: Pushing pressure inside a vessel that forces fluids and nutrients across a membrane.

hypercholesterolemia: Elevated serum cholesterol.

hyperdynamic: Increased contractility and ejection fraction (when referring to the left ventricle).

hyperhomocysteinemia: Elevated serum homocysteine.

hyperkalemia: Elevated serum potassium.

hyperlipidemia: Condition characterized by elevated total cholesterol (hypercholesterolemia), elevated low-density lipoprotein cholesterol, or elevated triglycerides.

hyperplasia: Excessive proliferation of normal cells.

hypersensitive carotid sinus: A reflex caused by increased parasympathetic tone when pressure is applied to the carotid sinus, resulting in a slowing of the heart rate.

hypertension: Condition characterized by a systolic or diastolic blood pressure above the normal range.

hyperthyroidism: Excessive secretion from the thyroid gland, resulting in increased basal metabolic rate.

hypertriglyceridemia: Elevated serum triglycerides.

hypertrophic cardiomyopathy (HCM): Cardiomyopathy characterized by hypertrophy of the myocardium, resulting in a decrease in ventricular filling and a decrease in cardiac output.

hypertrophic obstructive cardiomyopathy (HOCM): Hypertrophic cardiomyopathy with obstruction.

hypertrophy: Increased size.

hypokalemia: Low serum potassium.

hypomagnesemia: Low serum magnesium.

hypoperfusion: Decreased perfusion.

hypotension: A systolic or diastolic blood pressure below the normal range.

hypoventilation: Decreased ventilation (amount of inhaled oxygen).

hypovolemia: Diminished blood volume.

hypoxemia: Low level of oxygen in the blood.

hypoxia: Decreased oxygenation of the tissues.

idiopathic: Having no known cause.

idiopathic hypertrophic subaortic stenosis (IHSS): Previous name for hypertrophic cardiomyopathy.

implantable cardioverter-defibrillator (ICD): Device inserted into the heart that provides a defibrillation shock and other therapies to treat rapid heart rates in a variety of patients.

incentive spirometry: Procedure designed to mimic natural sighing by encouraging the patient to take long, slow, deep breaths using a device that provides visual or other positive feedback upon inhalation of a predetermined volume and sustained inflation for a minimum of 3 seconds.

inferior myocardial infarction: Myocardial infarction involving the inferior or bottom wall of the left ventricle.

inferior posterior myocardial infarction: Myocardial infarction involving the inferior and posterior walls of the left ventricle.

inferior vena cava: Principal vein that receives blood from below the level of the diaphragm, including the abdomen, pelvis, and lower extremities. The inferior vena cava empties into the right atrium.

innervation: Distribution of the nervous system.

inotrope: Medication used to increase heart rate.

inotropic: Influencing the force of contractility.

interatrial septum: A mass of connective tissue that separates the right and left atria.

intercalated disks: Disks that form a tight junction, allowing cardiac muscle cells to function as integrated units.

intermittent claudication: Severe pain in calf muscles with walking that is relieved by rest.

internal mammary artery graft: Most common arterial graft used in coronary artery bypass grafting. Has better long-term patency rates than vein grafts.

internal iliac arteries: Arteries that arise from the abdominal aorta and supply blood to the lower trunk, including the reproductive organs and the legs.

International Normalized Ratio (INR): A value that relates prothrombin time to the intensity of actual coagulation. Developed to correct problems with standardization of prothrombin time.

internodal pathways: Conduction pathways in the right atrium that allow conduction between the sinoatrial and atrioventricular nodes.

interstitial pneumonitis: Lung disease characterized by marked interstitial fibrosis. Has an insidious onset with slow, but severe, progression and a poor prognosis, with most patients dying of the disease.

interventricular septum: A mass of connective tissue that separates the right and left ventricles.

intima: The innermost wall of all arteries, which consists of a thin layer of endothelium.

intra-aortic balloon pump (IABP): An invasive catheter-based assistive device that uses counter-pulsation therapy. The balloon, located in the descending aorta, inflates during diastole and deflates during systole. The timing of balloon deflation just before systole reduces cardiac afterload, and balloon inflation during diastole increases myocardial perfusion.

intracoronary stent: Metal scaffold-type structure that is inserted into a coronary artery to help prevent elastic recoil and keep open the lumen of the vessel.

intracoronary (intravascular) ultrasound: A tiny ultrasound device that is threaded into an artery inside a millimeter-thick catheter. Ultrasound waves measure changes in wall thickness, providing a detailed cross section of the coronary artery.

intracranial hemorrhage: Bleeding inside the skull that encloses the brain.

intrinsic pathway (coagulation cascade): Pathway in the clotting cascade that is activated by damage to the red blood cells or the platelets. The intrinsic pathway can be assessed by monitoring activated partial thromboplastin time.

intubation: Placement of an endotracheal tube.

ischemia: Temporary lack of oxygen to the myocardium.

isolated systolic hypertension: A systolic blood pressure greater than 160 mm Hg that is accompanied by a normal diastolic blood pressure.

isovolumetric contraction: Contraction of the ventricle, occurring during the first phase of cardiac systole, when all cardiac valves are closed and the volume of blood in the ventricle remains constant. Also know as *isovolumic contraction.*

jugular venous pressure: Pressure in the jugular vein that increases or decreases in response to fluid status.

kinin: Substance that produces vasodilative effects.

lateral myocardial infarction: Myocardial infarction involving the lateral wall of the left ventricle.

left anterior descending artery (LAD): Coronary artery arising from the left main coronary artery that is responsible for supplying oxygenated blood to the anterior wall of the left ventricle.

left anterior hemiblock: Block of the anterior fascicle of the left bundle.

left atrial appendage: Appendage off the left atrium that is frequently the source of clot formation in atrial fibrillation.

left atrium: Chamber of the heart that receives oxygenated blood from the pulmonary veins.

left bundle branch: Conduction pathway that divides into the left posterior bundle branch and the left anterior bundle branch and carries impulses to the posterior, inferior, and anterior walls of the left ventricle.

left circumflex (LCX) artery: Coronary artery arising from the left main coronary artery that is responsible for supplying blood to the lateral wall of the left ventricle.

left common carotid artery: Artery that branches directly off the thoracic aorta and is one of two common carotid arteries that supply blood to the neck and head.

left main coronary artery: Major coronary artery arising from the left side of the aorta that supplies oxygenated blood to a major portion of the myocardium via the left anterior descending and left circumflex coronary arteries.

left subclavian artery: Artery that arises from the end of the aortic arch and is one of two subclavian arteries that supply blood to the upper extremities.

left ventricle: A thick-walled, high-pressure pump that receives oxygenated blood from the left atrium and pumps blood into the aorta.

left ventricular reduction surgery: Surgery in which a part of the left ventricle is cut out and the remaining walls are sewn together to decrease the size of the ventricle. Also called the *Batista procedure.*

leukocyte: White blood cell.

low-density lipoprotein cholesterol (LDL-C): A lipoprotein that is commonly referred to as the "bad" cholesterol because of its role in the development of atherosclerosis. LDL lipoprotein deposits cholesterol on the artery walls.

linear ablation: Catheter-based technique developed to achieve the same effect as with the surgical Maze procedure.

lipid: Fat or fat-like substance that is insoluble in water.

lipoprotein a: A lipoprotein similar to low-density lipoprotein cholesterol.

Löffler's endocarditis: Endomyocardial disease characterized by endomyocardial fibrosis, an unusually large number of eosinophils in the blood with infiltration of the heart.

lone atrial fibrillation: Atrial fibrillation in patients with normal cardiac and pulmonary function and with no known predisposing factors.

loop diuretic: An agent that works at the loop of Henle to increase sodium and water excretion.

low-molecular-weight heparin (LMWH): Heparin that is lower in molecular weight and smaller in size than unfractionated heparin.

lysis: Dissolution or decomposition (as in clot lysis).

Marfan's syndrome: Disorder characterized by abnormal length of the extremities, congenital anomalies of the heart, and other associated deformities.

mast cells: Connective tissue cell that plays a key role in the initiation of inflammation.

Maze procedure: Surgical procedure in which a series of incisions are made in the atria using radiofrequency or another form of energy to block reentrant pathways within the atrial tissue and to channel conduction in a more normal fashion.

media: The middle layer of an artery, which consists of smooth muscle and elastic connective tissue.

mediastinitis: Inflammation of the tissue of the mediastinum.

mediastinum: The space near the midline of the chest between the pleural sacs of the lungs that extends from the sternum to the spine. This space contains all the organs and tissues of the chest except the lungs.

medulla: The vasomotor center of the brain that interprets all information received from the baroreceptors.

metabolic syndrome: A grouping of lipid and nonlipid risk factors of metabolic origin.

metastatic cancer: Cancer that has spread beyond the site of origin.

metformin: Oral hypoglycemic agent that can potentially cause nephrotoxicity.

MET level: Metabolic equivalent unit used to estimate the amount of oxygen utilized by the body during physical activity.

mevalonic acid: A precursor to cholesterol.

microvascular: Related to very small vessels.

microvascular complications (of diabetes): Vision loss, nephropathy, neuropathy, and amputation.

minimally invasive coronary artery bypass (MIDCAB): Procedure performed on a beating heart without cardiopulmonary bypass and without the use of a median sternotomy.

mitral facies: Pinkish purple discoloration of the cheeks that is common in patients with severe mitral stenosis.

mitral regurgitation: Inadequate closure of the mitral valve that results in backward flow of blood from the left ventricle to the left atrium during ventricular systole. Also called *mitral insufficiency.*

mitral stenosis: Condition in which the mitral valve is unable to open normally, causing an obstruction of blood flow from the left atrium to the left ventricle during ventricular diastole.

mitral valve: Valve located between the left atrium and left ventricle.

mitral valve prolapse: Condition in which one or both of the mitral valve leaflets collapse into the atrium, sometimes allowing small amounts of blood to flow back into the atrium.

monophasic waveform defibrillators: Early generation defibrillators that use energy inefficiently and require higher amounts of energy for defibrillation or cardioversion shock.

monounsaturated fat: Beneficial fat in a heart-healthy diet that derives from a plant source and is liquid at room temperature. Examples include canola oil and olive oil.

murmur: An atypical sound produced by vibrations caused by turbulent blood flow. A cardiac murmur is typically associated with cardiac valve disease that creates turbulent blood flow through a valve that does not open or close properly.

muscarinic receptor: Type of parasympathetic, or cholinergic, receptor located in the heart and smooth muscle.

Musset's sign: Bobbing of the head with each heart beat.

myocardial imaging: Noninvasive studies utilized to assess various functions of the heart. These studies include cardiac echocardiography and radionuclide imaging and can be done individually or in combination with a stress test.

myocardial infarction (MI): Death or necrosis of myocardial tissue.

myocarditis: Inflammation of the myocardium.

myocardium: Thick middle layer of heart that contains cardiac muscle fibers.

myocyte: Contractile cardiac muscle cell.

myofibril: Small fiber that is the contractile element of muscle cells.

myoglobin: Sensitive cardiac biomarker that rises the earliest with myocardial damage.

natriuretic peptide: Hormones released by the heart during periods of volume overload. Increased production of these hormones causes vasodilation, both pulmonary and systemic, as well as diuresis. The release of these hormones is beneficial during periods of acute decompensated heart failure. Types of natriuretic peptides include atrial natriuretic peptide and brain natriuretic peptide.

necrosis: Accidental death of a portion of tissue.

nephrotoxic: Toxic to the kidneys.

nesiritide (Natrecor): A synthetic form of brain natriuretic peptide that is administered intravenously for patients in acute heart failure.

neurogenic atrial fibrillation: Atrial fibrillation caused by either increased vagal tone or increased adrenergic tone.

neurocardiogenic syncope: A loss of consciousness caused by overstimulation of the vagus nerve and a reduction in normal sympathetic activity resulting in hypotension, bradycardia, and peripheral vasodilation.

neurohormonal responses: Various hormonal and neurological responses that occur in heart failure to attempt to compensate for decreased cardiac output.

niacin: A B complex vitamin with additional dose-related pharmacological positive effects on lipid levels. Also called *nicotinic acid.*

nicotine: The physically addictive substance in tobacco.

nicotinic receptor: Type of parasympathetic, or cholinergic, receptor.

noncompliant ventricle: A ventricle that is unable to relax and fill properly during diastole.

nonvalvular atrial fibrillation: Atrial fibrillation in the absence of rheumatic heart disease that causes mitral stenosis or the absence of a prosthetic heart valve.

nonhomologous graft: Grafts from another species.

norepinephrine: A neurotransmitter of the sympathetic nervous system. Also called *nonadrenaline.*

nosocomial pneumonia: Pneumonia acquired in the hospital.

NPO: Nothing by mouth.

non-ST-segment elevation myocardial infarction (non-STEMI): A myocardial infarction diagnosis based on elevated cardiac biomarkers or enzymes. This type of myocardial infarction does not present with ST-segment elevation on the 12-lead ECG.

omega-3 fatty acid: Nonessential fatty acid contained in oily fish, such as salmon, lake trout, tuna, and herring.

oncotic pressure: The pulling pressure inside a vessel that draws fluid and other substances into the vessel.

off-pump coronary artery bypass (OPCAB): Coronary artery bypass surgery done without the use of a cardiopulmonary bypass machine. This approach to surgery does require an open chest procedure with a midline sternal incision.

opening snap: Abnormal sound made by the opening of a stenotic mitral or tricuspid valve.

opioid: Drug derived from an opium alkaloid. An example is morphine.

orthopnea: Shortness of breath when in a supine position.

orthostatic: Concerning an upright position.

ostium: Small opening in the aorta that gives rise to the right and left coronary artery systems.

oxidation: The process of a substance combining with oxygen.

pacemaker electrode: Electrode located at the end of a pacemaker lead wire that delivers the stimulus to the heart muscle to make it contract.

pacemaker generator: Lithium battery and the electrical microcircuitry necessary to operate a pacemaker. Also referred to as the *battery* or *can.*

pacemaker lead: Wire that travels from the pacemaker generator to the wall of the heart that carries the message to contract from the generator to the heart. Houses the pacemaker electrode at the end of the wire.

pacemaker pacing: The ability of a pacemaker to send an impulse through a lead wire to an electrode and stimulate the heart to contract.

pacemaker sensing: The ability of a cardiac pacemaker to recognize native cardiac activity that is occurring in a cardiac chamber that has a cardiac pacing electrode.

paclitaxel: An antiproliferative or antineoplastic agent used on drug-eluting stents that is also used as a chemotherapeutic agent.

papillary muscles: Muscle projections from the inner surface of the ventricles that attach to the chordae tendineae of the atrioventricular valves.

parasympathetic nervous system: Branch of the autonomic nervous system that helps the body conserve and restore resources.

parasympatholytic: Medication that lyses the parasympathetic nervous system.

parietal pericardium: Inner lining of the fibrous pericardium.

paroxysmal: Coming on suddenly and terminating without intervention. Used to describe tachydysrhythmias.

paroxysmal atrial fibrillation: Atrial fibrillation that comes on spontaneously and terminates itself. Cannot last longer than 7 days and usually lasts less than 24 hours.

paroxysmal nocturnal dyspnea: Awakening from a sleep state with sudden and intense shortness of breath.

pathological Q wave: Abnormally deep or wide Q wave that indicates necrosis of myocardial tissue.

percutaneous alcohol septal ablation (PASA): Procedure performed in a cardiac catheterization lab during which a catheter is inserted into a septal perforator branch (provides blood flow to the septum). Ethyl alcohol is then injected to produce a controlled septal myocardial infarction.

pedicle graft: Graft in which one end of an artery is left in its original position. Examples include internal mammary artery graft.

percutaneous left atrial appendage transcatheter occlusion (PLAATO): Procedure using a right cardiac catheterization in which a transseptal puncture is made and an occlusive device is placed in the left atrial appendage to prevent embolization of a thrombus.

percutaneous transluminal coronary angioplasty (PTCA): Catheter-based procedure in which a balloon is inflated at the site of coronary stenosis to increase the vessel lumen diameter.

pericardial knock: High-frequency heart sound heard in patients with restrictive pericarditis.

pericardiocentesis: Perforation of the pericardium via a needle for the purpose of removal of fluid from the pericardial space.

pericarditis: Inflammation of the pericardium.

pericardium: Thin fibrous sac that surrounds the heart.

perioperative: Period around surgery, which can include the preoperative, intraoperative, and postoperative periods.

peripartum cardiomyopathy: Cardiomyopathy associated with the last trimester of pregnancy or the postpartum period.

peritoneum: Membrane that lines the abdominal cavity.

permanent atrial fibrillation: Atrial fibrillation that is accepted as permanent or lasts longer than 1 year.

permanent pacemaker: Artificial device implanted in the heart that consists of a battery or generator, a lead wire, and an electrode that delivers a stimulus to the heart to maintain a normal heart beat.

persistent atrial fibrillation: Atrial fibrillation that lasts longer than 7 days.

pheochromocytoma: A tumor that produces catecholamines.

phrenic nerve: A motor and sensory nerve that provides innervation to the diaphragm, pericardium, and pleura.

plasmin: Fibrinolytic enzyme derived from plasminogen.

plasminogen: A protein important in preventing fibrin clot formation. The precursor to plasmin.

pleura: Membrane surrounding the lungs.

pneumothorax: Collection of air in the pleural cavity from a perforation through the chest wall or visceral pleura covering the lung.

plain old balloon angioplasty (POBA): Percutaneous transluminal coronary angioplasty (PTCA) done without the placement of an intracoronary stent.

polyneuropathy: Noninflammatory disorder that affects the peripheral nerves.

portal hypertension: Increased pressure in the portal vein (vein providing blood flow to the liver) caused by obstruction of blood flow through the liver.

posterior descending artery (PDA): Coronary artery arising from the right coronary artery in most people that supplies oxygenated blood to the posterior wall of the left ventricle.

posterior myocardial infarction: Myocardial infarction involving the posterior wall of the left ventricle.

postpericardiotomy syndrome: Inflammation of the pericardium late after coronary artery bypass graft surgery due to autoimmune response.

precordial leads: Chest leads on a 12-lead electrocardiogram; V_1 to V_6 or V_{1R} to V_{6R}.

preload: Stretch on the ventricular myocardial fibers caused by the volume in the ventricle at the end of ventricular diastole.

pressure gradient: Difference in pressure from one side of a valve to the other side of that valve.

prevalence: The number of cases of a disease in a specified population at a given time.

primary aldosteronism: Excessive excretion of aldosterone by the adrenal cortex.

primary coronary intervention (PCI): A procedure that treats coronary artery disease without the use of surgery. Most commonly, balloon angioplasty with or without stent placement. Also referred to as *percutaneous coronary intervention.*

primary prevention: Reducing risk in people without known coronary heart disease to prevent the development of disease.

proarrhythmic: Causing dysrhythmias.

procainamide: A potent class Ia antiarrhythmic agent used in the treatment of several cardiac dysrhythmias, including atrial fibrillation and ventricular tachycardia. A derivative of the local anesthetic procaine.

progesterone: A steroid hormone responsible for changes in the endometrium during the second half of the menstrual cycle, development of the maternal placenta, and development of the mammary glands.

progestin: Hormone that prepares the endometrium to receive a fertilized egg. Also a synthetic drug that has a progesterone-like effect on the uterus.

prolonged QT syndrome: A condition characterized by a prolonged QT interval on an electrocardiogram that predisposes a person to torsades de pointes.

prostaglandin I2: A chemical substance that produces vasodilation and inhibits platelet aggregation.

prothrombin: A circulating chemical substance that interacts with calcium salts to produce thrombin.

prothrombin time (PT): Coagulation test used to monitor the safety and effectiveness of warfarin.

protease: A protein-splitting enzyme.

pruritus: Severe itching.

pseudo: False.

pulmonary artery catheter: Catheter that is threaded through right heart and placed in the pulmonary artery. Has various ports that allow for measurement of various heart pressures and cardiac output.

pulmonary edema: Fluid in the pulmonary alveoli that interferes with gas exchange.

pulmonary embolus: Embolus in the pulmonary artery system that increases pulmonary pressure that can cause pulmonary infarction.

pulmonary vascular resistance: Resistance in the pulmonary system that the right ventricle must pump against. Also called *right-sided afterload.*

pulmonary vein ectopic foci ablation: Catheter-based procedure in which areas around the four pulmonary veins are isolated with radiofrequency energy to create a block and eliminate the ability of the foci to enter the left atrium.

pulmonary veins: Veins that carry oxygenated blood from the lungs to the left atrium.

pulmonic valve: Valve between the right ventricle and the pulmonary artery.

pulse pressure: Difference between systolic and diastolic blood pressure.

pulsus alternans: An alternation between weak and strong heart beats, with weak beats occurring every other beat.

Purkinje fibers: Conduction fibers located in the ventricles. Serve as the third option as a pacemaker for the heart, with the ability to pace at a rate of 20 to 40 beats per minute.

P wave: Wave on an electrocardiogram that represents atrial depolarization.

QRS complex: Complex on an electrocardiogram that represents ventricular depolarization.

Q wave: First negative deflection of the QRS complex.

radial artery: Artery along the thumb side of the wrist, which is used as a conduit for coronary artery bypass graft surgery.

recombinant deoxyribonucleic acid (DNA): DNA that has been artificially manipulated to combine DNA from one organism with DNA of another organism.

reentrant mechanism: Mechanism of a dysrhythmia whereby a wave of depolarization turns upon itself and reenters the tissue it just activated.

reflex tachycardia: Increased heart rate that occurs in response to a lowered blood pressure.

remodeling: A process of pathological growth whereby a ventricle hypertrophies and then dilates.

renin: An enzyme produced by the kidneys that, when released, stimulates activation of the renin-angiotensin-aldosterone system.

renin-angiotensin-aldosterone system (RAAS): Neurohormonal system that is activated in response to low cardiac output or low blood pressure. The end result is angiotensin II, a potent vasoconstrictor, and aldosterone, which causes sodium and water reabsorption.

renovascular disease: Disease of the renal arteries.

reperfusion: Restoration of oxygen to ischemic tissue.

repolarization: Return of a cardiac cell to a resting state.

resistant hypertension: Continued hypertension on full-dose therapy, including a diuretic.

restenosis: Renarrowing of the vessel lumen after a primary coronary intervention.

restrictive cardiomyopathy (RCM): Cardiomyopathy characterized by rigidity of the myocardial wall with decreased ability of the chamber walls to expand during cardiac filling.

retroperitoneal bleed: Bleeding into the space behind the peritoneum.

revascularization: Restoration, to the extent possible, of normal blood flow to the myocardium by surgical or percutaneous means.

rhabdomyolysis: Breakdown of muscle fibers with leakage of potentially toxic cellular contents into the systemic circulation.

rheumatic fever: A hemolytic streptococcal infection.

rheumatic heart disease: Damage to the heart that is the result of rheumatic fever. Normal cardiac complications include bacterial endocarditis with damage to the cardiac valves.

right atrium: Chamber of the heart that receives deoxygenated blood from the venous system.

right bundle branch: Conduction pathway that carries impulses to the right ventricle.

right coronary artery (RCA): Major coronary artery arising from the right side of the aorta that supplies blood to the inferior wall of the left ventricle.

right gastroepiploic artery: Artery that supplies blood to the greater curvature of the stomach and can be used as a conduit in coronary artery bypass graft surgery.

right ventricle: A thin-walled, low-pressure pump that receives deoxygenated blood from the right atrium and pumps blood into the pulmonary artery.

risk equivalent: Same risk as someone diagnosed with a disease, such as coronary heart disease.

risk factor: A characteristic found in a healthy person that is independently related to the future development of a disease, such as coronary heart disease.

Ross procedure: Procedure in which the pulmonic valve is placed in the aortic valve position and a tissue valve is placed in the pulmonic valve location.

rotational atherectomy: Use of high-speed rotating blades or burs to remove components of atherosclerotic plaque.

S_3: Third heart sound; heard immediately after the second heart sound; an indication of fluid overload.

S_4: Fourth heart sound; heard just before the first heart sound; an indication of a noncompliant ventricle.

saphenous vein graft: Vein graft taken from the greater saphenous vein of the leg. Most common vein graft material used in coronary artery bypass graft surgery.

sarcoidosis: Disease that causes inflammation or small lumps (also called nodules or granulomas) in the tissues.

sarcomere: A portion of the myofibril that contains protein units.

saturated fats: Fats that are usually solid at room temperature and typically come from animals.

secondary prevention: Method of reducing risk in people with known coronary heart disease to prevent future events.

second-degree heart block: A cardiac dysrhythmia that results when atrial impulses are not conducted normally through the AV node to the ventricle. Also referred to as *second-degree AV block.*

selective serotonin reuptake inhibitors (SSRIs): Class of antidepressant medications commonly used to treat depression in cardiac patients.

semilunar valves: The valves located between the ventricles and great vessels.

senile degenerative calcification: Progressive calcification of the valve leaflets.

serine: An amino acid found in many proteins.

sheath: Small, flexible catheter in a vascular access site. Guidewires and diagnostic and interventional devices are thread through the sheath during invasive and interventional procedures.

shoulder: Edge of a fibrous cap. A particularly vulnerable area that is frequently the location of ruptured plaque.

sick sinus syndrome (SSS): Rhythm marked by sinus node dysfunction (bradycardia or sinus arrest) alternating with periods of rapid atrial dysrhythmias. Also called *tachy-brady syndrome.*

single chamber pacemaker: A pacemaker that has an electrode for pacing in one chamber of the heart; traditionally, a ventricular pacemaker.

sinoatrial (SA) node: Natural pacemaker of the heart, which is located in the right atrium near the junction of the superior vena cava.

sirolimus: An immunosuppressive agent used on drug-eluting stents that is also used to prevent organ rejection during kidney transplantation.

ST-segment elevation myocardial infarction (STEMI): A myocardial infarction that produces ST-segment elevation on an electrocardiogram.

stable angina pectoris: Angina with a stable pattern that is brought on by exertion and relieved by rest or sublingual nitroglycerin.

stanol: A sterol that has been saturated.

statins (HMG-CoA reductase inhibitors): Another name for HMG-CoA reductase inhibitors; all drugs in this class end with the letters "statin."

stenosis: Narrowing of a passage.

sternotomy: The act of cutting through the sternum.

sterol: Compound found in the cell membranes of plants and animals. Plant sterols are used in the treatment of high cholesterol.

sternum: Flat bone in the middle of the thorax, or chest.

stress testing: Noninvasive assessment tool for coronary artery diseases that uses exercise or chemicals to stress the heart. May be done with or without myocardial imaging.

stroke volume: Volume of blood ejected by the left ventricle with each beat.

subendocardium: Middle myocardium.

substernal: Below the sternum.

superior vena cava: A principal vein that receives venous blood returning from the head, neck, upper extremities, and thorax and empties into the right atrium.

supraventricular dysrhythmia: dysrhythmia originating above the ventricles. Called *supraventricular tachycardia* when the heart rate is more than 100 beats per minute.

sympathetic nervous system (SNS): Branch of the autonomic nervous system that allows the body to function under stress.

sympathomimetic: A medication that mimics the sympathetic nervous system.

syncope: Transient lack of consciousness due to inadequate blood flow to the brain.

systemic lupus erythematosus (SLE): An autoimmune disease characterized by fever, skin rash, and arthritis, often with small hemorrhages in the skin and mucous membranes and inflammation of the pericardium.

systole: Contraction of the heart muscle that results in ejection of blood from the chamber.

systolic dysfunction: Left ventricular dysfunction involving a problem with ejection.

systolic ejection murmur: A murmur that occurs as blood is ejected through a stenotic aortic or pulmonic valve during early systole.

tachydysrhythmia: Cardiac dysrhythmias with a ventricular rate more than 100 beats per minute.

tachycardia: Heart rate greater than 100 beats per minute.

tachypnea: Increased respiratory rate.

tacrolimus: A potent immunosuppressant medication used to prevent and treat organ rejection.

thiazide diuretic: Diuretic that inhibits sodium and water reabsorption. Works in the ascending loop of Henle and the early distal tubule.

thiocyanate: Cyanide ions released into the system are converted to thiocyanate in the liver. Thiocyanate level should be monitored during infusions of nitroprusside because nitroprusside releases cyanide ions into the system.

thoracic aorta: Portion of aorta located in the thoracic cavity that contains the ascending aorta, the aortic arch, and the descending thoracic aorta.

thoracotomy: Surgical incision of the chest wall.

thrombin: An enzyme formed from prothrombin that converts fibrinogen to fibrin.

thrombocytopenia: Abnormal decrease in platelet number.

thromboembolus: Embolus that has broken away from a thrombus.

thrombolytic: Nonfibrin medication used to break down clots.

thrombophlebitis: Inflammation of a vein in conjunction with the formation of a thrombus.

thrombosis: Formation or existence of a blood clot.

thrombotic stroke: Ischemic stroke caused by a thrombus or an embolus from a thrombus.

thromboxane A2: Substance released with vascular injury that is a potent vasoconstrictor and platelet agonist.

thrombus: A blood clot that causes obstruction.

T lymphocyte: Lymphocyte cell that differentiates in the thymus and is responsible for cellular immunity.

torsades de pointes: A special ventricular tachycardia associated with a prolonged QT interval.

Traube's sign: Booming systolic and diastolic sounds heard over the femoral artery. Also called *pistol-shot sounds.*

transesophageal echocardiography (TEE): Placement of an ultrasound probe into the esophagus to view the aorta and cardiac structures. Eliminates the need to image through the chest wall.

transluminal extraction atherectomy: Procedure used for the extraction of visible thrombi within the coronary artery.

transmural: Full thickness of myocardium.

transmyocardial laser revascularization (TMLR): Form of revascularization whereby a series of transmural endomyocardial channels are created with lasers to improve myocardial blood supply.

transverse (T) tubules: Extensions of cell membranes in the cardiac muscle that allow calcium to enter the cells.

tricuspid valve: Valve located between the right atrium and right ventricle.

trifascicular block: A block of the normal conduction system involving simultaneous blockage of the right bundle branch, one of the two fascicles of the left bundle branch, and AV block.

triglyceride: Chemical compound of glycerol and three fatty acids that is a component of most animal and vegetable fats.

troponin I: Biomarker found only in cardiac muscle. The most sensitive indicator of myocardial damage.

T wave: Wave on an electrocardiogram that represents ventricular repolarization.

ulnar artery: Artery alongside the wrist, opposite the thumb.

unfractionated heparin (UFH): A commercially available anticoagulant produced from porcine or bovine tissue. Heparin prevents the extension of thrombus but does not lyse clots.

unstable angina pectoris: Angina at rest or with minimal exertion or an increased need for nitroglycerin.

urticaria: A vascular skin rash that produces papules or wheals and causes severe itching.

vagal: Response related to the stimulation of the parasympathetic nervous system, specifically the vagus nerve. A vagal response is characterized by a low heart rate, low blood pressure, light-headedness, and nausea.

Valsalva's maneuver: A maneuver that increases intrathoracic pressure, elicits the parasympathetic response, and decreases venous return to the heart.

valvuloplasty: Procedure in which a balloon is inflated in the cardiac valve orifice to fracture calcium deposits in the leaflets and stretch the annulus to return the valve to normal functioning.

vasoconstriction: Constriction of vessels.

vasodilation: Dilation of vessels.

vasopressor: Medication used to increase blood pressure and afterload.

vasospastic angina: Angina caused by spasm of a coronary artery. Also called *Prizmetal's angina*.

vasovagal response: Response of the parasympathetic nervous system that produces hypotension, bradycardia, diaphoresis, nausea, and vomiting.

Vaughan Williams classification system: Classification system for antiarrhythmic pharmacology that contains four classes.

venous oxygen saturation: The percent of oxygen saturation of venous blood after the tissues have extracted oxygen from the arterial blood. Normal range is 60% to 80%.

ventricular aneurysm: Localized dilation of the left ventricle at the site of infarction.

ventricular dysrhythmia: dysrhythmia originating from the ventricles. Called *ventricular tachycardia* when the heart rate is more than 100 beats per minute.

ventricular ectopy: Abnormal heart beats that originate from a ventricle rather than from the sinus node.

ventricular fibrillation: A quivering of the ventricles that results in a pulseless rhythm and cardiac arrest and is treated with immediate defibrillation.

ventricular outflow tract: The path the blood in a ventricle must follow when ejected from the ventricle.

ventricular pacemaker: Pacemaker that has a lead in the right ventricle and paces only the right ventricle.

ventricular septal myectomy: Surgical removal of a portion of a hypertrophied septum that is contributing to outflow obstruction.

viable: Capable of living.

visceral pericardium: Inner lining of the pericardium and outer lining of the heart and great vessels. Also called the *epicardium*.

vulnerable plaque: Atherosclerotic plaque that is prone to ulceration and rupture.

VVI pacemaker: Single chamber pacemaker with an electrode in the right ventricle that paces the right ventricle, senses normal activity in the left ventricle, and inhibits the pacemaker when the electrode senses normal cardiac activity.

wall motion abnormality: Abnormal movement of a wall of the left ventricle. Can be seen on echocardiogram.

warfarin: An oral anticoagulant agent that works indirectly through the liver by altering vitamin K–dependent clotting factors.

water-hammer pulse: A rapid rise and collapse of the pulse that can be felt upon palpation. Also called *Corrigan's pulse*.

Wolff-Parkinson-White (WPW) syndrome: Syndrome in which one or more accessory pathways connect the atria to the ventricles. Conduction over the accessory pathways causes preexcitation of the ventricles, predisposing the patient to tachydysrhythmias.

REFERENCES

Akashi, Y.J., Nakazawa, K., Kida, K., Ryu, S.,Takagi, A., Kishi, R., ... Miyake, F. (2003). Reversible ventricular dysfunction (takotsubo cardiomyopathy) following polymorphic ventricular tachycardia. *The Canadian Journal of Cardiology 19*(4), 449-451.

Akinpelu D. & Gonzalez, J.M. (2009). *Treadmill stress testing.* Retrieved from http://emedicine.medscape.com/article/160772-print

Akoum, N.W., Lowy, J., & Freedman, R.A. (2010). Pacemaker therapy. *ACP Medicine.* Available from https://www.acpmedicine.com/acp medicine/institutional/payPerAdd.action? chapterId=part01_ch07

American Association of Critical Care Nurses (AACN). (2010). *Practice alert: Oral care for patients at risk for ventilator-associated pneumonia.* Available at http://www.aacn.org/WD/Practice/Docs/PracticeAlerts/oral%20care% 2004-2010%20final.pdf

American Diabetes Association. (2010). Executive summary: Standards of medical care in diabetes. *Diabetes Care, 33*(Suppl 1), S4–S10.

American Heart Association. (n.d.) *Inflammation, heart disease and stroke: The role of C-reactive protein.* Available from http://www.american heart.org/presenter.jhtml?identifier=4648

American Heart Association. (2010). *Research facts, 2010.* Available from http://www.american heart.org/downloadable/heart/1265209045792 Research_Facts_2010.pdf

Anderson, J.L., Adams, C.D., Antman, E.M., Bridges, C.R., Califf, R.M., Casey, D.E., Jr., ... Wright, S. (2007). ACC/AHA 2007 guidelines for the management of patients with unstable angina/non-ST-elevation myocardial infarction: Executive summary. A report of the American College of Cardiology/American Heart Association Task Force on Practice Guidelines (Writing Committee to Revise the 2002 Guidelines for the Management of Patients With Unstable Angina/Non-ST-Elevation Myocardial Infarction). *Journal of the American College of Cardiology, 50*(7), 652–726.

Antman, E.M., Anbe, D.T., Armstrong, P.W., Bates, E.R., Green, L.A., Hand, M., ... Smith, S.C., Jr. (2004). *ACC/AHA guidelines for the management of patients with ST-elevation myocardial infarction: A report of the American College of Cardiology/American Heart Association Task Force on Practice Guidelines* (Committee to Revise the 1999 Guidelines for the Management of Patients With Acute Myocardial Infarction). Available at http://www.americanheart.org/download able/heart/1090338315100STEMIFinalFinal forposting.pdf

Aouizerat, B.E., Gardner, P.E., & Altman, G. (2010). Atherosclerosis, Inflammation, and Acute Coronary Syndrome. In S.L. Woods, E.S.S. Froelicher, S.U. Motzer, & E.J. Bridges (Eds.), *Cardiac nursing* (6th ed., pp. 111–131). Philadelphia, PA: Lippincott Williams & Wilkins.

Colucci, W.S (2004). Heart failure. In E. Braunwald (ed., *Essential atlas of heart diseases* (2nd ed., pp. 105-142). Philadelphia, PA: Current Medicine, Inc.

Arnett, D.K., Baird, A.E., Barkley, R.A., Basson, C.T., Boerwinkle, E., Ganesh, S.K., ... O'Donnell, C.J. (2007). Relevance of genetics and genomics for prevention and treatment of cardiovascular disease: A scientific statement from the American Heart Association Council on Epidemiology and Prevention, the Stroke Council, and the Functional Genomics and Translational Biology Interdisciplinary Working Group. *Circulation, 115*(22), 2878–2901.

Aultman Hospital. (2010). *Patient education booklet for implantable pacemakers and defibrillators.*

Balady, G.J., Williams, M.A., Ades, P.A., Bittner, V. Comoss, P., Foody, J.M., ... Southard, D. (2007). Core components of cardiac rehabilitation/secondary prevention programs: 2007 update: A scientific statement from the American Heart Association Exercise, Cardiac Rehabilitation, and Prevention Committee, the Council on Clinical Cardiology; the Councils on Cardiovascular Nursing, Epidemiology and Prevention, and Nutrition, Physical Activity, and Metabolism; and the American Association of Cardiovascular and Pulmonary Rehabilitation. *Circulation, 115*(20), 2675–2682.

Bashore, T.M., Granger, C.B., Hranitzky, P., & Patel, M.R. (2010). Heart disease. In S.J. McPhee, & M.A. Papadakis (Eds.), *Current medical diagnosis and treatment* (49th ed., pp. 294–386). New York, NY: McGraw-Hill.

Bene, S. & Vaughan, A. (2005). Acute coronary syndromes. In S.L.Woods, E.S.S. Froelicher, S.A. Motzer, & E.J. Bridges (Eds.), *Cardiac nursing* (5th ed., pp. 550–584). Philadelphia, PA: Lippincott Williams & Wilkins.

Bernstein, A.D., Daubert, J.C., Fletcher, R.D., Hayes, D.L., Luderitz, B., Reynolds, D.W., ... Sutton, R. (2002). The revised NASPE/BPEG generic code for antibradycardia, adaptive-rate, and multisite pacing. *Pacing and Clinical Electrophysiology, 25*(2), 260–264.

Berra, K.A. & Fair, J.M. (2010). Lipid management and cardiovascular disease. In S.L. Woods, E.S.S. Froelicher, S.U. Motzer, & E.J. Bridges (Eds.), *Cardiac nursing* (6th ed., pp. 823–841). Philadelphia, PA: Lippincott Williams & Wilkins.

Beyerbach, D.M. (2009). *Implantable cardiovderter-defibrillators.* Retrieved from http://emedicine.medscape.com/article/ 162245-overview

Blancher, S. (2010). Cardiac electrophysiology procedures. In S.L. Woods, E.S.S. Froelicher, S.U. Motzer, & E.J. Bridges (Eds.), *Cardiac nursing* (6th ed., pp. 400–419). Philadelphia, PA: Lippincott Williams & Wilkins.

Bojar, R.M. (2005). *Manual of perioperative care in adult cardiac surgery* (4th ed.), Malden, MA: Blackwell.

Bolooki, H.M. & Askari, A. (2009). *Acute myocardial infarction.* Retrieved from htps://www .clevelandclinicmeded.com/medicalpubs/ diseasemanagement/cardiology/acute-myo cardial-infarction

Bond, E.F. (2010). Anatomy and physiology. In S.L. Woods, E.S.S. Froelicher, S.U. Motzer, & E.J. Bridges (Eds.), *Cardiac nursing* (6th ed., pp. 1–41). Philadelphia, PA: Lippincott Williams & Wilkins.

Bonow, R.O., Carabello, B.A., Chatterjee, K., de Leon, A.C., Jr., Faxon, D.P., Freed, M.D., … Shanewise, J.S. (2008). 2008 focused update incorporated into the ACC/AHA 2006 guidelines for the management of patients with valvular heart disease: A report of the American College of Cardiology/American Heart Association Task Force on Practice Guidelines (Writing Committee to revise the 1998 guidelines for the management of patients with valvular heart disease). *Journal of the American College of Cardiology, 52*(13), e1–e142.

Boston Scientific. (2009). *Portable multimedia players and implantable pacemakers and defibrillators.* Available from http://www .bostonscientific.com/templatedata/imports/ HTML/CRM/A_Closer_Look/pdfs/ACL_ Portable_MultiMedia_Players_030609.pdf

Bott-Silverman, C. (2009). *Dilated and restrictive cardiomyopathies.* Available at http://www .clevelandclinicmeded.com/medicalpubs/ diseasemanagement/cardiology/dilated- restrictive-cardiomyopathy

Bozkurt, B. & Mann, D.L. (2007). Dilated cardiomyopathy. In J.T. Willerson, J.N. Cohn, H.J.J. Wellens, & D.R. Holmes, Jr. (Eds.), *Cardiovascular medicine* (3rd ed., pp. 1233–1260). London, England: Springer-Verlag.

Bradley, D.J., Bradley, E.A., Baughman, K.L., Berger, R.D., Calkins, H., Goodman, S.N., … Powe, N.R. (2003). Cardiac resynchronization and death from progressive heart failure: A meta-analysis of randomized controlled trials. *Journal of the American Medical Association, 289*(6), 730–740.

Braunwald, E., Antman, E.M., Beasley, J.W., Califf, R.M., Cheitlin, M.D., Hochman, J.S., et al. (2002). *ACC/AHA 2002 guideline update for the management of patients with unstable angina and non-ST-segment elevation myocardial infarction: A report of the American College of Cardiology/American Heart Association Task Force on Practice Guidelines* (Committee on the Management of Patients with Unstable Angina). Available from http://content.onlinejacc.org/cgi/content/long/ 40/7/1366

Bridges, C.R., Horvath, K.A., Nugent, W.C., Shahian, D.M., Haan, C.K., Shemin, R.J., … Edwards, F.H. (2004). The Society of Thoracic Surgeons practice guideline series: Transmyocardial laser revascularization. *Annals of Thoracic Surgery, 77*(4), 1494–1502.

Bridges, E.J. (2010). Regulation of cardiac output and blood pressure. In S.L. Woods, E.S.S. Froelicher, S.U. Motzer, & E.J. Bridges (Eds.), *Cardiac nursing* (6th ed., pp. 69–96). Philadelphia, PA: Lippincott Williams & Wilkins.

Bridges, E.J. & Schmelz, J.O. (2010). Systemic and pulmonary circulation and oxygen delivery. In S.L. Woods, E.S.S. Froelicher, S.U. Motzer, & E.J. Bridges (Eds.), *Cardiac nursing* (6th ed., pp. 42–68). Philadelphia, PA: Lippincott Williams & Wilkins.

Bristow, M.R. & Feldman, A.M. (2003). *COMPANION: Comparison of medical therapy, pacing, and defibrillation in chronic heart failure.* Retrieved from http://www.medscape .org/viewarticle/452023

Brunzell, J.D., Davidson, M., Furberg, C.D., Goldberg, R.B., Howard, B.V., Stein, J.H., & Witztum, J.L. (2008). Lipoprotein management in patients with cardiometabolic risk: Consensus conference report from the American Diabetes Association and the American College of Cardiology Foundation. *Journal of the American College of Cardiology, 51*(15), 1512–1524.

Bryg, R.J. (2009). Mitral stenosis. In M.H. Crawford (Ed.), *Current diagnosis and treatment in cardiology* (3rd ed., pp. 106–112). New York, NY: McGraw-Hill.

Buss, J. & Thompson, G. (Eds.). (2010). *Auscultation skills: Breath and heart sounds* (4th ed.). Philadelphia, PA: Lippincott Williams & Wilkins.

Calagan, J.L., Schachter, D.T., Kruger, M., Cameron, R.W., & Loghin, C. (2001). Diuretics and nitrates. In O.V. Adair (Ed.), *Cardiology secrets* (2nd ed., pp. 285-288). Philadelphia: Hanley & Belfus, Inc.

Calclasure, T.F., Kozlowski, C.M., Highfill, W.T., & Loghin, C. (2001). Angiotensin-converting enzyme inhibitors and other vasodilators. In O.V. Adair (Ed.), *Cardiology secrets* (2nd ed., pp. 275-279). Philadelphia: Hanley & Belfus, Inc.

Calhoun, D.A., Jones, D., Textor, S., Goff, D.C., Murphy, T.P., Toto, R.D., ... Carey, R.M. (2008). Resistant hypertension: Diagnosis, evaluation, and treatment: A scientific statement from the American Heart Association Professional Education Committee of the Council for High Blood Pressure Research. *Hypertension, 51*(6), 1403-1419.

Calkins, H., Brugada, J., Packer, D.L., Cappato, R., Chen, S.A., Crijns, H.J., ... Shemin, R.J. (2007). HRS/EHRA/ECAS expert consensus statement on catheter and surgical ablation of atrial fibrillation: Recommendations for personnel, policy, procedures and follow-up. A report of the Heart Rhythm Society (HRS) Task Force on Catheter and Surgical Ablation of Atrial Fibrillation. *Heart Rhythm, 4*(6), 816–861.

Cannon, C.P. (2000). Exploring the issues of appropriate dosing in the treatment of acute myocardial infarction: Potential benefits of bolus fibrinolytic agents. *American Heart Journal, 140*(6 Suppl), S154–S160.

Carabello. B.A. & Crawford, M.H. (2009). Aortic stenosis. In M.H. Crawford (Ed.), *Current diagnosis and treatment in cardiology* (3rd ed., pp. 82–94). New York, NY: McGraw-Hill.

Carroll, J.D. & Crawford, M.H. (2009). Restrictive cardiomyopathies. In M.H. Crawford (Ed.), *Current diagnosis and treatment in cardiology* (3rd ed., pp. 172–178). New York, NY: McGraw-Hill.

Centers for Disease Control and Prevention. (2009). *About BMI for adults.* Retrieved from http://www.cdc.gov/healthyweight/assessing/bmi/adult_bmi/index.html

Chan, P.S., Nallamothu, B.K., & Oral, H. (2009). *Amiodarone or dronedarone for atrial fibrillation: Too early to know the winner?* Retrieved from http://content.onlinejacc.org/cgi/content/full/54/12/1096

Cleveland Clinic. (n.d.). *Cardiovascular imaging.* Available from http://my.clevelandclinic.org/radiology/cardiovascular_imaging/default.aspx

Cooper, L.T., Baughman, K.L., Feldman, A.M., Frustaci, A., Jessup, M., Kuhl, U., ... Virmani, R. (2007). The role of endomyocardial biopsy in the management of cardiovascular disease. *European Heart Journal 28*(24), 3076-3093.

Corrado, D., Fontaine, G., Marcus, F.I., McKenna, W.J., Nava, A., Thiene, G., & Wichter, T. (2000). Arrhythmogenic right ventricular dysplasia/cardiomyopathy: Need for an international registry. *Circulation, 101*(11), e101–e106.

Cotter, G., Dittrich, H.C., Weatherley, B.D., Bloomfield, D.M., O'Connor, C.M., Metra, M., & Massie, B.M. (2008). The PROTECT pilot study: A randomized, placebo-controlled, dose-finding study of the adenosine A1 receptor antagonist rolofylline in patients with acute heart failure and renal impairment. *Journal of Cardiac Failure, 14*(8), 631–640.

Crawford, M.H. (2009). Mitral regurgitation. In M.H. Crawford (Ed.), *Current diagnosis and treatment in cardiology* (3rd ed., pp. 113–121). New York, NY: McGraw-Hill.

Curtin, R.J. & Griffin, B.P. (2009). Mitral valve disease. In W.D. Carey (Ed.), Cleveland Clinic: *Current Clinical Medicine* (2nd ed.) Philadelphia, PA: Saunders Elsevier

Darovic, G.O. (2002). *Hemodynamic monitoring: Invasive and noninvasive clinical application* (3rd ed.). Philadelphia, PA: Saunders.

Deelstra, M.H. (2010). Interventional cardiology techniques: Percutaneous coronary intervention. In S.L. Woods, E.S.S. Froelicher, S.U. Motzer, & E.J. Bridges (Eds.), *Cardiac nursing* (6th ed., pp. 537–554). Philadelphia, PA: Lippincott Williams & Wilkins.

Dennison, C.R., Miller, N.H., & Cunningham, S.G. (2010). Hypertension. In S.L. Woods, E.S.S. Froelicher, S.U. Motzer, & E.J. Bridges (Eds.), *Cardiac nursing* (6th ed., pp. 799–822). Philadelphia, PA: Lippincott Williams & Wilkins.

Dennison, R.D. (2007). *Pass CCRN* (3rd ed.). St. Louis, MO: Mosby/Elsevier.

Derrick, D. (2009). The "broken heart syndrome:" Understanding Takotsubo cardiomyopathy. *Critical Care Nurse 29*(1), 49-58.

Dima, C. & Desser, K.B. (2010). *Mitral stenosis.* Retrieved from http://emedicine.medscape.com/article/155724-overview

Dolgin, M., Fox, A.C., Gorlin, R., & Levin, R.I. (Eds.). (1994). *Nomenclature and criteria for diagnosis of diseases of the heart and great vessels* (9th ed., pp. 253–256). Boston, MA: Little, Brown & Co.

Dote, K., Sato, H., Tateishi, H., Uchida, T., & Ishihara, M. (1991). Myocaridal stunning due to simulatenous multivessel coronary spasms: A review of 5 cases. *Journal of Cardiology 21*(2), 203-214.

Dresing, T.J. & Schweikert, R.A. (2009). *Atrial fibrillation.* Retrieved from http://www.clevlandclinicmeded.com/medicalpubs/disease management/cardiology/atrial-fibrillation

Eagle, K.A., Guyton, R.A., Davidoff, R., Edwards, F.H., Ewy, G.A., Gardner, T.J., … Orszulak, T.A. (2004). *ACC/AHA 2004 guideline update for coronary artery bypass graft surgery: A report of the American College of Cardiology/American Heart Association Task Force on Practice Guidelines* (Committee to Update the 1999 Guidelines for Coronary Artery Bypass Graft Surgery). Available at http://circ.ahajournals.org/cgi/reprint/110/14/e340

Edwards, F.H., Engelman, R.M., Houck, P., Shahian, D.M., & Bridges, C.R. (2006). The Society of Thoracic Surgeons Practice Guideline Series: Antibiotic prophylaxis in cardiac surgery, Part I: Duration. *Annals of Thoracic Surgery, 81*(1), 397–404.

Ellenbogen, K.A. & Wood, M.A. (Eds.). (2008). *Cardiac pacing and ICDs* (5th ed.). West Sussex, UK: John Wiley & Sons.

Engelman, R., Shahian, D., Shemin, R., Guy, T.S., Bratzler, D., Edwards, F., ... Bridges, C. (2007). The Society of Thoracic Surgeons practice guideline series: Antibiotic prophylaxis in cardiac surgery, part II: Antibiotic choice. *Annals of Thoracic Surgery, 83*(4), 1569–1576.

Epstein, A.E., DiMarco, J.P., Ellenbogen, K.A., Estes, N.A.M., III, Freedman, R.A., Gettes, L.S., ... Sweeney, M.O. (2008). ACC/AHA/HRS 2008 guidelines for device-based therapy of cardiac rhythm abnormalities: A report of the American College of Cardiology/American Heart Association Task Force on Practice Guidelines (Writing Committee to Revise the ACC/AHA/NASPE 2002 Guideline Update for Implantation of Cardiac Pacemakers and Antiarrhythmia Devices). *Journal of the American College of Cardiology, 51*(21), e1–e62.

Ferraris, V.A., Ferraris, S.P., Moliterno, D.J., Camp, P., Walenga, J.M., Messmore, H.L., ... Despotis, G. (2005).The Society of Thoracic Surgeons practice guideline series: Aspirin and other antiplatelet agents during operative coronary revascularization (Executive summary). *Annals of Thoracic Surgery 79*(4), 1454–1461.

Ferraris, V.A., Ferraris, S.P., Saha, S.P., Hessel, E.A., 2nd, Haan, C.K., Royston, B.D., ... Body, S. (2007). Perioperative blood transfusion and blood conservation in cardiac surgery: The Society of Thoracic Surgeons and The Society of Cardiovascular Anesthesiologists Clinical Practice Guideline. *Annals of Thoracic Surgery, 83*(5-Suppl), S27–S86. Retrieved from http://ats.ctsnetjournals.org/content/vol83/5_Supplement

Fiore, M.C., Jaen, C.R., Baker, T.B., Bailey, W.C, Benowitz, N.L., Curry, S.J., et al. (2008). *Treating Tobacco Use and Dependence: 2008 Update. Clinical Practice Guideline.* Rockville, MD: U.S. Department of Health and Human Services. Public Health Service. May 2008.

Fischbach, F.T. & Dunning, M.B., III. (2009). *Manual of laboratory and diagnostic tests* (8th ed.). Philadelphia, PA: Lippincott Williams & Wilkins.

Folkeringa, R.J., Tieleman, R.G., & Crijns, H.J. (2004). Non-antiarrhythmic drugs to prevent atrial fibrillation. *Heart Rhythm, 1*(4), 516–518.

Fonseca, V., Bakris, G.L., Benjamin, E.M., Blonde, L., Boucher, J., Brancati, F.L., ... Clark, N.G. (2005). Summary of revisions for the 2005 clinical practice recommendations. *Diabetes Care, 28*(Suppl 1), S3.

Fraker, T.D., Jr. & Fihn, S.D. (2007). 2007 chronic angina focused update of the ACC/AHA 2002 guidelines for the management of patients with chronic stable angina: A report of the American College of Cardiology/American Heart Association Task Force on Practice Guidelines Writing Group to develop the focused update of the 2002 guidelines for the management of patients with chronic stable angina. *Journal of the American College of Cardiology, 50*(23), 2264–2274.

Fuster, V., Rydén, L.E., Cannom, D.S., Crijns, H.J., Curtis, A.B., Ellenbogen, K.A., …Wann, L.S. (2011). 2011 ACCF/AHA/HRS Focused updates incorporated into the ACC/AHA/ESC 2006 guidelines for the management of patients with atrial fibrillation: A report of the American College of Cardiology Foundation/ American Heart Association task force on practice guidelines developed in partnership with the European Society of Cardiology and in collaboration with the European Heart Rhythm Association and the Heart Rhythm Society. *Journal of the American College of Cardiology, 57*(11), e101-e198.

Ganz, L. (2004). *Implantable cardioverter-defibrillators.* Retrieved from http://www.emedicine.com/med/topic3386.htm

Gianni, M., Dentali, F., Grandi, A.M., Sumner, G., Hiralal, R., Lonn, E. (2006). Apical ballooning syndrome or takotsubo cardiomyopathy: A systematic review. *European Heart Journal 27*(13), 1523-1529.

Gibbons, R.J., Abrams, J., Chatterjee, K., Daley, J., Deedwania, P.C., Douglas, J.S., … Williams, S.V. (2002). *ACC/AHA 2002 guideline update for the management of patients with chronic stable angina: A report of the American College of Cardiology/American Heart Association Task Force on Practice Guidelines* (Committee to update the 1999 Guidelines for the Management of Patients with Chronic Stable Angina). Available at http://www.american heart.org/downloadable/heart/1044991838085 StableAnginaNewFigs.pdf

Gidding, S.S., Lichtenstein, A.H., Faith, M.S., Karpyn, A., Mennella, J.A., Popkin, B., … Whitsel, L. (2009). Implementing American Heart Association pediatric and adult nutrition guidelines: A scientific statement from the American Heart Association Nutrition Committee of the Council on Nutrition, Physical Activity and Metabolism, Council on Cardiovascular Disease in the Young, Council on Arteriosclerosis, Thrombosis and Vascular Biology, Council on Cardiovascular Nursing, Council on Epidemiology and Prevention, and Council for High Blood Pressure Research. *Circulation, 119*(8), 1161–1175.

Gimbel, J.R. (2004). When should patients be allowed to drive after ICD implantation? *Cleveland Clinic Journal of Medicine, 71*(2), 125–128. Available at http://www.iranep.org/ Articles/ICD%20Driving%20Cleveland.pdf

GlaxoSmithKline. (2005). *Argatroban clinical monograph.* Retrieved from http://www. argatroban.com/anticoagulant_clinic_01.htm

Gold Standard/Elsevier. (2010). *Clinical pharmacology database.* Retrieved from http://www .clinicalpharmacology.com/?epm=2_1

Goswami, V.J. (2008). *Cardiomyopathy, restrictive.* Retrieved from http://emedicine.medscape .com/article/153062-overview

Grady, D., Herrington, D., Bittner, V., Blumenthal, R., Davidson, M., Hlatkey, M., … Wenger, N. (2002). Cardiovascular Disease Outcomes During 6.8 Years of Hormone Therapy. *The Journal of the American Medical Association 288*(1), 49-57.

Gregoratos, G., Abrams, J., Epstein, A.E., Freedman, R.A., Hayes, D.L., Hlatky, M.A., ... Winters, S.L. (2002). *ACC/AHA/NASPE 2002 Guideline update for implantation of cardiac pacemakers and antiarrhythmia devices: Summary article: A report of the American College of Cardiology/American Heart Association Task Force on Practice Guidelines* (ACC/AHA/NASPE Committee to Update the 1998 Pacemaker Guidelines). Available at http://circ.ahajournals.org/cgi/content/short/106/16/2145

Greinacher, A., Lubenow, N., & Eichler, P. (2003). Anaphylactic and anaphylactoid reactions associated with lepirudin in patients with heparin-induced thrombocytopenia. *Circulation, 108*(17), 2062–2065.

Grundy, S.M., Becker, D., Clark, L.T., Cooper, R.S., Denke, M.A., Howard, W.J., ... Van Horn, L. (2002). *Third report of the National Cholesterol Education Program (NCEP) Expert Panel on: Detection, evaluation, and treatment of high blood cholesterol in adults* (Adult Treatment Panel III) (NIH publication No. 02-5215). Available at http://www.nhlbi.nih.gov/guidelines/cholesterol/atp3full.pdf

Grundy, S.M., Cleeman, J.I., Merz, C.N.B., Brewer, H.B., Jr., Clark, L.T., Hunninghake, D.B., ... Stone, N.J. (2004). Implications of recent clinical trials for the National Cholesterol Education Program Adult Treatment Panel III Guidelines. *Circulation, 110*(2), 227–239.

Harris, W.S., Mozaffarian, D., Rimm, E., Kris-Etherton, P., Rudel, L.L., Appel, L.J., ... Sacks, F. (2009). Omega-6 fatty acids and risk for cardiovascular disease: A science advisory from the American Heart Association Nutrition Subcommittee of the Council on Nutrition, Physical Activity, and Metabolism; Council on Cardiovascular Nursing; and Council on Epidemiology and Prevention. *Circulation, 119*(6), 902–907.

Haskell, W.L., Lee., I.M., Pate, R.R., Powell, K.E., Blair, S.N., & Franklin, B.A., ... Bauman, A. (2007). Physical activity and public health: Updated recommendations for adults from the American College of Sports Medicine and the American Heart Association. *Circulation, 116*(9), 1081–1093.

Heart Failure Society of America. (2004). Implications of recent trials for heart failure performance measures. *Journal of Cardiac Failure, 10*(1), 4–5.

Heart Rhythm Society. (n.d.). *Implantable Cardioverter Defibrillators (ICD).* Available from http://www.hrsonline.org/PatientInfo/Treatments/ICD/index.cfm

Hirsh, J. & Bhatt, D.L. (2004). Comparative benefits of clopidogrel and aspirin in high-risk patient populations: Lessons from the CAPRIE and CURE studies. *Archives of Internal Medicine, 164*(19), 2106–2110.

Hobbs, R. & Boyle, A. (2009). *Heart failure.* Retrieved from http://www.clevelandclinicmeded.com/medicalpubs/diseasemanagement/cardiology/heart-failure

Howie, J. (2008). Cardiomyopathy and myocarditis. In D.K. Moser & B.Riegel (Eds.), *Cardiac nursing: A companion to Braunwald's heart disease* (pp.1110-1123). St. Louis, MO: Saunders/Elsevier.

Hughes, J. & Platt, K. (2010). Minimally invasive cardiac surgery. In *Cardiac Surgery Essentials for Critical Care Nursing.* (Hardin, S.R. & R. Kaplow, Eds.). Sudbury, MA: Jones & Bartlett Publishers, LLC.

Hunt, S.A., Abraham, W.T., Chin, M.H., Feldman, A.M., Francis, G.S., Ganiats, T.G., ... Yancy, C.W. (2009). 2009 focused update incorporated into the ACC/AHA 2005 Guidelines for the Diagnosis and Management of Heart Failure in Adults: A report of the American College of Cardiology Foundation/American Heart Association Task Force on Practice Guidelines. *Journal of the American College of Cardiology* 53(15), e1–e90.

Jacobson, C. (2010). Arrhythmias and conduction disturbances. In S.L. Woods, E.S.S. Froelicher, S.U. Motzer, & E.J. Bridges (Eds.), *Cardiac nursing* (6th ed., pp. 333–387). Philadelphia, PA: Lippincott Williams & Wilkins.

Jacobson, C. & Gerity, D. (2010). Pacemakers and implantable defibrillators. In S.L. Woods, E.S.S. Froelicher, S.U. Motzer, & E.J. Bridges (Eds.), *Cardiac nursing* (6th ed., pp. 655–704). Philadelphia, PA: Lippincott Williams & Wilkins.

Jacobson, C., Marzlin, K., & Webner, C. (2007). *Cardiovascular nursing practice: A comprehensive resource manual and study guide for clinical nurses.* Aliso Viejo, CA: American Association of Critical Care Nurses

Jessup, M. (2004). Resynchronization therapy is an important advance in the management of congestive heart failure: View of an antagonist. *Journal of Cardiovascular Electrophysiology,* 14(9 Suppl.), S30–S34.

Jessup, M., Abraham, W.T., Casey, D.E., Feldman, A.M., Francis, G.S., Ganiats, T.G., ... Yancy, C.W. (2009). 2009 focused update: ACCF/AHA Guidelines for the Diagnosis and Management of Heart Failure in Adults: A report of the American College of Cardiology Foundation/American Heart Association Task Force on Practice Guidelines. *Circulation, 119*(14), 1977–2016.

Jones, D.W., Peterson, E.D., Bonow, R.O., Masoudi, F.A., Fonarow, G.C., Smith, S.C., Jr., ... Gibbons, R.J. (2008). Translating research into practice for healthcare providers: The American Heart Association's strategy for building healthier lives, free of cardiovascular diseases and stroke. *Circulation, 118*(6), 687–696.

King, S.B., III, Smith, S.C., Jr., Hirshfeld, J.W., Jr., Jacobs, A.K., Morrison, D.A., & Williams, D.O. (2007). 2007 focused update of the ACC/AHA/SCAI 2005 Guideline Update for Percutaneous Coronary Intervention. *Journal of the American College of Cardiology, 51*(2), 172–209.

Kurisu, S., Inoue, I., Kawagoe, T., Ishihara, M., Shimatani, Y., Nishioka, K., ... Yoshida, M. (2002). Does coronary stenting affect microvascular circulation in patients with anterior acute myocardial infarction? Comparison with balloon angioplasty. *Circulation Journal* 66(10), 917-920.

Kramer, M.K., Newton, K.M., & Froelicher, E.S.S. (2010). Coronary heart disease risk factors. In S.L. Woods, E.S.S. Froelicher, S.U. Motzer, & E.J. Bridges (Eds.), *Cardiac nursing* (6th ed., pp. 753–768). Philadelphia, PA: Lippincott Williams & Wilkins.

Kumanyika, S.K., Obarzanek, E., Stettler, N., Bell, R., Field, A.E., Fortmann, S.P., ... Hong, Y. (2008). Population-based prevention of obesity: The need for comprehensive promotion of healthful eating, physical activity, and energy balance: A scientific statement from American Heart Association Council on Epidemiology and Prevention, Interdisciplinary Committee for Prevention (formerly the Expert Panel on Population and Prevention Science). *Circulation, 118*(4), 428–464.

Kushner, F.G., Hand, M., Smith, S.C., Jr., King, S.B., 3rd, Anderson, J.L., Antman, E.M., ... Williams, D.O. (2009). 2009 focused updates: ACC/AHA guidelines for the management of patients with ST-elevation myocardial infarction (updating the 2004 guideline and 2007 focused update) and ACC/AHA/SCAI guidelines on percutaneous coronary intervention (updating the 2005 guideline and 2007 focused update): A report of the American College of Cardiology Foundation/American Heart Association Task Force on Practice Guidelines. *Journal of the American College of Cardiology, 54*(23), 2205–2241.

Lauck, S., Mackay, M., Galte, C., & Wilson, M. (2008). A new option for the treatment of aortic stenosis: Percutaneous aortic valve replacement. *Critical Care Nurse, 28*(3), 40–51.

Lazar, H.L., McDonnell, M., Chipkin, S.R., Furnary, A.P., Engelman, R.M., Sadhu, A.R., ... Shemin, R.J. (2009). The Society of Thoracic Surgeons practice guideline series: Blood glucose management during adult cardiac surgery. *Annals of Thoracic Surgery, 87*(2), 663–669.

Ledoux, D. (2010). Acquired valvular heart disease. In S.L. Woods, E.S.S. Froelicher, S.U. Motzer, & E.J. Bridges (Eds.), *Cardiac nursing* (6th ed., pp. 705–721). Philadelphia, PA: Lippincott Williams & Wilkins.

Ledoux, D. & Luikart, H. (2010). Cardiac surgery. In S.L. Woods, E.S.S. Froelicher, S.U. Motzer, & E.J. Bridges (Eds.), *Cardiac nursing* (6th ed., pp. 595–622). Philadelphia, PA: Lippincott Williams & Wilkins.

Leeper, B. (2009). Valvular disease and surgery. In K.K. Carlson (Ed.), *AACN Advanced critical care nursing* (pp. 322–346). St. Louis, MO: Saunders.

Levine, B.S. (2002). *Cardiac/vascular nursing review and resource manual.* Washington, D.C.: American Nurses Credentialing Center.

Lewis, S.M., Heitkemper, M.M., & Dirksen, S.R. (2004). *Medical-surgical nursing: Assessment and management of clinical problems* (6th ed.). St. Louis: Mosby.

Lichtman, J.H., Bigger, J.T., Jr., Blumenthal, J.A., Frasure-Smith, N., Kaufmann, P.G., Lespérance, F., ... Froelicher, E.S. (2008). Depression and coronary heart disease: Recommendations for screening, referral, and treatment: A science advisory from the American Heart Association Prevention Committee of the Council on Cardiovascular Nursing, Council on Clinical Cardiology, Council on Epidemiology and Prevention, and Interdisciplinary Council on Quality of Care and Outcomes Research: Endorsed by the American Psychiatric Association. *Circulation, 118*(17), 1768–1775.

Lloyd-Jones, D., Adams, R., Carnethon, M., De Simone, G., Ferguson, T.B., Flegal, K., ... Hong, Y. (2009). Heart disease and stroke statistics – 2009 update: A report from the American Heart Association Statistics Committee and Stroke Statistics Subcommittee. *Circulation, 119*(3), e21–e181.

Lorenz, R.A., Lorenz, R.M., & Codd, J.E. (2005). Perioperative blood glucose control during adult coronary artery bypass surgery. *AORN Journal, 81*(1), 126–144.

Maden, S.K. & Froelicher, E.S.S. (2010). Psychosocial risk factors: Assessment and management interventions. In S.L. Woods, E.S.S. Froelicher, S.U. Motzer, & E.J. Bridges (Eds.), *Cardiac nursing* (6th ed., pp. 769–782). Philadelphia, PA: Lippincott Williams & Wilkins.

Malouf, J.F., Edwards, W.D., Tajik, A.J., & Seward, J.B. (2008). Functional anatomy of the heart. In V. Fuster, R.A. O'Rourke, R.A. Walsh, & P. Poole-Wilson (Eds.), *Hurst's the Heart* (12th ed., pp. 45-86). New York, NY: McGraw Hill Medical.

Mangano, D.T., Miao, Y., Vuylsteke, A., Tudor, I.C., Juneja, R., Filipescu, D., ... Levin, J. (2007). Mortality associated with aprotinin during 5 years following coronary artery bypass graft surgery. *Journal of the American Medical Association, 297*(5), 471–479.

Maron, B.J., McKenna, W.J., Danielson, G.K., Kappenberger, L.J., Kuhn, H.J., Seidman, C.E., ... Torbicki, A. (2003). American College of Cardiology/European Society of Cardiology clinical expert consensus document on hypertrophic cardiomyopathy: A report of the American College of Cardiology Foundation Task Force on Clinical Expert Consensus Documents and the European Society of Cardiology Committee for Practice Guidelines. *Journal of the American College of Cardiology, 42*(9), 1687–1713.

Maron, B.J., Towbin, J.A., Thiene, G., Antzelevitch, C., Corrado, C, Arnett, D., ... Young, J.B. (2006). Contemporary definitions and classification of the cardiomyopathies. *Circulation 113*(14), 1807-1816.

Martin, K. & Froelicher, E.S. (2005). Smoking cessation: A systematic approach to managing patients with heart disease. In S.L. Woods, E.S. Froelicher, S.A. Motzer, & E.J. Bridges (Eds.), *Cardiac nursing* (5th ed., pp. 838-855). Philadelphia: Lippincott Williams & Wilkins.

Mayo Clinic. (2010.) *Ranolazine.* Available from http://www.mayoclinic.com/health/drug-information/DR602019

McCance, K.L. (2006). Structure and function of the cardiovascular and lymphatic systems. In K.L. McCune & S.E. Huether (Eds.), *Pathophysiology: The biologic basis for disease in adults and children* (5th ed., pp. 1029–1080). St. Louis, MO: Elsevier Mosby.

McPherson, J.A. (2010). *Aortic Stenosis.* Retrieved from http://emedicine.medscape.com/article/150638-overview

McRae, A.T., 3rd, Chung, M.K., & Asher, C.R. (2001). Arrhythmogenic right ventricular cardiomyopathy: A cause of sudden death in young people. *Cleveland Clinic Journal of Medicine, 68*(5), 459–467.

McRae, M.E., Rodger, M., & Bailey, B.A. (2009). Transcatheter and transapical aortic valve replacement. *Critical Care Nurse, 29*(1), 22–37.

MedlinePlus. (2008). Paclitaxel injection. Available at http://www.nlm.nih.gov/medlineplus/druginfo/meds/a607070.html

MedlinePlus. (2010). *Sirolimus.* Available at http://www.nlm.nih.gov/medlineplus/druginfo/meds/a602026.html

Medtronic, Inc. (2010). *Our story: Our first pacemakers.* Available from http://www.medtronic.com/about-medtronic/our-story/our-first-pacemakers/index.htm

Mendoza, R. & Loghin, C. (2001). Calcium channel antagonists. In O.V. Adair (Ed.), *Cardiology secrets* (2nd ed., pp. 285-288). Philadelphia: Hanley & Belfus, Inc.

Miller, J. (2010). Cardiopulmonary bypass and off pump coronary artery bypass. In *Cardiac Surgery Essentials for Critical Care Nursing.* (Hardin, S.R. & R. Kaplow, Eds.). Sudbury, MA: Jones & Bartlett Publishers, LLC.

Moons, P., Canobbio, M.M., Nickolaus, M.J., Verstappen, A. (2008). Care of adults with congenital heart disease. In D.K. Moser & B. Riegel (Eds.), *Cardiac nursing: A companion to Braunwald's heart disease* (pp. 1085-1109). St. Louis, MO: Saunders/Elsevier.

Moore, K.L. & Dalley, A.F., II. (1999). *Clinically oriented anatomy* (4th ed.). Philadelphia, PA: Lippincott Williams & Wilkins.

Morrison, L.J., Verbeek, P.R., McDonald, A.C., Sawadsky, B.V., & Cook, D.J. (2000). Mortality and prehospital thrombolysis for acute myocardial infarction: A meta-analysis. *Journal of the American Medical Association, 283*(20), 2686–2692.

Mosca, L., Appel, L.J., Benjamin, E.J., Berra, K., Chandra-Strobos, N., Fabunmi, R.P., ... Williams, C.L. (2004). Evidence-based guidelines for cardiovascular disease prevention in women. *Journal of the American College of Cardiology, 43*(5), 900–921.

Mosca, L., Banka, C.L., Benjamin, E.J., Berra, K., Bushnell, C., Dolor, R.J., ... Wenger, N.K. (2007). Evidence-based guidelines for cardiovascular disease prevention in women: 2007 update. *Circulation, 115*(11), 1481–1501.

Moser, D.K. & Riegel, B. (2008). *Cardiac nursing: A companion to Braunwald's heart disease.* Philadelphia, PA: Saunders Elsevier.

Myers, J. (2010). Exercise and activity. In S.L. Woods, E.S.S. Froelicher, S.U. Motzer, & E.J. Bridges (Eds.), *Cardiac nursing* (6th ed., pp. 842–860). Philadelphia, PA: Lippincott Williams & Wilkins.

Nelson, G.D. (1993). Historical perspectives: A brief history of cardiac pacing. *Texas Heart Institute Journal, 20*(1), 12–18. Retrieved from http://www.ncbi.nlm.nih.gov/pmc/articles/PMC325046/pdf/thij00040-0032.pdf

Niinami, H., Ogasawara, H., Suda, Y., & Takeuchi, Y. (2005). Single-vessel revascularization with minimally invasive direct coronary artery bypass: Minithoracotomy or ministernotomy? *Chest, 127*(1), 47–52.

Nishimura, R.A, Carabello, B.A., Faxon, D.P., Freed, M.D., Lytle, B.W., O'Gara, P.T., ... Shah, P.M. (2008). ACC/AHA 2008 guideline update on valvular heart disease: Focused update on infective endocarditis: A report of the American College of Cardiology/American Heart Association Task Force on Practice Guidelines. *Journal of the American College of Cardiology, 52*(8), 676–685.

Nishimura, R.A. & Holmes, D.R., Jr. (2004). Clinical practice: Hypertrophic obstructive cardiomyopathy. *New England Journal of Medicine, 350*(13), 1320–1327.

Nishizaki, K. & Seki, T. (2005). Early results of aortic connector system for proximal anastomosis of the saphenous vein graft. *Annals of Thoracic and Cardiovascular Surgery, 11*(2), 98–103.

Novaro, G.M. (2009). *Aortic valve disease.* Retrieved from http://www.clevelandclinicmeded.com/medicalpubs/diseasemanagement/cardiology/aortic-valve-disease

O'Donnell, J.K., Mehta, L., & Faulhaber, P.F. (2008). Pharmacologic stress testing: A new selective vasodilator. In *Hurst's the Heart: Manual of Cardiology* (R.A. O'Rourke, R.A. Walsh, & V.V. Fuster, Eds.). New York: McGraw-Hills, Companies, Inc.

Opie, L.H. (2004). *Heart physiology: From cell to circulation* (4th ed.). Philadelphia, PA: Lippincott Williams & Wilkins.

Opie, L.H. & Gersh B.J. (Eds.). (2009). *Drugs for the heart* (7th ed.). Philadelphia, PA: Saunders Elsevier.

Nelson, M.E., Rejeski, W.J., Blair, S.N., Duncan, P.W., Judge, J.O., King, A.C., Macera, C.A., & Castaneda-Sceppa, C. (2007). *Physical activity and public health in older adults: Recommendation from the American College of Sports Medicine and the American Heart Association.* Retrieved from http://circ.aha journals.org/cgi/reprint/116/9/1094.pdf

Pickering, T.G., Hall, J.E., Appel, L.J., Falkner, B.E., Graves., J., Hill, M.N., ... Roccella, E.J. (2005). *Recommendations for blood pressure measurement in humans and experimental animals: Part 1: Blood pressure measurement in humans: A statement for professionals from the subcommittee of Professional and Public Education of the American Heart Association Council on High Blood Pressure Research.* Retrieved from http://hyper.ahajournals.org/cgi/content/full/45/1/142

Porth, C.M. (2005). *Pathophysiology: Concepts of altered health states* (7th ed.). Philadelphia, PA: Lippincott Williams & Wilkins.

Potter, L. & Martin, C. (2005). *Health literacy fact sheets.* Available at http://www.chcs.org/publications3960/publications_show.htm?doc_id=291711

Prasad, A., Lerman, A., & Rihal,C.S (2008). Apical ballooning syndrome (Tako-Tsubo or stress cardiomyopathy): A mimic of acute myocardial infarction. *American Heart Journal; 155*(3), 408-417.

Racz, M.J., Hannan, E.L., Isom, O.W., Subramanian, V.A., Jones, R.H., Gold, J.P., ... Rose, E.A. (2004). A comparison of short- and long-term outcomes after off-pump and on-pump coronary artery bypass graft surgery with sternotomy. *Journal of the American College of Cardiology, 43*(4), 557–564.

Raghavan, M. & Marik, P.E. (2005). Anemia, allogenic blood transfusion, and immunomodulation in the critically ill. *Chest, 127*(1), 295–307.

Rahitoomla, S.H. (2008). Aortic valve disease. In V. Fuster, R.A. O'Rourke, R.A. Walsh, P. Poole-Wilson (Eds.), *Hurst's the heart* (12th ed. pp 1697–1730). New York, NY: McGraw Hill Medical.

Raible, E. (2008). ENHANCE: Imaging study did not show clinical benefit. Cardiology Today (February 1, 2008). Available from http://www.cardiologytoday.com/view.aspx?rid=29541

Richardson, P., McKenna, W., Bristow, M., Maisch, B., Mautner, B., O'Connell, J., ... Nordet, P. (1996). Report of the 1995 World Health Organization/International Society and Federation of Cardiology Task Force on the Definition and Classification of Cardiomyopathies. *Circulation, 93*(5), 841–842.

Ridker, P.M., Danielson, E., Fonseca, F.A., Genest, J., Gotto, A.M., Kastelein, J.J., ... Glynn, R.J. (2008). Rosuvastatin to prevent vascular events in men and women with elevated C-reactive protein. *New England Journal of Medicine, 359*(21), 2195-2207. Retrieved from http://www.nejm.org/doi/full/10.1056/NEJMoa0807646

Rimmerman, C.M. (2010). *Coronary Artery Disease.* Available at https://www.cleveland clinicmeded.com/medicalpubs/diseasemanage ment/cardiology/coronary-artery-disease

Rochester Medical Center. (n.d.). *Permanent pacemakers.* Retrieved from http://www.rochester medicalcenter.com/permanent_pacemakers.htm

Rosendorff, C., Black, H.R., Cannon, C.P., Gersh, B.J., Gore, J., Izzo, J.L. Jr., ... Oparil, S. (2007). Treatment of hypertension in the prevention and management of ischemic heart disease: A scientific statement from the American Heart Association Council for High Blood Pressure Research and the Councils on Clinical Cardiology and Epidemiology and Prevention. *Circulation, 115*(21), 2761–2788.

Rosenthal, L. & McManus, D.D. (2008). *Atrial fibrillation.* Available from http://emedicine. medscape.com/article/151066-overview

Rosenthal, L. (2011). *Atrial fibrillation.* Retrieved http://emedicine.medscape.com/article/ 151066-overview

Salberg, L. (2004). *How to choose a septal reduction method: Issues you should know when it is time to choose.* Retrieved from http://www .enewsbuilder.net/hypertrophic/e_article 000222719.cfm

Schoen, F.J. & Mitchell, R.N. (2010). The heart. In V. Kumar, A.K. Abbas, N. Fausto, & J.C. Aster (Eds.), *Robbins and Cotran pathologic basis of disease* (8th ed., pp. 529–588). Philadelphia, PA: Saunders Elsevier.

Sen-Chowdhry, S., Syrris, P., McKenna, W.J. (2005). Genetics of right ventricular cardiomyopathy. *Journal of Cardiovascular Electrophysiology 16*(8), 927-935.

Shah, P.M. (2009). Hypertrophic cardiomyopathies. In M.H. Crawford (Ed.), *Current diagnosis and treatment in cardiology* (3rd ed., pp. 164–171). New York, NY: McGraw-Hill.

Shoulders-Odom, B. (2008). Management of patients after percutaneous coronary interventions. *Critical Care Nurse 28*(5), 28-40.

Skyler, J.S., Bergenstal, R., Bonow, R.O., Buse, J., Deedwania, P., Gale, E.A., ... Sherwin, R.S. (2009). Intensive glycemic control and the prevention of cardiovascular events: Implications of the ACCORD, ADVANCE, and VA diabetes trials: A position statement of the American Diabetes Association and a Scientific Statement of the American College of Cardiology Foundation and the American Heart Association. *Circulation, 119*(2), 351–357.

Smith, S.C., Jr., Allen, J., Blair, S.N., Bonow, R.O., Brass, L.M., Fonarow, G.C., ... Taubert, K.A. (2006). AHA/ACC Guidelines for Secondary Prevention for Patients With Coronary and Other Atherosclerotic Vascular Disease: 2006 update: Endorsed by the National Heart, Lung, and Blood Institute. *Circulation 113*(19), 2363–2372.

Smith, S.C., Jr., Feldman, T.E., Hirshfeld, J.W., Jr., Jacobs, A.K., Kern, M.J., King, S.B., III, ... Riegel, B. (2006). ACC/AHA/SCAI 2005 guideline update for percutaneous coronary intervention: Summary article: A report of the American College of Cardiology/American Heart Association Task Force on Practice Guidelines (ACC/AHA/SCAI Writing Committee to Update the 2001 Guidelines for Percutaneous Coronary Intervention). *Journal of the American College of Cardiology, 47*(1), 216–235.

Smith, S.W., Zvosec, D.L., Sharkey, S.W., & Henry, T.D. (2002). *The ECG in acute MI: An evidence-based manual of reperfusion therapy.* Philadelphia, PA: Lippincott Williams & Wilkins.

Sohn, M., Hawk, M., Martin, K., & Froelicher, E.S.S. (2010). Smoking cessation and relapse prevention. In S.L. Woods, E.S.S. Froelicher, S.U. Motzer, & E.J. Bridges (Eds.), *Cardiac nursing* (6th ed., pp. 783–798). Philadelphia, PA: Lippincott Williams & Wilkins.

Soine, L.A. (2010). Heart failure and cardiogenic shock. In S.L. Woods, E.S.S. Froelicher, S.U. Motzer, & E.J. Bridges (Eds.), *Cardiac nursing* (6th ed., pp. 555–594). Philadelphia, PA: Lippincott Williams & Wilkins.

Steinke, E.E., Gill-Hopple, K., Valdez, D., & Wooster, M. (2005). Sexual concerns and educational needs after implantable cardioverter defibrillator. *Heart & Lung: The Journal of Acute and Critical Care 34*(5), 299-308.

Sweeney, M.O. & Prinzen, F.W. (2006). A new paradigm for physiologic ventricular pacing. *Journal of the American College of Cardiology, 47*(2), 282-288.

The Medicines Company. (2009). *Product monograph: Angiomax (bivalirudin) for injection.* Available at http://www.themedicines company.com/pdf/ANG-PMN-011-06_ Product_Monograph.pdf

Theobald, K. & McMurray, A. (2004). Coronary artery bypass graft surgery: Discharge planning for successful recovery. *Journal of Advanced Nursing, 47*(5), 483–491.

Thomassian, B.D. (2010). Diabetes mellitus and metabolic syndrome. In S.L. Woods, E.S.S. Froelicher, S.U. Motzer, & E.J. Bridges (Eds.), *Cardiac nursing* (6th ed., pp. 876–888). Philadelphia, PA: Lippincott Williams & Wilkins.

U.S. Department of Health and Human Services. (2004). *The seventh report of the Joint National Committee on Prevention, Detection, Evaluation, and Treatment of High Blood Pressure* (NIH publication No. 04-5230). Available at http://www.nhlbi.nih.gov/ guidelines/hypertension/jnc7full.pdf

U.S. Food and Drug Administration. (2009). *FDA announces new warning on Plavix: Avoid use with Prilosec/Prilosec OTC.* Retrieved from http://www.fda.gov/NewsEvents/Newsroom/ PressAnnouncements/2009/ucm191169.htm

U.S. Food and Drug Administration. (2010). *Plavix (clopidogrel): Reduced effectiveness in patients who are poor metabolizers of the drug.* Retrieved from http://www.fda.gov/Safety/Med Watch/SafetyInformation/SafetyAlertsfor HumanMedicalProducts/ucm204256.htm

Verrier, J.M.B. & Deelstra, M.H. (2010). Acute coronary syndromes. In S.L. Woods, E.S.S. Froelicher, S.U. Motzer, & E.J. Bridges (Eds.), *Cardiac nursing* (6th ed., pp. 511–536). Philadelphia, PA: Lippincott Williams & Wilkins.

Vohra, H.A., Levine, A., & Dunning, J. (2005). Can ventilation while on cardiopulmonary bypass improve post-operative lung function for patients undergoing cardiac surgery? *Interactive Cardiovascular and Thoracic Surgery, 4*(5), 442–446.

Wang, S.S. (2010). *Aortic regurgitation.* Retrieved from http://emedicine.medscape.com/article /150490-overview

Wiegand, D.L., Preuss, T., & Hambach, C. (2008). Care of Patients with Acquired Valvular Heart Disease. In D.K. Moser & B.Riegel (Eds.), *Cardiac nursing: A companion to Braunwald's heart disease* (pp. 1030–1051). St. Louis, MO: Saunders/Elsevier.

Wittstein, I.S., Thiemann, D.R., Lima, J.A., Baughman, K.L., Schulman, S.P., Gerstenblith, G., … Champion, H.C. (2005). *New England Journal of Medicine 352*(6), 539-548.

Wilson, W., Taubert, K., Gewitz, M., Lockhart, P.B., Baddour, L.M., Levison, M., … Durack, D.T. (2007). Prevention of infective endocarditis. Guidelines from the American Heart Association: A guideline from the American Heart Association Rheumatic Fever, Endocarditis, and Kawasaki Disease Committee, Council on Cardiovascular Disease in the Young, and the Council on Clinical Cardiology, Council on Cardiovascular Surgery and Anesthesia, and the Quality of Care and Outcomes Research Interdisciplinary Working Group. *Circulation, 116*(15), 1736–1754.

Wohl, B., Peters, R.W., Carliner, N., Plotnick, G., & Fisher, M. (1982). Late unheralded pacemaker pocket infection due to staphylococcus epidermidis: A new clinical entity. *Pacing and Clinical Electrophysiology, 5*(2), 190–195.

Woods, S.E., Smith, J.M., Sohail, S., Sarah, A., & Engle, A. (2004). The influence of type 2 diabetes mellitus in patients undergoing coronary artery bypass graft surgery: An 8-year prospective cohort study. *Chest, 126*(6), 1789–1795.

Wyse, D.G., Waldo, A.L., DiMarco, J.P., Domanski, M.J., Rosenberg, Y., Schron, E.B., … Corley, S.D. (2002). A comparison of rate control and rhythm control in patients with atrial fibrillation. *New England Journal of Medicine, 347*(23), 1825–1833.

Yeo, T.P. & Berg, N.C. (2004). Counseling patients with implanted cardiac devices. *Nurse Practitioner, 29*(12), 58–65.

Zevitz, M. (2010). *Cardiomyopathy, hypertrophic.* eMedicine Cardiology retrieved from http://emedicine.medscape.com/article/152913-overview

Zipes, D.P., Camm, A.J., Borggrefe, M., Buxton, A.E., Chaitman, B., Fromer, M., … Tracy, C. (2006). ACC/AHA/ESC 2006 guidelines for management of patients with ventricular arrhythmias and the prevention of sudden cardiac death. *Circulation 114*(10), e385-e484.

Zoghbi, W.A. & Afridi, I. (2003). Aortic regurgitation. In M.H. Crawford (Ed.), *Current diagnosis and treatment in cardiology* (2nd ed., pp. 121-130). New York: McGraw-Hill.

Zoghbi, W.A. & Crawford, M.H. (2009). Aortic regurgitation. In M.H. Crawford (Ed.), *Current diagnosis and treatment in cardiology* (3rd ed., pp. 95–105). New York, NY: McGraw-Hill.

INDEX

Page references followed by *fig* indicate an illustrated figure; followed by *t* indicate a table; followed by *b* indicate a box.

A

abciximab (ReoPro), 57, 58

ACC/AHA
aortic balloon valvuloplasty recommendations, 216*b*
aortic valve replacement recommendations, 217*b*, 222*b*
cardiac catheterization recommendations by, 94-95
chronic mitral regurgitation medical therapy recommended by, 237
consumption of omega-3 recommended by, 76
heart disease staging, 179*t*
Heart Failure Guidelines, 153, 161-162*t*
indications for cardiac pacing, 263-264
mitral balloon valvotomy recommendations, 233*b*
mitral valve repair or replacement recommendations, 233*b*
no longer recommending antibiotics for native valve disease, 231
vasodilator therapy guidelines by, 221

ACC/AHA/NASPE Guidelines for Implantation of Cardiac Pacemakers and Antiarrhythmia Devices, 263-264, 278, 279

ACE (angiotensin-converting enzyme), 22

ACE inhibitors
ACS therapy using, 109, 112
acute mitral regurgitation, 239
aortic stenosis treated with, 215
chronic aortic regurgitation treated with, 222
description and benefits of, 32, 34-35
heart failure treatment using, 163, 164*t*, 165*t*
hypertension treatment using, 71
hypertrophic cardiomyopathy (HCM) treated with, 198
major side affects of, 35
mitral regurgitation, 238
predisposing patients to hyperkalemia, 161
specific medications listed, 35*b*
takotsubo cardiomyopathy treated with, 205

ACS (acute coronary syndrome)
cardiac biomarkers used in the evaluation of, 105-106*t*
continuum of, 97*fig*
definition of, 87

inflammation process in, 88-89
overview of, 97-98
supportive medical therapy used for, 107-109
UA (unstable angina), 87, 90, 98
See also non-STEMI; STEMI

ACS management
activity and daily walking, 113-114
anxiety and stress reduction, 114
cardiac rehabilitation, 114-116
medications used as part of, 111-112, 113
patient education, 112-113
psychosocial issues, 116-117
three objectives of discharge medical, 112

ACS medical therapy
ACE inhibitors, 109
anticoagulants, 107-108
aspirin, 107
beta-blockers, 108
clopidogrel/prasurgrel, 107
morphine sulfate, 108
nitroglycerin, 108
oxygen, 107

action potential, 14

acute aortic regurgitation
clinical presentation and physical examination of, 223
diagnosis of, 223
medical therapy for, 223
outcomes for, 223
pathophysiology of, 222-223
surgical replacement for, 223

acute coronary event
EMS (emergency response) to, 112-113
patient education recognizing, 112-113

acute decompensated heart failure
BNP (brain natriuretic peptide) levels and, 167
diuretics strategy for treating, 167-168
inotropic therapy for, 168
patient monitoring and care, 168
precipitating factors of, 167
ultrafiltration for treating, 168
vasodilator therapy for, 168

acute mitral regurgitation
clinical presentation of, 239
diagnosis of, 239

Western Schools® offers over 2,000 hours to suit all your interests – and requirements!

Cardiovascular

- Cardiovascular Nursing: A Comprehensive Overview (2nd ed.)
- Cardiovascular Pharmacology (2nd ed.)
- **A** The 12-Lead ECG in Acute Coronary Syndromes (3rd ed.)

Clinical Conditions/Nursing Practice

- **A** Advanced Assessment (2nd ed.)
- Ambulatory Surgical Care (2nd ed.)
- Arterial Blood Gases: A Systematic and Easy Approach
- Asthma: Nursing Care Across the Lifespan
- Clinical Care of the Diabetic Foot (2nd ed.)
- **A** Complete Nurses Guide to Diabetes Care (2nd ed.)
- Chronic Obstructive Lung Disease
- Death, Dying, & Bereavement (2nd ed.)
- Diabetes Essentials for Nurses (2nd ed.)
- Essentials of Patient Education
- Fibromyalgia in Women
- Genetic & Inherited Disorders of the Pulmonary System
- Helping the Obese Patient Find Success
- Holistic & Complementary Therapies
- Home Health Nursing (3rd ed.)
- Humor in Health Care: The Laughter Prescription (2nd ed.)
- IV Therapy: Essentials for Safe Practice
- Management of Systemic Lupus Erythematosus
- Multiple Sclerosis: Nursing Strategies to Improve Patient Outcomes
- Orthopedic Nursing: Caring for Patients with Musculoskeletal Disorders (2nd ed.)
- Ostomy Management
- Pain & Symptom Management
- Pain Management: Principles and Practice
- **A** Palliative Practices: An Interdisciplinary Approach
- Pharmacologic Management of Asthma
- Pneumonia in Adults
- Pulmonary Rehabilitation
- Rotator Cuff Injury and Recovery
- Seizures: A Basic Overview
- Wound Management and Healing (2nd ed.)

Critical Care/ER/OR

- Acute Respiratory Distress Syndrome (ARDS)
- Adult Acute Respiratory Infections (UPDATED 1st ed.)
- Auscultation Skills (4th ed.)
  - — Heart Sounds
  - — Breath Sounds
- Basic Trauma Nursing
- Critical Care & Emergency Nursing
- Fire Risk Reduction for Operative and Invasive Procedures
- Hemodynamic Monitoring
- Lung Transplantation
- **A** Practical Guide to Moderate Sedation/Analgesia
- Traumatic Brain Injury

Geriatrics

- Alzheimer's Disease: A Complete Guide for Nurses
- Alzheimer's Disease and Related Disorders
- Cognitive Disorders in Aging
- Depression in Older Adults
- Early-Stage Alzheimer's Disease
- Geriatric Assessment
- Healthy Aging
- Nursing Care of the Older Adult (2nd ed.)
- Psychosocial Issues Affecting Older Adults (2nd ed.)
- Substance Abuse in Older Adults

Infectious Diseases

- Avian (H5N1) Influenza (2nd ed.)
- H1N1 Flu (2nd ed.)
- Hepatitis C: The Silent Killer (2nd ed.)
- HIV/AIDS
- Infection Prevention for Healthcare Professionals
- Influenza: A Vaccine-Preventable Disease (UPDATED 2nd ed.)
- MRSA
- Pertussis: Diagnosis, Treatment, and Prevention
- Tuberculosis Across the Lifespan
- West Nile Virus (3rd ed.)

Oncology

- Cancer in Women (2nd ed.)
- Cancer Nursing
- Chemotherapy and Biotherapies
- Lung Cancer (UPDATED 2nd ed.)
- Skin Cancer

Pediatrics/Maternal-Child/Women's Health

- **A** Assessment and Care of the Well Newborn
- Birth Control Methods and Reproductive Choices
- Birth Defects Affecting the Respiratory System
- Childhood Obesity
- Diabetes in Children (2nd ed.)
- Effective Counseling Techniques for Perinatal Mood Disorders
- Fetal and Neonatal Drug Exposure
- Induction of Labor
- Manual of School Health (3rd ed.)
- Maternal-Newborn Nursing
- Menopause: Nursing Care for Women Throughout Mid-Life
- **A** Obstetric and Gynecologic Emergencies (4th ed.)
  - — Obstetric Emergencies
  - — Gynecologic Emergencies
- Pediatric Abusive Head Trauma
- Pediatric Health & Physical Assessment
- Perinatal Mood Disorders: An Overview
- Pregnancy Loss
- Respiratory Diseases in the Newborn
- Women's Health: Contemporary Advances and Trends (3rd ed.)

Professional Issues/Management/Law

- Ethical Issues in Children's Health Care
- Ethical Practices with Older Adults
- Protecting Patient Safety: Preventing Medical Errors
- Management and Leadership in Nursing
- Ohio Nursing Law Affecting Daily Practice
- Surviving and Thriving in Nursing

Psychiatric/Mental Health

- **A** ADHD in Children and Adults
- Adoptive Families: Trends and Therapeutic Interventions
- Asperger's Syndrome
- Attention Deficit Hyperactivity Disorders Throughout the Lifespan
- Behavioral Approaches to Treating Obesity
- Best Practices With Lesbian, Gay, and Bisexual Youth and Their Families
- **A** Bipolar Disorder
- Bullies, Victims, and Bystanders: From Prevalence to Prevention
- Caring for Patients with Mental Health Issues: Strategies for All Nurses
- **A** Child/Adolescent Clinical Psychopharmacology (2nd ed.)
- **A** Childhood Maltreatment
- Childhood Trauma
- **A** Clinical Psychopharmacology Made Simple (7th ed.)
- Clinical Neuropsychology: Applications in Practice
- **A** Collaborative Therapy with Multi-stressed Families
- Counseling Substance Abusing or Dependent Adolescents
- Depression: Prevention, Diagnosis, and Treatment
- Disaster Mental Health
- **A** Ethnicity and the Dementias
- **A** Evidence-Based Mental Health Practice
- Evidence-Based Practice: What Every Nurse Needs to Know
- Grief, Bereavement, and Mourning in Children and Adults
- **A** Growing Up with Autism
- Identifying and Assessing Suicide Risk in Adults
- Identifying and Treating Young and Adult Children of Alcoholics
- **A** Integrative Treatment for Borderline Personality Disorder
- Intimate Partner Violence: An Overview
- Major Depression in Adults: Signs, Symptoms & Treatment Strategies
- **A** Mental Disorders in Older Adults
- **A** Mindfulness and Psychotherapy
- **A** Multicultural Perspectives in Working with Families
- Multidimensional Health Assessment of the Older Adult
- **A** Obsessive Compulsive Disorder
- Post-Divorce Parenting: Mental Health Issues and Interventions
- Posttraumatic Stress Disorder: An Overview
- **A** Problem and Pathological Gambling
- Psychiatric Nursing: Current Trends in Diagnosis (2nd ed.)
- Psychopharmacology for Nurses
- **A** Psychosocial Aspects of Disaster
- **A** Schizophrenia
- Schizophrenia: Signs, Symptoms, and Treatment Strategies
- Serious Mental Illness: Comprehensive Case Management
- Sexual Health Counseling
- Substance Abuse (UPDATED 1st ed.)
- Suicide
- **A** Trauma Therapy
- **A** Treating Explosive Kids
- **A** Treating Substance Use Problems in Psychotherapy Practice
- **A** Treating Victims of Mass Disaster and Terrorism
- Understanding Attachment Theory
- Understanding Loss & Grief: Implications for Healthcare Professionals

Visit our website at www.WesternSchools.com

for course descriptions and additional CE offerings!